Progress in Epileptic Disorders
Volume 2

Generalized Seizures:
From clinical phenomenology
to underlying systems and networks

Progress in Epileptic Disorders
International Advisory Board

Aicardi Jean, *France*
Arzimanoglou Alexis, *France*
Baumgartner Christoph, *Austria*
Brodie Martin, *UK*
Cross Helen, *UK*
Duchowny Michael, *USA*
Elger Christian, *Germany*
French Jacqueline, *USA*
Glauser Tracy, *USA*
Gobbi Giuseppe, *Italy*
Guerrini Renzo, *Italy*
Hirsch Edouard, *France*
Kahane Philippe, *France*
Luders Hans, *USA*
Meador Kimford, *USA*
Moshé Solomon L., *USA*
Noachtar Soheyl, *Germany*
Noebels Jeffrey, *USA*
Palmini André, *Brazil*
Perucca Emilio, *Italy*
Pitkanen Asla, *Finland*
Ryvlin Philippe, *France*
Scheffer Ingrid, *Australia*
Schmitz Bettina, *Germany*
Schmidt Dieter, *Germany*
Serratosa José, *Spain*
Shorvon Simon, *UK*
Tinuper Paolo, *Italy*
Thomas Pierre, *France*
Tuxhorn Ingrid, *Germany*
Wolf Peter, *Denmark*

Progress in Epileptic Disorders
Volume 2

Generalized Seizures:
From clinical phenomenology to underlying systems and networks

Edouard Hirsch
Frederick Andermann
Patrick Chauvel
Jerome Engel
Fernando Lopes da Silva
Hans Luders

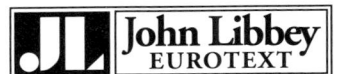

ISBN: 2-7420-0621-4
ISSN: 1777-4284
Vol. 2.

Published by
Éditions John Libbey Eurotext
127, avenue de la République, 92120 Montrouge, France
Tél. : 01 46 73 06 60
Site internet : http://www.jle.com

John Libbey Eurotext
42-46 High Street
Esher, Surrey
KT10 9KY
United Kingdom

© 2006, John Libbey Eurotext. All rights reserved.

Unauthorized duplication contravenes applicable laws.
Il est interdit de reproduire intégralement ou partiellement le présent ouvrage sans autorisation de l'éditeur ou du Centre Français d'Exploitation du Droit de Copie, 20, rue des Grands-Augustins, 75006 Paris.

Contents

Foreword IX

Workshop participants XI

Section I:
Generalized seizures and epilepsies: a bilateral "focal" dysfunction?

What is a generalized seizure?
  Patrick Chauvel 3

What is a Generalized epilepsy?
  Frederick Andermann 23

Section II:
Tonic seizures and brainstem systems

From brainstem to forebrain in generalized animal models of seizures and epilepsies
  Phillip C. Jobe, Ronald A. Browning 33

Systems and networks in tonic seizures and epilepsies in humans
  Warren T. Blume 53

Comments from participants
  Ajay Gupta 69
  Pavel Mares 70

Section III:
Absence seizures and cortico-thalamic systems

Propagation and dynamic processing of cortical paroxysms in the basal ganglia networks during absence seizures
  Jeanne T. Paz, Pierre-Olivier Polack, Seán J. Slaght, Jean-Michel Deniau,
  Séverine Mahon, Stéphane Charpier 75

Cortical control of absence seizures: focal initiation, spreading and modulation
  Gilles van Luijtelaar, Evbenia Y. Sitnikova, Inna S. Midzyanovskaya 93

Systems and networks in absence seizures and epilepsies in humans
  Edouard Hirsch, Maria-Paola Valenti 119

Spike-wave seizures in corticothalamic systems
  Mircea Steriade 127

Section IV:
Myoclonic seizures and the frontal lobe

Animal models of myoclonic seizures and epilepsies
  Jana Velíškova, Libor Velíšek 147

Systems and networks in myoclonic seizures and epilepsies
  Matthias J. Koepp, Khalid Hamandi 163

Connections between primary reading epilepsy and juvenile myoclonic epilepsy?
  Thomas A. Mayer, Peter T. Wolf, Frauke Shroeder, Theodor W. May 183

Section V:
Primary versus Secondary Tonic-clonic seizures

Behavior, neural circuits and plasticity in acute and chronic animal models of generalized tonic-clonic seizures
  Norberto Garcia-Cairasco 197

The semiology and pathophysiology of the secondary generalized tonic-clonic seizures
  Samden Lhatoo, Hans Lüders 229

Tonic-clonic and clonic-tonic-clonic seizures in human primary generalized epilepsies
  Reyna M. Durón, Julia N. Bailey, Marco T. Medina, Iris E. Martinez-Juàrez, Miyabi Tanaka, María Elisa Alonso, Ramón H. Castro Ortega, Katerina Tanya Perez-Gosiengfiao, Ignacio Pascual-Castraviejo, Adriana Ochoa, Aurelio Jara-Prado, Jesus Machado-Salas, Lizardo Mija, Antonio V. Delgado-Escueta 247

Section VI:
The "cortical" and "centrencephalic" theories revisited

Cortical trigger in generalized seizures
  Fernando Lopes da Silva 271

Section VII:
Phenomenology versus networks: clinical consequences

Why can some antiepileptic drugs control certain types of seizures and aggravate others?
Dieter Schmidt 285

Section VIII:
Concluding remarks

Can we replace the terms "focal" and "generalized"?
Jerome Engel 305

Foreword

"Generalized Seizures: From clinical phenomenology to underlying systems and networks" is the second volume in the *"Progress in Epileptic Disorders"* book series, edited in collaboration with the journal *"Epileptic Disorders"* and published by John Libbey Eurotext.

A *"Generalized seizure"* corresponds to an ictal manifestation whose initial semeiology indicates, or is consistent with, more than minimal involvement of both cerebral hemispheres. A *network* is a functionally and anatomically connected set of cortical and subcortical brain regions where activity in any one part affects the activity in all others. A *system* is a group of independent but interrelated elements (networks) comprising a unified whole. A considerable amount of evidence supports the existence of specific cortical and subcortical networks in the genesis, expression and control of generalized seizures. Animal and human data suggest that the so-called generalized seizures involve selective networks while sparing others. A greater understanding of those systems and networks will ultimately lead to improved targeted therapies for these forms of epilepsy.

The book is the fruit of a workshop, designed as a discussion forum, with the participation of experts from all over the world, to extensively review available clinical, neurophysiological and basic research data in order to generate new avenues and hypotheses for research, clinical practice and care.

The first section traces back to the definitions and concepts underlying the terms "generalized seizures and epilepsies". Section II reviews human and animal data suggesting that the brainstem network plays an important role in tonic seizures generation. The third and fourth sections analyze recent knowledge on cortico-thalamic and basal ganglia networks involved in absence and myoclonic seizures, both in animal models and in human. The fifth section compares the phenomenology of "Primary *versus* Secondary Tonico-clonic seizures", including animal data, clinical expression in human and genetics. Section VI returns to the discussion "Cortical" *versus* "Centrencephalic" theories. The last two chapters review in detail the clinical applications of current knowledge, to pharmacological and clinical care.

On behalf of the scientific committee of the workshop we sincerely thank all the participants for their valuable contributions and UCB for having accepted to collaborate in this project of the journal *Epileptic Disorders* and support it throughout, with an unrestricted educational grant.

Edouard Hirsch, Frederick Andermann, Patrick Chauvel,
Jerome Engel Jr., Fernando Lopes da Silva, Hans Luders

Mircea Steriade, MD, DSc

Mircea Steriade, M.D., D.Sc., a renowned investigator in the fields of generalized epilepsy and sleep died on Friday April 14, 2006 of cancer at the age of 81. He was Professor of Anatomy and Physiology and Head of the Laboratory of Neurophysiology at Laval University in Quebec.

Laden with honors, always curious, and imaginative he was a prodigious worker to the end. Although finally obliged to cancel his participation at the Rome workshop in February 2006, he was the first to send us his chapter as a contribution to the debate on the pathophysiology of generalized seizures.

Probably his most important contributions in research were the demonstration of facilitatory actions exerted by the brainstem reticular formation on responsiveness of thalamocortical neurons, the demonstration that the GABAergic thalamic reticular nucleus is crucially involved in the generation of sleep spindles, the identification of a new sleep oscillation, the slow cortical oscillation which has the virtue of grouping other sleep rhythms, showing that some epileptic seizures may develop without discontinuity from sleep oscillations and that neocortex is the minimal substrate of such seizures. He demonstrated in vivo two distinct modes of discharge of thalamic neurons, one related to the waking state, the other to sleep. He also showed, using intracerebral recordings in behaving animals, that the proportion and firing patterns of different neuronal classes in neocortex are dependent on the behavioral state of vigilance.

His work constructed a solid base for our understanding of diffuse or generalized epilepsies and this chapter is a tribute to this view. Mircea Steriade was a warm, friendly colleague and an outstandingly affectionate father. He will be missed not only by his family, but also by the world of sleep and epilepsy research worldwide.

This volume is a tribute to his memory.

The Scientific Committee

Workshop on *"Generalized Seizures: From clinical phenomenology to underlying systems and networks"* Rome, February 2006

Scientific Committee:
Fred Andermann (Canada), Alexis Arzimanoglou (France), Patrick Chauvel (France), Jerome Engel (USA), Edouard Hirsch (France), Philippe Kahane (France), Fernando Lopes da Silva (The Netherlands), Hans Luders (USA), Philippe Ryvlin (France)

Editors:
Edouard Hirsch, Fred Andermann, Patrick Chauvel, Jerome Engel, Fernando Lopes da Silva, Hans Luders

List of Participants

Andermann Frederick, Neurology and Pediatrics, McGill University, Epilepsy Service, Montreal Neurological Institute and Hospital, 3801 University Street, Montreal, Quebec H3A 2B4, Canada
frederick.andermann@mcgill.ca

Andermann Eva, Departments of Neurology & Neurosurgery and Human Genetics; Director, Neurogenetics Unit, Montreal Neurological Institute & Hospital, McGill University, Montreal, Quebec H3A 2B4, Canada
eva.andermann@mcgill.ca

Arzimanoglou Alexis, Neurologist, Child Neurologist, Head of the Epilepsy Program, Child Neurology & Metabolic Diseases Department, University Hospital Robert Debré, 48 Boulevard Sérurier, 75935 Paris Cedex 19, France
alexis.arzimanoglou@rdb.aphp.fr

Avanzini Giuliano, Research Director, Istituto Nazionale Neurologico C. Besta, Via Celoria 11, 20133 Milano, Italy
avanzini@istituto-besta.it

Blume Warren, University Campus, 339 Windermere Road, London, Ontario, Canada N6A 5A5
warren.blume@lhsc.on.ca

Blumenfeld Hal, MD, PhD, Director of Medical Studies in Clinical Neuroscience, Yale University School of Medicine, LCI 1007; Box 208108, 333 Cedar Street, New Haven, CT 06520-8018
hal.blumenfeld@yale.edu

Browning Ronald A, Department of Physiology, Southern Illinois University School of Medicine, Carbondale, Illinois 62901 – 6512, USA

Bureau, Michelle, 505 avenue du Prado, 13008 Marseille, France
michelle-bureau@wanadoo.fr

Carreno Mar, MD, PhD, Servicio de Neurología, Hospital Clínic,
c/Villarroel, 170, 08036 Barcelona, Spain
mcarreno@clinic.ub.es

Charpier Stéphane, Institut National de la Santé et de la Recherche Médicale U 667,
Collège de France, 75231 Paris, France
stephane.charpier@college-de-france.fr

Chauvel Patrick, Professor of Neurology, Service de Neurophysiologie Clinique et INSERM U751,
Hôpital de la Timone et Faculté de Médecine, 13005 Marseille, France
patrick.chauvel@mail.ap-hm.fr

Cossette Patrick, MD, MSc, FRCPC, Département de médecine, Université de Montréal,
CHUM-Hôpital Notre-Dame, 1560 Sherbrooke est, Montréal, Qc H2L 4M1
patrick.cossette@umontreal.ca

D'Antuono Margherita, PharmD, PhD, Dept of Neuroscience, University of Rome "Tor Vergata",
Via di Montpellier 1, 00133 Rome, Italy
dantuono@uniroma2.it

Delgado-Escueta Antonio, Epilepsy Center, Suite 3405, Bldg 500, VA Glahs,
West LA Medical Center, 11301 Wilshire Blvd, Los Angeles, CA 90073, USA
escueta@ucla.edu

Depaulis Antoine, PhD – Directeur de recherche, INSERM, Université Joseph Fournier
UFR Biologie – Bâtiment B, 2280 rue de la Piscine Grenoble, France
antoine.depaulis@ujf-grenoble.fr

Deransart Colin, PhD, INSERM U.704 – UJF, Grenoble, France
colin.deransart@ujf-grenoble.fr

Engel Jerome, Jr., Reed Neurological Research Center, UCLA School of Medicine
710 Westwood Plaza, CA 90024-1769 Los Angeles, USA
engel@ucla.edu

Gale Karen, 4453 Volta Pl NW, Washington DC 20007, USA
galek@georgetown.edu

Garcia-Caraisco Norberto, Director of the Neurophysiology and Experimental Neuroethology
Laboratory, Ribeirão Preto School of Medicine-University of São Paulo,
Avenida Bandeirantes 3900, CEP 14049-900 Ribeirão Preto, São Paulo, Brazil
ngcairas@fmrp.usp.br

Gil-Nagel Antonio, MD, Servicio de Neurologia, Programa de Epilepsia,
Hospital Ruber Internacional, La Maso 38, Mirasierra, 28034 Madrid, Spain
agnagel@ya.com; agnagel@ruberinternacional.es

Grisar Thierry, Chairman, University of Liège-Faculty of Medicine, Vice-chairman of the Department of Preclinical Sciences BP, Servive of Human Neurophysiology and Biochemistry
Chair of the CNCM, Avenue de l'Hopital,1, bâtiment B36 4000, Liège, Belgium
tgrisar@ulg.ac.be

Gupta Ajay, MD, Cleveland Clinic Lerner College of Medicine/Case Western Reserve University,
Section of Pediatric Epilepsy, S-51/Neurology, Cleveland Clinic Foundation,
9500 Euclid Avenue, Cleveland OH 44195, USA
guptaa1@ccf.org

Hirsch Edouard, Neurologist-Neurophysiologist, Epileptology Service, Neurology Department,
University Hospitals, 1 Place de l'Hôpital, 67091 Strasbourg Cedex, France
edouard.Hirsch@chru-strasbourg.fr

Inoue Yushi, MD. PhD, National Epilepsy Center, Shizuoka Institute of Epilepsy and Neurological Disorders, Urushiyama 886, Aoi-ku, Shizuoka 420-8688, Japan
yushi@szec.hosp.go.jp

Jaladyan Varsine, Child Neurologist, Child Neurology Department & Children's Epileptology Center, "Arabkir" Joint Medical Center and Institute of Child and Adolescent Health, Mamikoniants 30, 375014 Yerevan, Armenia
vjaladyan@yahoo.com

Jobe Phillip, Department of Biomedical and Therapeutic Sciences, University of Illinois College of Medicine, PO Box 1649, Peoria, Illinois 61656-1649, USA
jobe252@insightbb.com

Kahane Philippe, MD, PhD, Head of the Epilepsy Unit, Neurology Department and INSERM U704, University Hospital, BP 217X, 38043 Grenoble, France
philippe.kahane@ujf-grenoble.fr

Koepp Matthias, MD PhD, Department of Clinical and Experimental Epilepsy, Institute of Neurology, University College London, London, UK
mkoepp@ion.ucl.ac.uk

Lemieux Louis, Professor of Physics Applied to Medical Imaging, Department of Clinical and Experimental Epilepsy, Institute of Neurology, University College London, Queen Square, London WC1N 3BG, UK
l.lemieux@ion.ucl.ac.uk

Lhatoo Samden, S51, Cleveland Clinic Foundation, 9500 Euclid Ave, Cleveland, OHIO 44195, USA
lhatoos@ccf.org; slhatoo@aol.com

Lopes da Silva Fernando, University of Amsterdam, Amsterdam, The Netherlands
silva@science.uva.nl

Lüders Hans O., Director, S-91, Cleveland Clinic Epilepsy Center, Cleveland Clinic Foundation, 9500 Euclid Ave, Cleveland, OHIO 44195, USA
ludersh@ccf.org

Mares Pavel, M.D., D.Sc., Professor of Pathophysiology, Department of Developmental Epileptology, Institute of Physiology, Academy of Sciences of the Czech Republic, Videnska 1083, CZ-14220 Prague 4, Czech Republilc
maresp@biomed.cas.cz

Mayer Thomas, Saxonian Epilepsy Center Radeberg, Wachauerstr. 30, 01465 Radeberg, Germany
t.mayer@kleinwachau.de

Minassian Berge A., MD, The Hospital for Sick Children, 555 University Ave, Toronto, ON M5G 1X8, Canada
bminass@sickkids.ca

Montavont Alexandra, MD, Neurological Hospital, Lyon, France
a_montavont@yahoo.fr

Nair Dileep R., M.D., Director of Clinical Neurophysiology/Epilepsy Fellowship and Intraoperative Neurophysiology Monitoring, The Cleveland Clinic Foundation, Section of Adult Epilepsy/ Desk S51, 9500 Euclid Avenue, Cleveland, Ohio 44145, USA
NAIRD@ccf.org

Ozkara Cigdem, Cerrahpasa Tip Fakultesi, Noroloji ABD, Kocamustafapasa, Istanbul, Turkey
cigdemoz@istanbul.edu.tr

Ryvlin Philippe, Department of Functional Neurology and Epileptology, Neurology University Hospital, 59 Boulevard Pinel, 69003 Lyon, France
ryvlin@cermep.fr

Schmidt Dieter, M.D., Emeritus Professor of Neurology, Free University of Berlin, Epilepsy Research Group, Geothe Strasse 5, 14163 Berlin, Germany
dbschmidt@t-online.de

Seeck Margitta, Médecin adjointe agrégée, Clinique de Neurologie, Unité d'évaluation préchirurgicale d'épilepsie, rue Micheli-du-Crest 24, CH-1211 Genève 14, Switzerland
margitta.seeck@hcuge.ch

Serratosa Jose, MD, PhD, Jefe Asociado, Unidad de Epilepsia, Servicio de Neurologia, Fundacion Jimenez Diaz, Universidad Autonoma de Madrid, Avda Reyes Catolicos 2, 28040 Madrid, SPAIN
serratosa@telefonica.net

Shields Donald, Neurology and Pediatrics, David Geffen School of Medicine at UCLA, Los Angeles, USA
wshields@mednet.ucla.edu

Tassinari Carlo Alberto, MD, Neurologist, Dept. of Neurological Sciences, University of Bologna, 40139 Bologna, Italy
carloalberto.tassinari@ausl.bologna.it

Thomas Pierre, MD, PhD, UF EEG-Epileptologie, Service Neurologie Pav. D, Hôpital Pasteur, 30 Voie Romaine, 06002 NICE Cedex 01, France
piertho@wanadoo.fr

Valenti Maria-Paola, Neurology Department, University Hospitals, 1 Place de l'Hôpital, 67091 Strasbourg, France

Van Luijtelaar Gilles, Dr, Biological Psychology, Nijmegen Institute for Cognition and Informatics, Radboud University Nijmegen, PO Box 9104, 6500 HE Nijmegen, The Netherlands
g.vanluijtelaar@nici.ru.nl

Veliskova Jana, AECOM, K 312, 1410 Pelham Pkwy. SO., Bronx, NY 10461, USA
jvelisko@aecom.yu.edu

Vezzani Annamaria, PhD, Head of Exp. Neurol. Lab., Dept Neurosci, Mario Negri Inst. for Pharmacol. Res., Milano, Italy
vezzani@marionegri.it

Wyllie Elaine, Head, Pediatric Epilepsy Program, The Cleveland Clinic Foundation, 9500 Euclid Avenue, 44195 Cleveland, Ohio, USA
WYLLIEE@ccf.org

Workshop supported by an unrestricted educational grant from UCB

Section I:
Generalized seizures and epilepsies: a bilateral "focal" dysfunction?

What is a generalized seizure?

Patrick Chauvel

Service de Neurophysiologie Clinique, Hôpital de la Timone, APHM ;
Laboratoire de Neurophysiologie & Neuropsychologie, INSERM U 751 ;
Faculté de Médecine, Université de la Méditerranée, Marseille, France

To question the nature of a generalized seizure is to pose the question of its localization, which is itself an oxymoron. H.Gastaut appears to have been the first to propose this term to describe epileptic seizures "without focal onset", in a confidential publication published in Marseille Médical in 1955. The term was used verbally in meetings and in EEG labs, but it was Gastaut who decided to use it in the classification of seizures.

The term appeared officially in the first international classification of epileptic seizures in 1970, and was defined as follows: "Generalized seizures, bilateral symmetrical seizures or seizures without local onset [are] seizures in which the clinical features do not include any sign or symptom referable to an anatomical and/or functional system localized in one hemisphere, and usually consist of initial impairment of consciousness, motor changes which are generalized or at least bilateral and more or less symmetrical and may be accompanied by an 'en masse' autonomic discharge; in which the electroencephalographic patterns from the start are bilateral, grossly synchronous and symmetrical over the two hemispheres; and in which the responsible neuronal discharge takes place, if not throughout the entire grey matter, then at least in the greater part of it and simultaneously on both sides" (Classification, Epilepsia, 1970).

With the advances of insight to basic mechanisms of epilepsies derived from the study of experimental models, as well as a better understanding the pathophysiology of seizures recorded in patients with modern EEG techniques or with depth electrodes, the term "generalized" currently appears outdated. However, the use of this expression to describe a concept represented real progress in the second half of the last century, essentially because it coincided with the first electrophysiological characterization of human epilepsies by EEG. The influence of EEG, and of underlying cerebral mechanisms in states of vigilance and attention was directly inspired by the discovery of the physiology of the Reticular Formation by Magoun and Moruzzi in the 50s. Their influence was so strong that the clinical phenomenology was interpreted less in terms of localization than in terms of the EEG pattern distribution.

The following definition by Gastaut and Broughton (1972) is a good summary: "Generalized epileptic seizures [...] share the common features of impairment of consciousness and en masse mobilization of autonomic phenomena, often associated with bilaterally symmetrical motor signs, either positive (convulsions) or negative (hypotonia). The electroencephalographic discharge is also bilateral, synchronous, and symmetrical".

■ "Universal" convulsions

The term "generalized" had not been used before the advent of EEG. A distinction between "partial" and "generalized" seizures was not actually made in 19th century literature. Though the approach to seizures was essentially descriptive, and despite the fact that the quality of the observations of those times remain unequalled, separation between the two types of seizures did not appear evident from a clinical perspective. Gowers (1881), who provided the first detailed description of the Grand Mal seizure, distinguished between severe and minor attacks. Jackson attempted to bridge the gap between the symptoms and their anatomical basis; the beginnings of his classification tended to rest on hierarchical (and parallel) levels and according to degrees of intensity understood as manifesting discharge propagation. That is why, for Jackson, there is a difference of degree between Petit Mal and Grand Mal, not a difference of type: "The facts that those very epilepsies in which consciousness is *first* lost, or is lost very early, are the cases in which the convulsion is nearly universal, in which the two sides are more nearly equally convulsed; and that it is in these cases that there is at the very first much pallor of the face, tend to confirm the conclusion that the sensori-motor processes concerned in consciousness are evolved out of and potentially contain all other (lower) series. It is, indeed, most significant, whatever the explanation may be, that there are slight cases (*petit mal*) in which, with transient loss of consciousness, there is deep pallor of the face (and body?) and a slight wave of universal movement" (Jackson, 1873).

Even though the so-called "universal" convulsions were reported as bilateral, Gowers, and then Jackson mentioned that an asymmetry was very often observed, especially in the initial adversion of head and eyes to one side. The very sophisticated descriptions of Jackson and their theoretical arguments are well-known: it is remarkable that he seemed never to be preoccupied by the search for a synchronizing mechanism unifying the discharge of the two hemispheres (because no clinical data made this necessary). No confusion was made between the "universalisation" of the convulsions and loss of consciousness; rather, a distinction was drawn between the "epileptiform" convulsions of rolandic origin, and the "epileptic" seizures (epilepsy proper or genuine epilepsy) with a more anterior ("prefrontal") onset. The question of consciousness was approached in a rather cautious manner (according to Spencer). The notion of degrees of alteration of consciousness as a function of discharge duration, and therefore of propagation towards regions which receive and treat "heterogeneous" information, was preferred to the notion of centre. Jackson would have localized the seizures which are nowadays named "generalized" in cortical areas hierarchically superior to the motor cortex, *i.e.* in front of it ("prefrontal"), which corresponded to his "highest level". As seen above, he did not differentiate between Grand Mal and Petit Mal by their anatomical origin, but by the intensity of the discharge.

■ The "centrencephalic" concept

Penfield was preoccupied by the mechanisms of consciousness in relation to memory integration. The conditions of stimulation of the awake patient in the operating theatre were poorly adapted to the study of seizures, especially convulsive seizures. However, the question of alteration of consciousness in epilepsy was an underlying theme in Penfield's work, and he was in search of Jackson's "highest level". His collaboration with Jasper provided a model which was to support most of Penfield's hypotheses, for memory integration as well as for the location of the "stream of consciousness".

In 1935 Gibbs *et al.* had described the EEG pattern characteristic of Petit Mal (PM) absences (bilateral, synchronous and symmetrical spike-and-waves, at 3 Hz). Jasper and Drooglever-Fortuyn (1947), addressing the functional anatomy of Petit Mal (PM), had experimentally reproduced this in the cat by 3Hz stimulation of the thalamic intra-laminar nuclei, considered as the rostral part of the ascending activating system. They claimed that their model could explain seven of the characteristics of PM EEG. In fact, this experiment was not easily reproducible, and direct stimulation of traversing thalamo-cortical fibers could not be excluded. Later, under the supervision of Jasper, Perot studied the relations of mesencephalon and thalamus in the genesis of this pattern and its links with the level of barbiturate anaesthesia, and Pollen (1964) demonstrated that the wave of the spike-and-wave was generated by a prolonged inhibitory post-synaptic potential in pyramidal neurons of the cortex.

However, Jasper later attributed the centrencephalic concept to Penfield saying that, in parallel with the experimental demonstration of the functional importance of the ascending reticular activating system and of its reciprocal interactions with the cerebral cortex, Penfield had developed the concept of a "centrencephalic system" on the basis of his surgical experience (Jasper, 1969). In Penfield's mind, this integrating system was supposed to be a materialization of Jackson's "highest level", which had cautiously not been anatomically defined, stating only that it encompassed the "nonspecific" frontal and/or parietal cortex. In fact, "centrencephalon" and "highest level" shared the same anatomical imprecision. The definitions of the centrencephalon were given by Penfield in 1950 and 1957. Placed within the brain stem and also including the diencephalon, it was responsible for integration of the function of the two cerebral hemispheres. For this reason, it was considered functionally unseparable from the cortex (Penfield, 1957).

From the centrencephalic system to centrencephalic seizures. The question of centrencephalic seizures was an attempt to explain the "dramatic and remarkable" electrical manifestation of Petit Mal absence, sometimes associated with convulsive seizures that were generalized from the onset. Jasper and Kershman (1941) established a difference between patients with a diffuse encephalopathy, and those without evident cerebral damage, which they termed "idiopathic or cryptogenic". The latter were considered to be "centrencephalic", without any cortical lesion. These two classes were expected to be distinguished by the electrical features of their seizures during EEG recording. A common central pacemaker was postulated to account for synchronization of the bilateral discharge.

As an electroencephalographer, Gastaut found the centrencephalic concept most appealing; as a physician, he developed a pathophysiological hypothesis that could account for the clinical features of the different types of generalized seizures. He elucidated these hypotheses in his book with Broughton in 1972. For instance, the generalized tonic-clonic seizure was said to involve the participation of both thalamus and brain stem reticular formation. The "recruiting" EEG pattern was compared to similar rhythms obtained by Dempsey and Morrison (1942) in stimulating thalamic nuclei, and its interruption by slow rhythmic waves was explained by an inhibitory thalamo-caudate loop. The motor and autonomic signs of the Grand Mal seizure were the consequence of activation of reticulo-spinal and sympathetic efferents from the brain stem modulated by thalamo-reticular connections. In the same way, the whole clinical spectrum of generalized seizures (tonic, myoclonic, clonic generalized, absence, and atonic seizures) was explained in terms of various excitatory/inhibitory interplays between brain stem reticular formation, thalamus and caudate nucleus (*Figure 1*).

■ Secondary bilateral synchrony and the role of the frontal cortex

In the same period during which the centrencephalic theory was developed, Jasper had also clearly shown that lesions within the mesial cortex of the frontal lobe ("parasagittal lesions") could give rise to interictal spike-and-wave discharges resembling those of generalized epilepsies (Tükel and Jasper, 1952). They remarked that the discharges might occur bilaterally but were restricted and asymmetrical over the midline, and that from time to time they would be more widepread and symmetrical bursts were triggered. These were less rhythmic than in Petit Mal, and electro-clinical correlations were not observed. They called this phenomenon "secondary bilateral synchrony" to differentiate it from the "primary bilateral synchrony" of PM absences (*Figure 2*). They postulated that this type of synchrony between the two hemispheres was also under the control of the centrencephalic synchronizing system triggered by the cortical lesional area.

The observation of this mode of interaction between cortex and thalamus in the generation of spike-and-wave patterns later prompted Gloor, having observed the effects of intra-carotid injection of metrazol in patients (Gloor, 1969), to create an experimental model in the cat by systemic injection of penicillin (Gloor *et al.*, 1977; Quesney *et al.*, 1977). In contrast with the dominant opinion at the Montreal Neurological Institute (MNI), Gloor was the first to note the discrepancies between experimental and human studies: "If the experimental studies in animals [...] are considered as strongly in favour of the centrencephalic hypothesis, pharmacological studies, especially those employing the intracarotid injection of Metrazol and Sodium Amytal, are those militating against it, tending to support instead the alternative

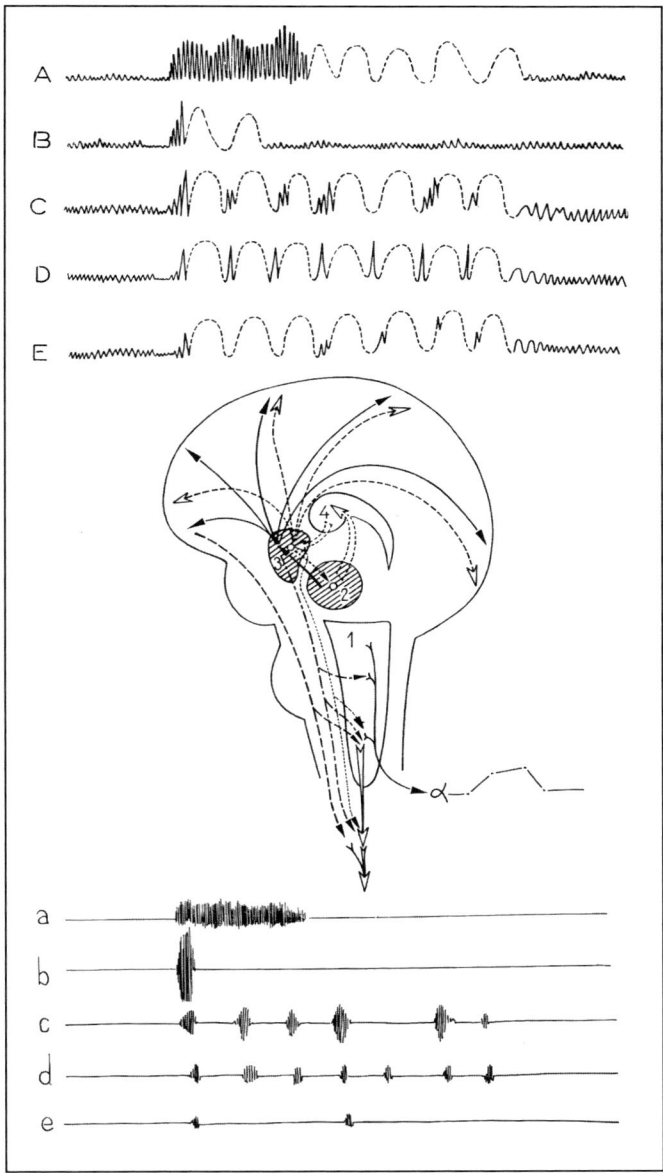

Figure 1. Gastaut's hypothesis for generalized seizures (adapted from Gastaut & Broughton, 1972). The recruiting system (thalamic reticular formation-shaded areas) is responsible for a EEG recruiting discharge, but can be antagonized by the thalamocaudate inhibitory system (caudate nucleus in clear, labelled 4). Depending on the relative effectiveness and the time lag between the two systems, five schematic situations can be encoutered, exemplified in A, B, C, D, E (EEG patterns) with a, b, c, d, e, being the corresponding motor patterns. The recruiting systems activity is illustrated by full arrows and traces, the inhibitory activity by dotted arrows and traces. A is the model of tonic seizures, B of bilateral myoclonus, C of clonic generalized seizures, D of petit mal absence, and E of atonic and myoclonic-atonic seizures. The clear structure labelled 1 is the brain stem reticular formation with its autonomic efferents.

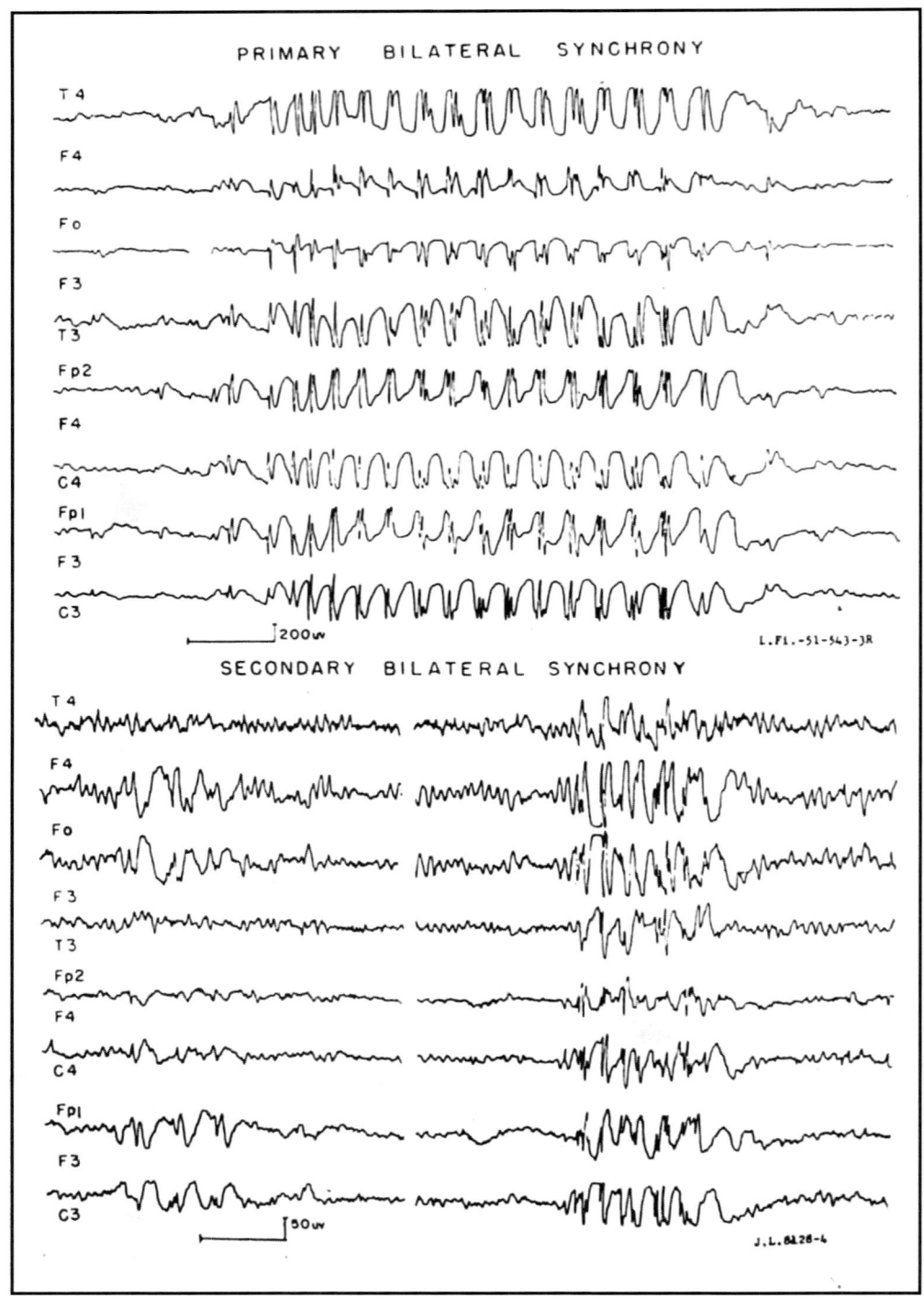

Figure 2. Secondary Bilateral Synchrony (from Tükel & Jasper, 1952). Explanations in the text.

notion of a cortical origin of centrencephalic epilepsy" (Gloor, 1969). Following the previous observations of Bennett (1953), he confirmed that injection of Metrazol in one or the other of the carotids could reproduce the electrographic and clinical manifestations of Petit Mal at a very low threshold. Arguing about the cerebral distribution of the carotid system, and the incapacity for a vertebral injection to produce the same effect, he concluded an initial responsibility of the cortex in producing this pattern, without eliminating the role of a subcortical relay in the bilateral synchronization of the discharge. Hence Gloor's concept of "generalized cortico-reticular" or "generalized cortico-centrencephalic epilepsies" *(Figure 3)*.

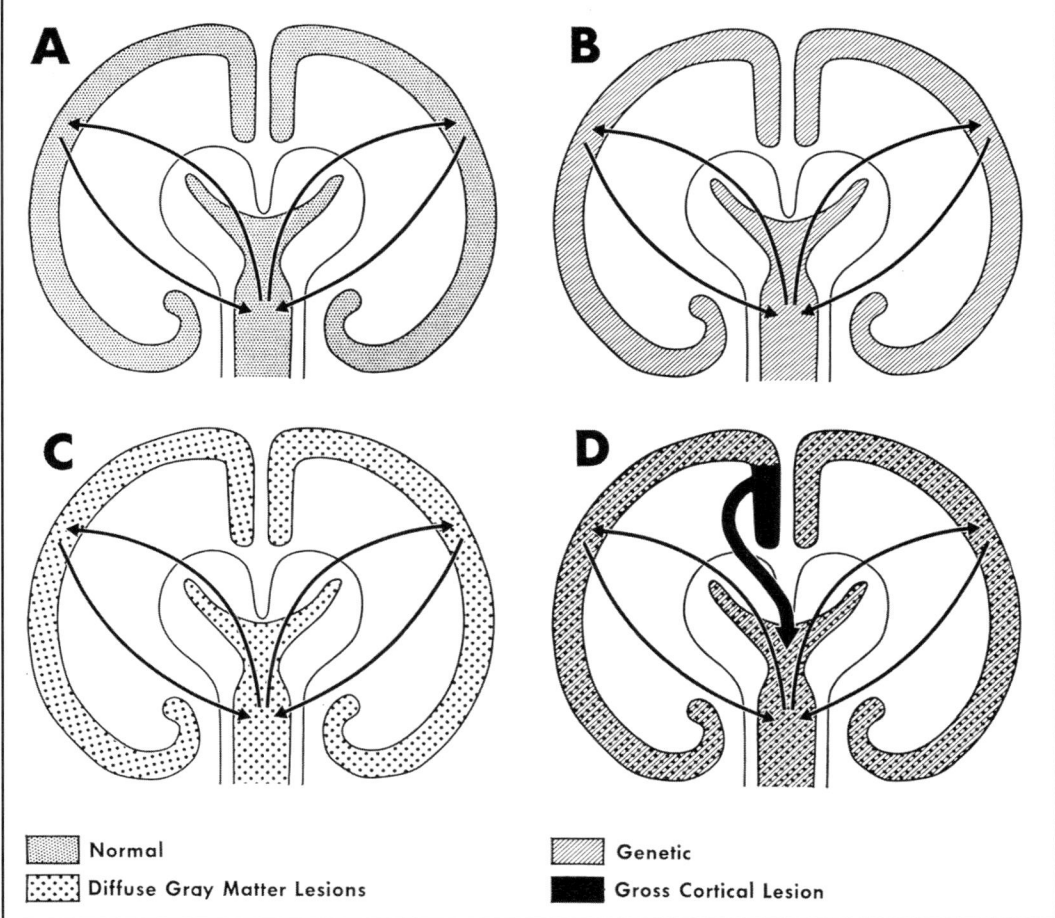

Figure 3. Subtypes of cortico-centrencephalic epilepsies (Gloor, 1969). This schematic drawing of interactions between cerebral cortex and reticular formation in the upper brain stem illustrates three possible conditions of bilateral synchronous paroxysmal discharges being triggered. In B, a genetically determined disturbance is present in cortex and in brain stem ("classical" centrencephalic epilepsy); in C, there is a diffuse encephalopathy; in D, a cortical parasagittal lesion is responsible for bilateral synchronous discharges, because there is a predisposition either genetic of organic.

Talairach and Bancaud were the first to investigate patients who were candidates for epilepsy surgery with intra-cerebral electrodes implanted according to a stereotaxic method based on precise anatomy (Talairach *et al.*, 1967). They had the opportunity to investigate patients who presented with "atypical absences" with abrupt and clear-cut loss of contact, followed or not by subtle motor signs or automatisms, and sometimes secondary generalization initiated by adversion of head and eyes (Bancaud *et al.*, 1965). The coincident EEG discharge consisted of irregular spike-and-waves around 3 Hz, bilateral but asymmetrical *(Figure 4)*.

When recording such seizures with intra-cerebral electrodes during SEEG, they noted that (i) the ictal discharge which correlated with clinical absence was actually composed of rhythmical spike-and-waves localized in premotor and prefrontal cortex, and (ii) the

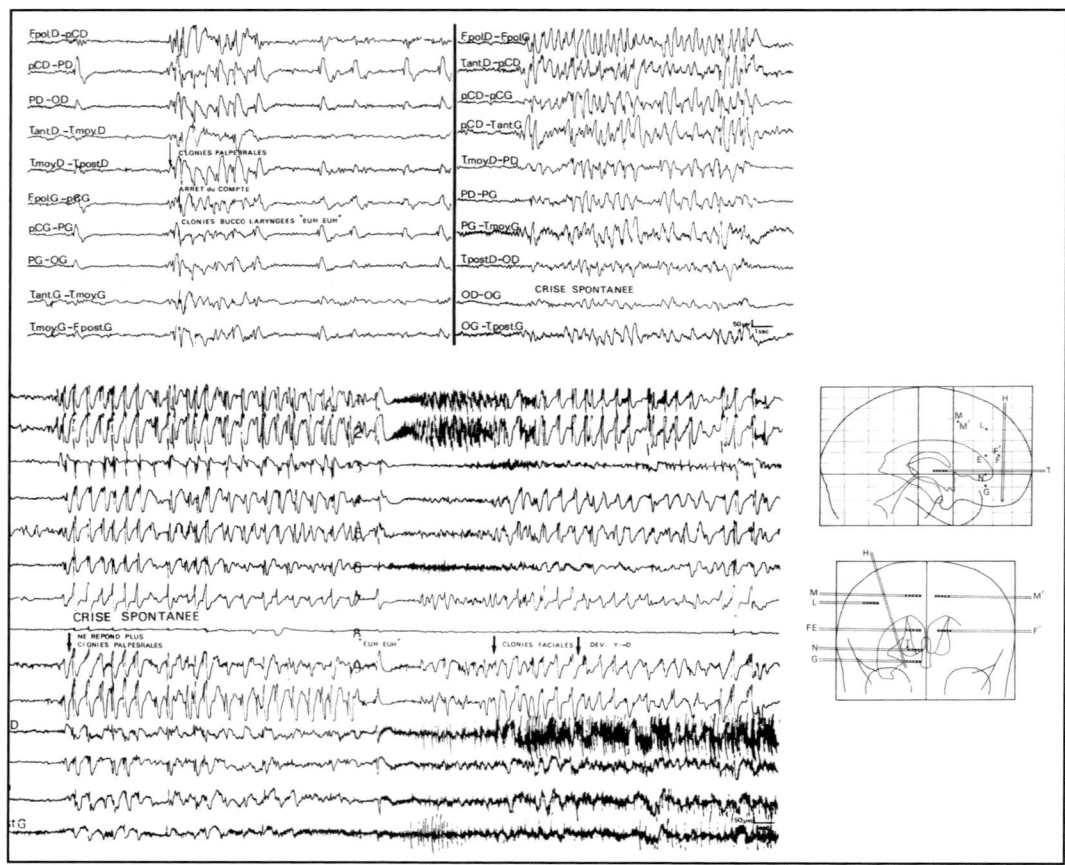

Figure 4. Intra-cerebral recording (SEEG) of a frontal absence (adapted from Bancaud *et al.*, 1973). Explanation in the text. Top traces represent EEG and bottom traces SEEG in the same patient. Capital letters refer to the name of the intracerebral electrodes, as indicated in the schema of the implantation (bottom right). Same time calibration for EEG and SEEG. Time calibration is 1 s.

motor manifestations (eyelid myoclonia, adversion) associated with or following the initial loss of contact were due to a fast discharge originating in the very same areas as the "negative" symptoms (Bancaud *et al.*, 1973).

Another interesting observation was the common anatomical origin of spike-and-wave discharge and tonic-clonic generalized seizures in the border area between prefrontal-and premotor cortex. In a patient presenting with absence seizures, stimulation of one or the other anterior premotor mesial cortex could provoke discharges of high-frequency and high-amplitude spikes that spread very rapidly to the contralateral homotopic regions and to the precentral cortex, correlated with generalized tonic-clonic seizures *(Figure 5)*.

The bulk of these earlier studies by Bancaud and Talairach took the opposite view from the previous defenders of the centrencephalic hypothesis, in demonstrating that the frontal cortex in front of the primary motor area could be responsible for seizures perfectly mimicking generalized seizures. Moreover, these data had been obtained in epileptic patients, whereas direct evidence for subcortical generators was obviously still lacking. Nevertheless, the epilepsies investigated with SEEG could have been diagnosed at least as symptomatic or cryptogenic generalized, but not as idiopathic epilepsies, and it was not yet established that the premotor areas in question could generate a 3Hz pattern of spike-and-wave by themselves without being driven by a remote thalamic generator. Bancaud *et al.* contributed this evidence in 1974. In a group of 10 patients stimulated at 3Hz in various areas of the frontal lobe, spike-and-wave could be triggered at the same frequency in mesial premotor and prefrontal regions, associated with clinical features of Petit Mal absence *(Figure 6)*.

■ Absence seizures studied with fMRI-EEG

Recent developments in NMR-based imaging have allowed correlation of paroxysmal interictal activities with BOLD activation (Waites *et al.*, 2005). This method has been applied to the question of absence seizure brain topography. In a first study, Salek-Haddadi *et al.* (2003) demonstrated a clear thalamic activation with hypoactivation bilaterally in the frontal lobe. Aghakhani *et al.* (2004) then emphasized hyperactivation in both thalami, while hyper- as well as hypoactivations were evident in mesial and lateral prefrontal and premotor regions. Labate *et al.* (2005) in a single case, and Gotman *et al.* (2005) in a series of patients showed a combined thalamo-cortical activation with a complex set of hyperactivations in some parts of the frontal lobe and hypoactivations in other, adjacent, areas. These data are in good agreement with Gloor's concept of a cortico-reticular network in absence seizures.

■ Viewing generalized as partial seizures: can the frontal cortex generate all the electro-clinical patterns termed "generalized"?

These data gathered from intracerebral recordings help in understanding the overestimation of the extent of a generator by standard EEG, which led to the notion of "generalized" epilepsies, whereas their clinical tableau had not rendered this

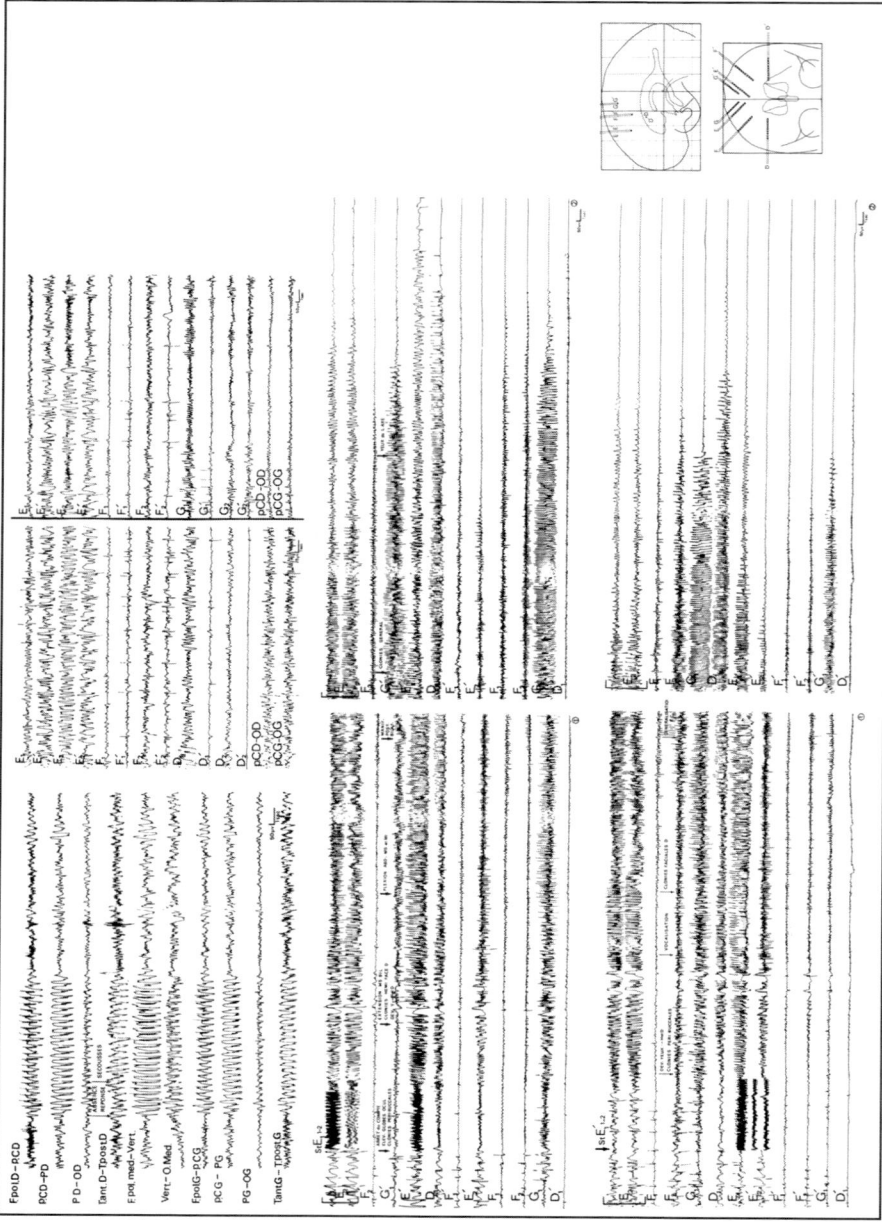

Figure 5. Intracerebral recordings (SEEG) in a patient with absences and tonic-clonic generalized seizures. Direct stimulation of either premotor cortex could induce generalized seizures, from the same region generating spike-and-waves correlated with absences. From Bancaud et al., 1973. EEG recording of an absence (top left) and intracerebral localisation of the spike-and-wave discharge in both electrodes E and E' (as shown in the schema of implantation at the bottom, E is in the right premotor and E' in the left premotor cortex). St e and St E' indicate time of stimulation (50 Hz) applied to these electrodes (stimulation artifact is visible on the traces. Time calibration (at the bottom of the traces) is 1 s.

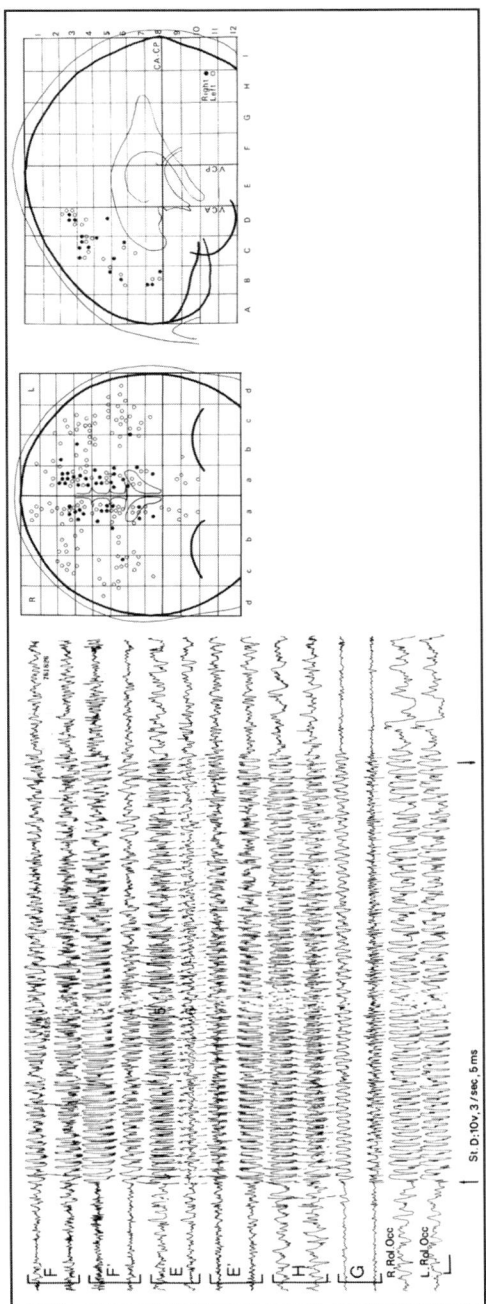

Figure 6. Reproduction of PM absences by 3Hz stimulation of frontal mesial cortex (from Bancaud *et al.*, 1974). E-E' and F-F' are two symmetrical electrodes in the dorsal premotor cortex, whereas H and G are situated in the right ventral premotor cortex with inner leads in the cingulate gyrus. The two bottom traces are simultaneous EEG. Positive (full dots) and negative (clear dots) sites are represented in Talairach's grid. Time calibration (bottom left) is 1 s.

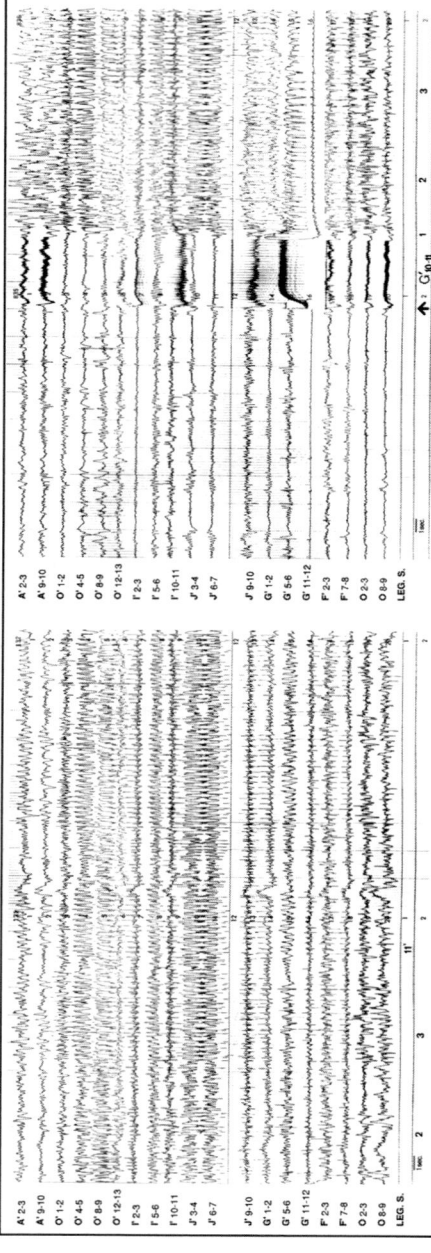

Figure 7. A seizure characterized by focal and sustained spike-and-wave discharge in the dominant (left) inferior frontal gyrus and clinically expressed by an arrest of speech without comprehension deficit. A direct electrical train stimulation (50 Hz) applied to the seizure onset area triggers the same clinical phenomenon with spike-and-wave discharge from the onset (without preceding fast discharge). O' is situated in the left orbito-frontal cortex, G' and J' in two different sites of the left inferior frontal gyrus. The other electrodes are in other parts of the left and right (O) frontal lobe. Time calibration is 1 s.

designation necessary. The anatomical location of the spike-and-wave (or fast discharge) generators in the dorsal and medial frontal lobe makes their projection over the entire anterior scalp likely, and with parietal spread, over almost all the suprasylvian electrodes (Gavaret et al., 2006).

So, as outlined above, the concept of "generalized" came from EEG descriptions before the era of source localization. Most of the publications on this type of seizures were "electroencephalographic" and their clinical manifestations were, within their subcategories, considered as rather monomorphic. Attempts to apply the same clinical tools used for localising diagnosis of partial seizures to these particular seizures were rare. Curiously, the subtle motor signs observed in association with arrest and loss of consciousness were not interpreted in terms of cerebral localisation. Likewise, the frequent overlap between clinical forms of seizures in the same patient seemed to be discussed in terms of entities, not in anatomo-functional relations. These considerations do not aim to minimize the difficulties inherent in these bilateral epilepsies. The immediate impairment of consciousness and the post-ictal amnesia have limited access to a possible subjective content. The localization issue has undoubtedly been hampered by the difficult problems that remain to be solved with EEG, all the more confusing as bilateral and widespread discharges were considered to mean generalized.

A very careful analysis of absence attacks semiology was performed by Penry, Porter and Dreifuss in 1975. In 48 patients with recurring absence seizures, 374 clinical absence attacks were recorded by video-EEG and analyzed independently by two observers. Only one patient experienced an attack comprising only "blank staring" accompanied by unawareness and amnesia, but 40 per cent of patients exhibited this type of attack in addition to more complex absence attacks. Simple absences were actually very rare. The others most often contained, in order of prevalence, either automatisms (88%), mild clonic components (71%), decreased postural tone (41%), or a combination of two or more of these features. The relationship between increased duration of the seizures and the occurrence of automatisms was significant. Using similar techniques, Stefan (1983) studied the temporal structure of absence symptoms in 59 patients (528 seizures). The ratios between clonic signs and automatisms, as well as between increase and decrease of tone were inverted, in comparison with Penry's work. He described a global functional course of motor activity from cranial parts of the body – such as the ocular region – towards more caudal regions. "In analogy to the Jacksonian march of partial elementary motor seizures these findings were interpreted as a march of generalizing seizure activity of absence type. Its recognition allows us to understand many motor as well as so-called 'automatic' absence symptoms as correlated elements of a general organization plan. The development of a nuclear-layer model explains the fact, that in short-lasting absences often only ocular symptoms occur, whereas in long lasting absences oral automatisms or motor activities of the extremities as well as gestural automatisms become manifest". In these two studies, clinical semiology appears to be much more structured than expected, and could be soundly interpreted as revealing a frontal cortical organization.

Niedermeyer, who had had the opportunity to perform intracerebral recordings in patients with generalized spike-and-waves and more specifically Lennox-Gastaut syndrome, was readily convinced by Bancaud's hypothesis of a frontal origin

(Niedermeyer *et al.*, 1970; Laws *et al.*, 1969). In addition to the preceding arguments, he added an interpretation of sudden arrest and fast recovery in absence seizures as a consequence of a brisk suspension of working memory, which is elaborated in the dorso-lateral frontal cortex (Pavone & Niedermeyer, 2000).

Holmes *et al.* (2004) recorded twenty-five absence seizures in five subjects with primary generalized epilepsy with dense-array, 256-channel scalp EEG to determine whether specific regions of cerebral cortex are activated at the onset and during the propagation of the seizures. They used source analysis methods to localize the spike components of each spike-wave burst in each seizure, with sources visualized with standard brain models. The onset of seizures was typically associated with activation of discrete, often unilateral areas of dorsolateral frontal or the orbital frontal lobe. Consistently across all seizures, the negative slow wave was maximal over frontal cortex, and the spike that appeared to the follow the slow wave was highly localized over frontopolar regions of the orbital frontal lobe. In addition, sources in dorsomedial frontal cortex were engaged for each spike-wave cycle. They concluded that absence seizures are not truly "generalized", with immediate global cortical involvement, but rather involve selective cortical networks, including orbital frontal and mesial frontal regions, in the propagation of ictal discharges.

The situation of the frontal eye field (FEF) and the eyelid projection in the dorso-lateral premotor region (Koyama *et al.*, 2004; Gong *et al.*, 2005) could explain why eyelid flutter and eyeball elevation or deviation represent the nuclear (minimal) motor symptomatology in Stefan's model, followed, with spread, by arrest of speech and movement (pre-SMA) and loss of contact and impairment of consciousness (dorsolateral premotor-prefrontal cortex bilaterally). The FEF in man is located at the cross section of the precentral sulcus and the superior frontal sulcus, in a region supporting the connections between multimodality afferents and initiation of action and gesture.

In the thread of this hypothesis, there exists for most of the cardinal manifestations of generalized seizures an anatomo-functional interpretation with the same basis as that of partial seizures.

One important parameter that directly determines the sense of clinical semiology is the mode of discharge and its frequency. A tonic, or a clonic, or a spike-and-wave discharge firing in a given cortical area will not produce the same clinical effect.

As anticipated by Pollen, a spike-and-wave discharge can induce inhibitory (or negative) signs, without necessarily being bilateral and synchronous. This phenomenon has been observed in non-convulsive status epilepticus, or in the few case reports of seizures characterized by unilateral spike-and-wave discharges (*Figure 7*).

Such cases (Niedermeyer *et al.*, 1979) demonstrate that the frontal cortex can host a generator of ictal spike-and-waves responsible for negative symptoms.

Cases of myoclonic-astatic, or tonic-atonic seizures, which are the cause of frequent falls, share common features with the drop-attacks of bilateral frontal lobe epilepsies. These drop-attacks are surgically remediable with anterior callosotomy. The EEG pattern associated with these atonic seizures, which are often preceded by axial or rhizomelic myoclonic jerks, is generally composed of irregular spike-and-wave (with or without subsequent flattening) followed by high-amplitude slow waves. Such seizures have rarely been recorded in depth studies. As exemplified in *figure 8*, they actually consist of a brief spike-and-wave burst from arising as a high-frequency discharge followed by slow waves; these activities are located in medial and lateral parts of the dorsal and ventral premotor cortex. In the illustrated case, rising of the arms in extension was observed at the end of the fast discharge, and the fall occurred just after it, during the slowing phase of the activities.

As has been underlined on several occasions in this chapter, the presence of fast discharges has been noticed as a component of the majority of electrical patterns in these seizures, as well as in the interictal periods. This EEG trait has certainly been underestimated in scalp recordings, because of the shielding effect of the skull and meninges. Interrelation between spike-and-wave and fast discharges is a key point, necessary for understanding the transition (first reported by Bancaud *et al.*, 1973) from absence type to tonic-clonic seizures. The question is whether certain cortical structures such as premotor cortex are more susceptible than others to generate these patterns under specific conditions.

This observation reproduces Bancaud's previous findings on 3 Hz stimulation of the anterior frontal lobe, and reinforces the hypothesis of a specific role of this cortical region in determining the electrical patterns of the so-called generalized seizures.

■ Discussion and Hypothesis

As in every seizure involving the cortex, a network is operating, and as such, most of the time, the thalamus forms part of this. What is special in the so-called generalized seizures is their bilaterality early from the onset, and their synchrony, associated with impairment of consciousness. These features, added to the relative monomorphism of their clinical tableau, could simply indicate that all of these attacks involve the same cortical/subcortical systems. Given that their clinical manifestations are mainly motor, positive and/or negative, and autonomic, with initial loss of consciousness, the first-line candidate structure would be the frontal cortex.

The experience of intracerebral recordings (with the bias that the epilepsies investigated through this method are not idiopathic) teaches us that:

– clinical semiology analogous to what has been described under the category of "generalized" seizures may be correlated with the presence of ictal discharges starting and (rapidly) spreading in premotor or premotor/prefrontal, or prefrontal/premotor/precentral/parietal areas;

– a focal or lateralized onset may be noticed, with fast spread to both premotor mesial and lateral areas;

– what is not seen over the scalp (except in certain cases with prominent involvement of dorsolateral cortex) is the very frequent presence of oscillatory high-frequency ("fast" or "tonic") discharges and their close interrelations with spike-and-wave discharges. These may sometimes appear in short bursts at the top or on the slope of the slow wave (see *Figure 4*). At seizure onset, these fast discharges often seem to be

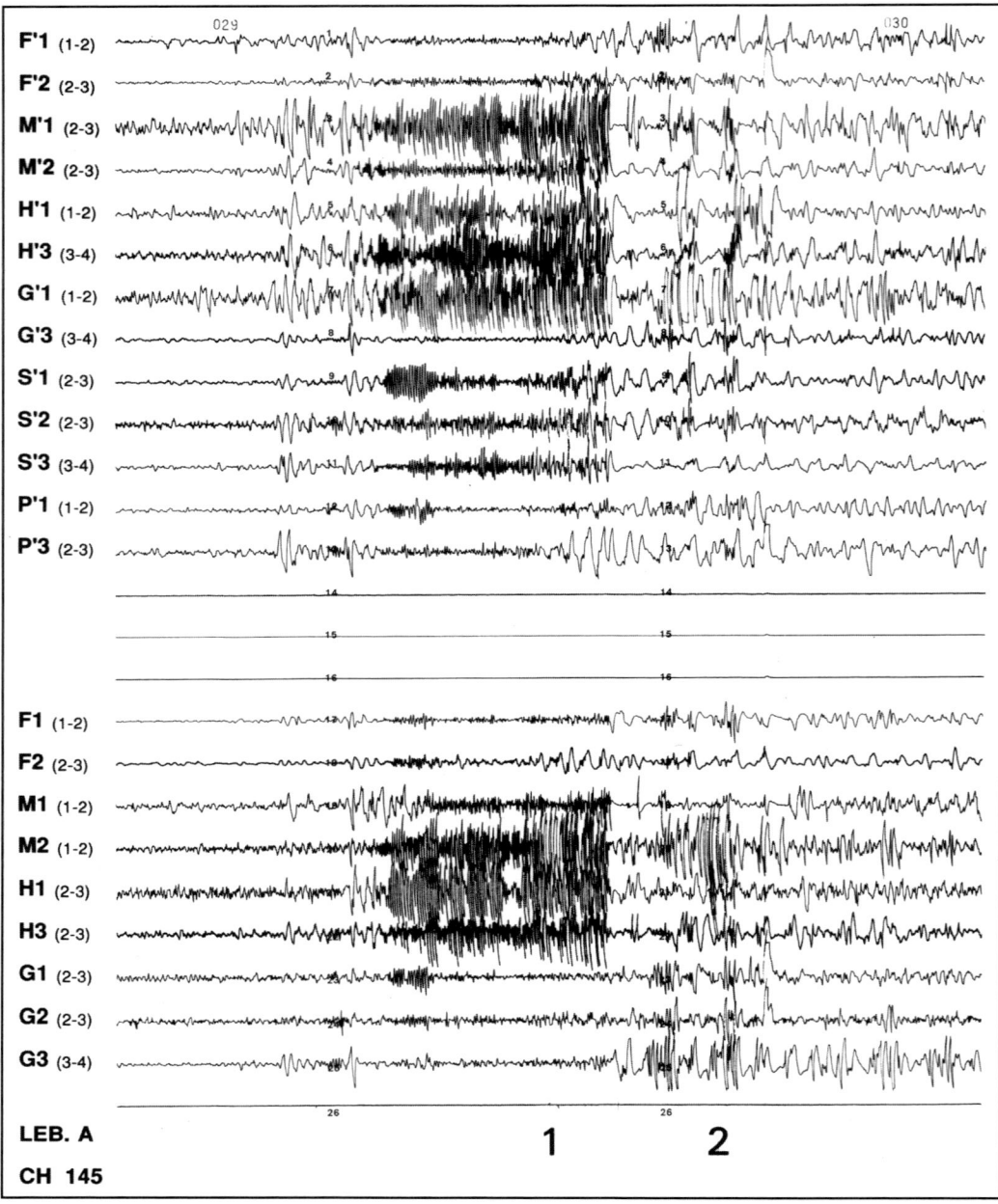

Figure 8. Intracerebral recording of an epileptic drop-attack. 1: slow raising of both arms, slight vocalization; 2: axial hypotonia and fall. Top traces are SEEG recording of the left frontal (F' to S') and parietal (P') cortex, while bottom traces (F to G) are simultaneous SEEG recording of the right frontal cortex. Same letter symbols represent symmetrical electrodes. Indices correspond to depth of the leads of the orthogonal latero-medial multilead electrodes: 1 indicates the more medial and 3 the more lateral leads, and 2 the intermediate. Total duration of the trace: 20 s.

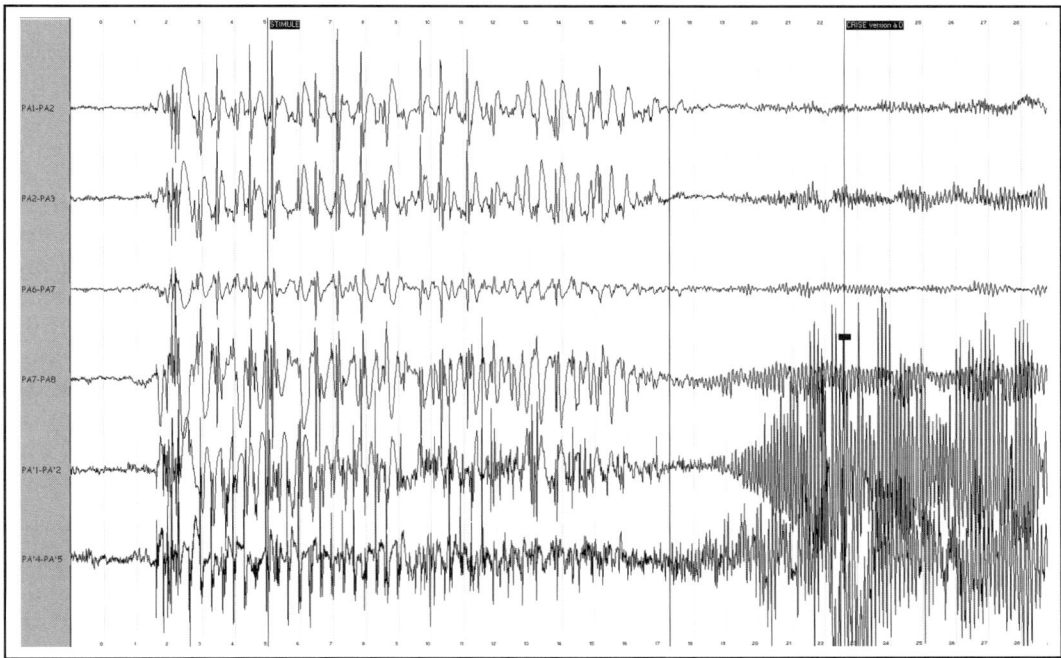

Figure 9. Stimulation of the lateral premotor cortex at 3 Hz. Stimulation (1mA) at 3Hz is applied between two successive leads of an intracerebral electrode passing latero-medially through area 8, then area 6 to reach the pre-SMA with its more medial leads. Lateral and medial premotor cortices are activated by each shock, which generates a spike-and-wave. However, the spike-and-wave immediately spreads to homotopic areas of the opposite side. After 14 s, a fast discharge with increasing amplitude relays the spike-and-wave and similarly spreads to the opposite hemisphere. What should be remarked is that high-frequency bursts are triggered from the start of the stimulation, mostly in the lateral parts of the stimulated left premotor cortex, and merge into a continuous fast discharge. Clinically, the patient stops reading, then deviates eye and head to the right, then presents a bilateral tonic-clonic generalized seizure. Four upper traces: medial and lateral right premotor cortex from top to bottom; two lower traces: medial (pre-SMA) and lateral (junction area 6-FEF) left premotor cortex. Calibration: time between two vertical line is 1 s (total divation 30 s).

triggered by a huge synchronizing slow wave-spike, but they may also be occur without a preceding event, then increase in amplitude and decrease in frequency ("recruiting" discharge);

– the anatomo-electro-clinical correlations are interesting to consider:

• spike-and-waves (spW), which may obviously be interictal most of the time, are the ictal electrical pattern of seizures characterized by arrest and negative motor signs in general. Different conditions in the transition from interictal to ictal spW are encountered: increased rhythmicity and spread with augmented synchronization between several structures, especially bilateral homotopic areas, but unilateral extended spW discharges may well lead to clinical arrest (Niedermeyer, 1979).

- Tonic discharges are responsible for different semiological patterns depending on their location, their spread and their frequency. As mentioned above, bursts of fast discharges intermingled with spikes or spW may be observed interictally, especially during slow-wave sleep. They may appear as triggered by spindles, or even as amplification of spindles. Ictal fast discharges are components of tonic, tonic-clonic, tonic/atonic, and myoclonic seizures. Gastaut's hypothesis of interplay between excitatory/tonic fragmented by inhibitory/slow wave activities in building-up a "generalized" seizure is in agreement with refinding from depth recordings. The motor tonic correlations of fast discharges are observed when they are located in premotor and premotor-motor regions and occur at certain frequencies. However, electro-clinical correlations are often not so strict with positive motor semiology. This can lag behind the fast discharge by seconds. In tonic/atonic seizures, increased tone in proximal upper limb is delayed and builds up until the end of the discharge, and the brisk loss of postural tone occurs during the final high-amplitude slow waves. It is therefore easy to conceive that a fast discharge developing in "negative" premotor areas produces no overt clinical sign at the onset but does so later as spread occurs.

- It is quite possible that fast bilateral discharges impair consciousness by interfering with dorsolateral prefrontal/premotor functions and simultaneously produce arrest of speech and gesture just as stimulation of the pre-SMA would do. As a final remark, discharges originating in these regions of the frontal cortex are not confined to the frontal lobe, but systematically spread to anterior parietal cortex from pre-SMA and to anterior occipital cortex from prefrontal regions. An alternative hypothesis could also be elaborated based on initial discharges in the parieto-occipital mesial regions with fast spread forward to prefrontal and premotor areas, with a similar clinical appearance. This is one of the possible reasons for failure of anterior two-third callosotomies.

So, what is a generalized seizure? This is one of the most difficult questions in epileptology. As a working hypothesis, we could propose that its clinical semiology, whatever the type, would be directly determined by the localization, the initial extent and the systemic organization of the discharge in the cerebral cortex, particularly the frontal lobe. Its peculiarity in modulation and synchronization mechanisms pertains very likely to thalamo-cortical oscillatory networks. Even in the case of subcortical triggers, all the components of these networks, cortex included, should be abnormally excitable in order for this system to produce these types of seizures. The classic idea of a "transfer" of spike-and-waves driving remote target areas should be revisited (Ono *et al.*, 2002a, b).

References

Aghakhani Y, Bagshaw AP, Benar CG, Hawco C, Andermann F, Dubeau F, Gotman J. fMRI activation during spike and wave discharges in idiopathic generalized epilepsy. *Brain* 2004; 127 (Pt 5): 1127-44.

Bancaud J, Talairach J, *et al.* La StéréoElectroEncephalographie dans l'Épilepsie. Paris: Masson, 1965: 321.

Bancaud J. Physiopathogenesis of generalized epilepsies of organic nature (stereoelectroencephalographic study). In: Gastaut H, Jasper H, Bancaud J, Waltregny A, eds. *The physiopathogenesis of the epilepsies*. Springfield, Illinois: Charles C. Thomas, publisher, 1969: 158-85.

Bancaud J, Talairach J, Geier S, Scarabin JM. *EEG et SEEG dans les tumeurs cérébrales et dans l'épilepsie.* Paris: 1973: 351.

Bancaud J, Talairach J, Morel P, Bresson M, Bonis A, Geier S, Hemon E, Buser P. "Generalized" epileptic seizures elicited by electrical stimulation of the frontal lobe in man. *Electroencephalogr Clin Neurophysiol* 1974; 37 (3): 275-82.

Bennett FE. Intracarotid and intravertebral Metrazol in petit mal epilepsy. *Neurology* 1953; 3: 668-73.

Clinical and electroencephalographical classification of epileptic seizures. *Epilepsia* 1970; 11: 102-13.

Fisher RS, Niedermeyer E. Depth EEG studies in the Lennox-Gastaut syndrome. *Clin Electroencephalogr* 1987; 18 (4): 191-200.

Gastaut H, Gastaut Y, Roger A, Roger J. Étude statistique des différents types électro-cliniques d'épilepsie. *Marseille Médical* 1955 : 553-562.

Gastaut H, Broughton R. Epileptic Seizures. Charles C Thomas publisher, Springfield, Illinois. 1972, 286 pp.

Gavaret M, Badier JM, Marquis P, McGonigal A, Bartolomei F, Regis J, Chauvel P. Electric Source Imaging in Frontal Lobe Epilepsy. *J Clin Neurophysiol* (in press).

Gibbs FA, Gibbs EL. Epilepsy. In: *Atlas of Electroencephalography* Cambridge: Addison-Wesley, 1952: vol. 2.

Gloor P. Neurophysiological bases of generalized seizures termed centrencephalic. In: Gastaut H, Jasper H, Bancaud J, Waltregny A, eds. *The physiopathogenesis of the epilepsies.* Springfield, Illinois: Charles C Thomas, publisher, 1969: 209-36.

Gloor P, Quesney LF, Zumstein H. Pathophysiology of generalized penicillin epilepsy in the cat: the role of cortical and subcortical structures. II. Topical application of penicillin to the cerebral cortex and to subcortical structures. *Electroencephalogr Clin Neurophysiol* 1977; 43 (1): 79-94.

Gong S, DeCuypere M, Zhao Y, LeDoux MS. Cerebral cortical control of orbicularis oculi motoneurons. *Brain Res* 2005; 1047 (2): 177-93.

Gotman J, Grova C, Bagshaw A, Kobayashi E, Aghakhani Y, Dubeau F. Generalized epileptic discharges show thalamocortical activation and suspension of the default state of the brain. *Proc Natl Acad Sci USA* 2005; 102 (42): 15236-40.

Gowers WR. *Epilepsy and other chronic convulsive disorders.* New York: William Wood and company, 1881: 255.

Hamandi K, Salek-Haddadi A, Fish DR, Lemieux L. EEG/functional MRI in epilepsy: The Queen Square Experience. *J Clin Neurophysiol* 2004; 21 (4): 241-8.

Holmes MD, Brown M, Tucker DM. Are "generalized" seizures truly generalized? Evidence of localized mesial frontal and frontopolar discharges in absence. *Epilepsia* 2004; 45 (12): 1568-79.

Jackson JH. On the anatomical, physiological, and pathological investigation of epilepsies. *West Riding Lunatic Asylum Medical Reports* 1873; 3: 315.

Jasper HH, Droogleever-Fortuyn J. Experimental studies on the functional anatomy of petit mal epilepsy. *Res Publ Assoc Nerv Ment Dis* 1947; 26: 272-98.

Jasper HH, Kershman J. Electroencephalographic classification of the epilepsies. *Arch Neurol Psychiat (Chicago)* 1941; 45: 903-43.

Jasper HH. Introduction. In: Gastaut H, Jasper H, Bancaud J, Waltregny A, eds. *The physiopathogenesis of the epilepsies.* Springfield, Illinois: Charles C Thomas, publisher, 1969: 201-8.

Koyama M, Hasegawa I, Osada T, Adachi Y, Nakahara K, Miyashita Y. Functional magnetic resonance imaging of macaque monkeys performing visually guided saccade tasks: comparison of cortical eye fields with humans. *Neuron* 2004; 41 (5): 795-807.

Labate A, Briellmann RS, Abbott DF, Waites AB, Jackson GD. Typical childhood absence seizures are associated with thalamic activation. *Epileptic Disord* 2005; 7 (4): 373-7.

Laws E, Niedermeyer E, Walker AE. Depth EEG findings in epileptics with generalized spike-wave complexes. *Electroencephalogr Clin Neurophysiol* 1970; 28 (1): 94-5.

Morison RS, and Dempsey EW. Study of thalamocortical relations. *Amer J Physiol* 1942; 135: 281-92.

Moruzzi G, Magoun HW. Brain stem reticular formation and activation of the EEG. 1949. *J Neuropsychiatry Clin Neurosci* 1995; 7 (2): 251-67.

Niedermeyer E, Laws ER Jr, Walker EA. Depth EEG findings in epileptics with generalized spike-wave complexes. *Arch Neurol* 1969; 21 (1): 51-8.

Niedermeyer E, Fineyre F, Riley T, Uematsu S. Absence status (petit mal status) with focal characteristics. *Arch Neurol* 1979; 36 (7): 417-21.

Ono T, Matsuo A, Baba H, Ono K. Is a cortical spike discharge "transferred" to the contralateral cortex via the corpus callosum? An intraoperative observation of electrocorticogram and callosal compound action potentials. *Epilepsia* 2002a; 43 (12): 1536-42.

Ono T, Fujimura K, Yoshida S, Ono K. Suppressive effect of callosotomy on epileptic seizures is due to the blockade of enhancement of cortical reactivity by transcallosal volleys. *Epilepsy Res* 2002b; 51 (1-2): 117-21.

Pavone A, Niedermeyer E. Absence seizures and the frontal lobe. *Clin Electroencephalogr* 2000; 31 (3): 153-6.

Penfield W. *Consciousness and centrencephalic organization*. Premier Congrès International des Sciences Neurologiques. Brussels, 1957: 7-18.

Penfield W. The interpretive cortex; the stream of consciousness in the human brain can be electrically reactivated. *Science* 1959; 129 (3365): 1719-25.

Penry JK, Porter RJ, Dreifuss RE. Simultaneous recording of absence seizures with video tape and electroencephalography. A study of 374 seizures in 48 patients. *Brain* 1975; 98 (3): 427-40.

Perot P. *Mesencephalic-thalamic relations in wave and spike mechanisms*. Montreal, McGill University: PhD thesis, 1963.

Pollen DA. Intracellular studies of cortical neurons during thalamic induced wave and spike. *Electroenceph Clin Neurophysiol* 1964; 17: 398-404.

Quesney LF, Gloor P, Kratzenberg E, Zumstein H. Pathophysiology of generalized penicillin epilepsy in the cat: the role of cortical and subcortical structures. I. Systemic application of penicillin. *Electroencephalogr Clin Neurophysiol* 1977; 42 (5): 640-55.

Salek-Haddadi A, Lemieux L, Merschhemke M, Friston KJ, Duncan JS, Fish DR. Functional magnetic resonance imaging of human absence seizures. *Ann Neurol* 2003; 53 (5): 663-7.

Stefan H. Epileptic absences. Studies on the structure, pathophysiology and clinical course of the seizure. *Fortschr Med* 1983; 101 (21): 996-8.

Talairach J, Szikla G, et al. *Atlas d'Anatomie Stéréotaxique du Télencéphale*. Paris: Masson, 1967: 323.

Tükel K, Jasper HH. The electroencephalogram in parasagittal lesions. *Electroencephalogr Clin Neurophysiol Suppl* 1952; 4 (4): 481-94.

Waites AB, Shaw ME, Briellmann RS, Labate A, Abbott DF, Jackson GD. How reliable are fMRI-EEG studies of epilepsy? A nonparametric approach to analysis validation and optimization. *Neuroimage* 2005; 24 (1): 192-9.

What is Generalized Epilepsy?

Frederick Andermann

Neurology and Pediatrics, McGill University Epilepsy Service, Montreal Neurological Institute, Quebec, Canada

There was, for many generations, a great deal of uncertainty about the causes and significance of different forms of epilepsy. One must remember that before Berger's development of the electroencephalogram there was much discussion as to whether childhood absence attacks were actually epileptic manifestations or a phenomenon sui generis (Friedmann, 1906). It was the recognition of the diffuse nature of the spike and wave discharge, as opposed to the focal or localized discharges which led to firming up the concept of a generalized epileptic process. This is now generally accepted, despite many observations of various focal phenomena in patients with generalized spike and wave. These arguments continue to preoccupy clinical and basic epileptologists to this day. As an example, one can quote the ongoing stream of publications discussing the frontal electrographic and neuropsychological manifestations in patients with diffuse spike and wave as a manifestation of juvenile myoclonic epilepsy (Devinsky, 1997; Simister, 2003a).

The recognition of epileptic syndromes has raised the issue of the varying seizure patterns, or "components" e.g., absences, myoclonus, generalized tonic clonic or clonic tonic seizures found in different combinations in different syndromes. The description of syndromes has also highlighted the now classical observations of the age and maturation dependent forms of generalized idiopathic epilepsies who are, to a large extent, genetically determined *(Figure 1)* (Janz, 1994). The reasons for the pathophysiology and coexistence in this group of syndromes of absences, myoclonic jerks, tonic clonic attacks, clonic tonic clonic seizure patterns are still insufficiently clarified, and represent a continuing challenge for the basic investigators. The demonstration of generalized spike and wave, common to these patients, clearly indicated a close relationship between these different epileptic patterns, though the spike and wave itself may show considerable variation. Recognition of the systems and networks involved in the largely genetic, multifactorial generalized epilepsies, greatly contributed to our understanding of the mechanisms that might then lead to an improved and more rational definition of this group of epileptic disorders.

One of the first issues addressed was the frequency of the discharges and the recognition of what used to be called "atypical spike and wave", or slow spike and wave. This was eventually recognized as the hallmark of a group of disorders where

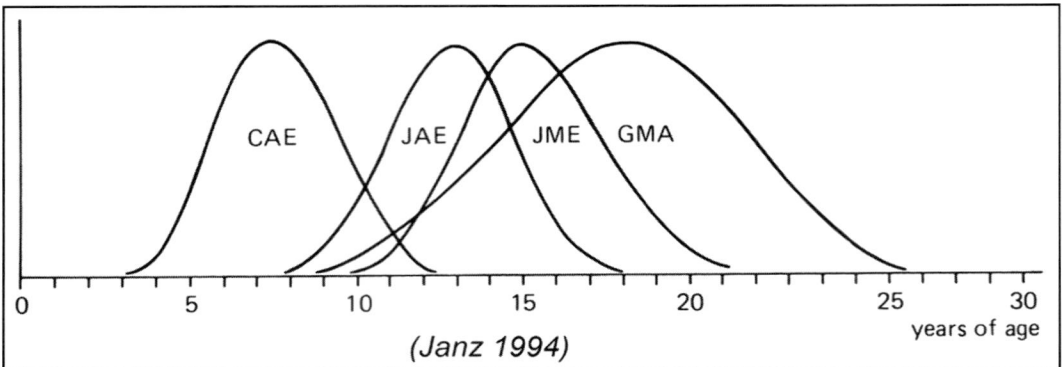

Figure 1. The age related forms of idiopathic generalized epilepsies and their overlap.

intelligence was limited, background activity abnormal, deterioration the rule, and the clinical patterns different, though sharing some of the features seen in patients with primary generalized idiopathic epilepsy (Lennox, 1950; Gastaut, 1966).

In the early days of widespread availability of the EEG the slow spike and wave pattern was found to be associated with important cognitive disabilities, deterioration and great unresponsiveness to therapeutic agents. This has led to the pioneering descriptions of Henri Gastaut and William Lennox, whose names have remained eponymically attached to at least one of the syndromes with generalized epileptic discharge. In early life recognition of a combination of seizure patterns with myoclonus, falling attacks, and absences, led to the identification by Hermann Doose of myoclonic astatic epilepsy, sometimes but not always refractory and associated with cognitive deficits (Doose, 1970). Even earlier in life infantile spasms with their dismal prognosis were perceived as a generalized process. The recognition of the role of focal or regional changes and the subsequent development of surgical treatment in children with this form has highlighted the relationship between focal and generalized abnormalities indicating a process of secondary generalization and a favourable response to surgical treatment pioneered by the group of Chugani, Shields, and Shewmon (Chugani, 1900). Dissection of these features illustrates that despite the diffuse nature of the interictal epileptic discharge, focal or regional features may be present and one may then ask what are the predominating characteristics, and how should such forms of epilepsy be perceived. It seems clear that both regional and generalized aspects may coexist, but one has to take into account, in addition to these features, the genetic aspects, natural history, coexistence of different ictal manifestations and the response to treatment. Diffuse widespread or indeed generalized features seem most significant and thus inclusion in the group of generalized epilepsies seems appropriate.

The relationship of focal cortical areas and manifestations to the generalized electrographic changes and seizure patterns seen in some of the reflex epilepsies has permitted development of a unified concept of activation of a generalized process by areas of regional or focal cortical hyperexcitability (Ferlazzo et al., 2005) in response to such stimuli as reading, calculating, measuring, thinking, visual flashes, viewing patterns or praxis. Patterns with both features of localized cortical function and widespread epileptic manifestation may include quite typical generalized patterns such as seen in juvenile myoclonic epilepsy. This highlights a form of interaction which makes classification difficult. Attributing different orders of value to the focal and to the generalized aspects leads to a somewhat arbitrary conceptualization of some of these forms of reflex epilepsy. One is swayed to emphasize the generalized or diffuse features despite activation by initial focal mechanisms. Most important however remains the recognition of the interaction of the focal or regional symptoms with the generalized features in these epilepsies.

The advent of modern imaging has also led to some difficulties in distinguishing between focal and generalized epileptic processes. As an example, one may look at patients with band heterotopia or double cortex. In these individuals the anatomical changes are often generalized and so are many of the electrographic abnormalities. Some of these patients however may have a predominantly focalized abnormality as well, which has encouraged attempts at surgical treatment despite the widespread developmental abnormality. Results of resections of the electrographically most active area have, with rare exceptions, led to poor results (Bernasconi et al., 2001). On the other hand, recognition of the anatomical basis of mesial temporal epilepsy has been a major factor in encouraging selective resections often limited to the amygdala and the hippocampus. Despite evidence for more widespread and contralateral dysfunction such limited resections may lead to very good surgical results (Arruda et al., 1996). Obviously the concept of a pinpoint or highly circumscribed origin of the seizures does not explain all the clinical, neuropsychological and psychiatric manifestations of this disorder.

The progressive myoclonus epilepsies serve as an illustration of the concept of systems and networks underlying clinical patterns. Almost 20 different pathological processes produce a very similar, though not quite identical clinical pattern. Unverricht Lundborg disease, Lafora, neuronal ceroid lipofuscinosis, sialidosis, and many others share the key features of myoclonus, tonic-clonic, or clonic-tonic-clonic seizures, ataxia, and mental deterioration, albeit in varying clinical degrees (Berkovic et al., 1986). Yet, the anatomical basis of these different pathological processes is not well recognized and progress in their understanding on a molecular level has far outstripped recognition of the pathological changes. One may postulate a common anatomical system involving cortical, brainstem and cerebellar structures but this has not been clearly identified. What is clear is that a variety of pathological changes can produce similar clinical patterns, related, though not identical, to the generalized or diffuse epilepsies across life.

The recognition of the genetic basis of some partial epilepsies in the absence of identifiable structural changes points to regional mechanisms in contrast to the diffuse nature of the more common generalized epilepsies, which have multifactorial or polygenic inheritance (Andermann et al., 2005).

The natural urge to construct a framework which is widely accepted and on which new findings can be superimposed, new treatments developed and new insights reached, leads to the establishment of classifications of biological or medical phenomena. These are, by definition, temporary, to be replaced and updated as new knowledge becomes available. Great care must be taken not to introduce confusion leading to counterproductive results. Identification of epileptic syndromes has led to improvements in diagnosis and in treatment of the epilepsies. At the same time one must always be aware that syndromes represent somewhat forced constructs and that because of the individuality of the subjects one must always be aware of the neurobiological continuum on which individuals must be placed.

The bilateral and diffuse nature of the spike and wave discharge with sudden onset and offset, and without perceptible warnings, has prompted Penfield and Jasper to speculate on the existence of a system projecting from subcortical structures to diffuse cortical regions, the so-called centrencephalic system (*Figure 2*) (Penfield and Jasper, 1954). This concept, though it accounted for many of the clinical features, was criticized, notably by Walsh, also on theoretical grounds, but it has continued to linger in the epileptological literature (Walsh, 1957). Gloor's work on experimental generalized epilepsy has led to the concept of corticoreticular mechanisms and to this day studies have centered on the relationship of cortical to subcortical structures in the genesis of these forms of seizures and epilepsies (Gloor, 1968). The concept will no doubt continue to evolve as more data become available, clarifying not only the genesis of different clinical patterns, but also their evolution throughout life. The characteristic coexistence of the different clinical patterns, and also their evolution over time, has been well recognized and defined by Janz. This overlap has been graphically illustrated in a series of diagrams which have stood the test of time (Janz, 1994).

The progression from spike and wave to the multiple spike pattern is age dependent, as Gibbs and his group have recognized early (Gibbs, 1935). The patterns of change in the electrographic manifestations over life, with the demonstration of multiple sharp wave discharges, originally termed as the "grand mal" pattern by Gibbs, replacing the spike and wave discharge, is still a phenomenon not sufficiently explained by modern neuroscience.

One may then say that primary generalized epilepsy includes a group of clinical syndromes which share genetic background, clinical patterns, the absence of gross pathology, compatibility with normal cognitive development, normal EEG background activity, age dependency, and responsivity to some antiepileptic medications. One must also recognize that this definition is incomplete, that it does not take into account a variety of focal features, transition to forms with greater severity, and imperfect correspondence with all the above-mentioned factors. These syndromes are subserved by neuronal networks and systems which are being increasingly identified.

Secondary generalized epilepsy also emerged as an identifiable concept, subsuming a number of epileptic syndromes. The distinction between primary and secondary epilepsy is by no means always easy, and this was beautifully illustrated by the late Peter Gloor as a continuum of electrical and clinical patterns ranging across a spectrum of epileptic disorders (*Figure 3*) (Gloor, 1979). In addition, asymmetries, both in spike and wave and even in clinical manifestations, have increasingly been recognized, and here too, the distinction between what is an essentially generalized discharge from a primarily focal process may be far from easy.

Whether hemigeneralized seizures, as encountered in children, deserve to be enshrined as a specific epileptic syndrome has never been fully settled.

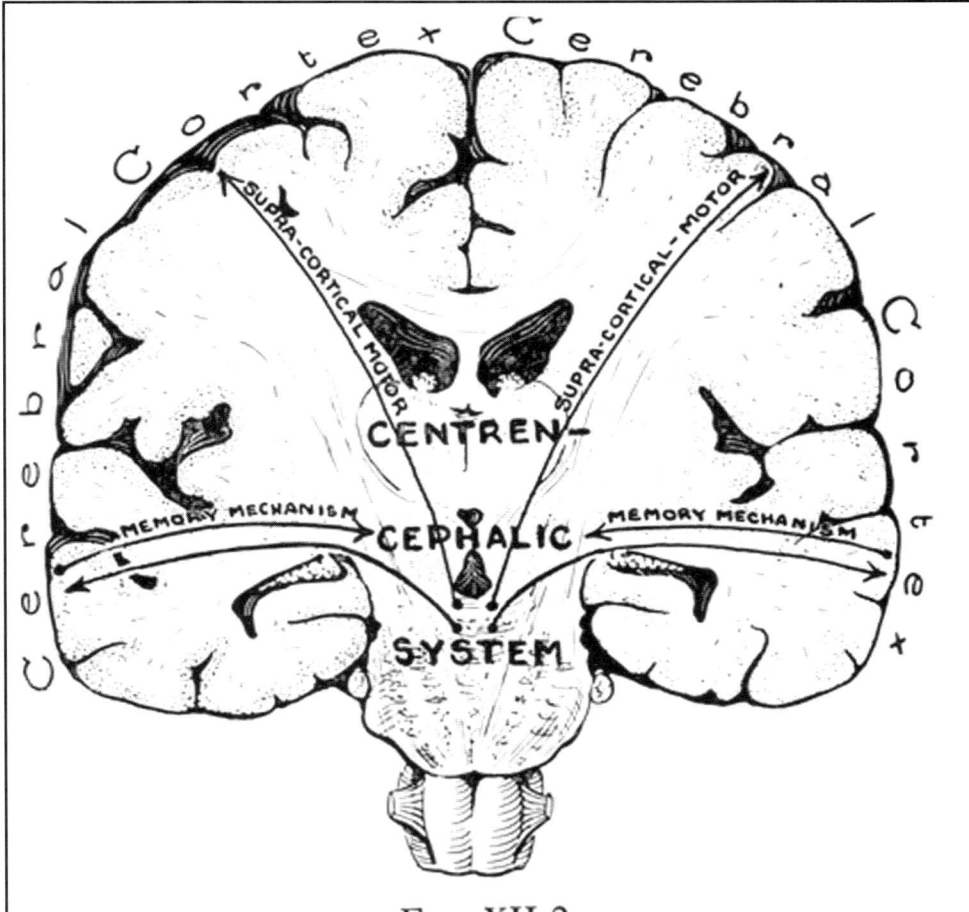

FIG. XII-2

FIG. XII-2. The centrencephalic system may be defined as that neurone system, centering in the higher brain stem, which has been up to the present, or may be in the future, shown to have equal functional relationships with the two cerebral hemispheres. It forms the chief central integrating mechanism for various areas of cortex. The to-and-fro projection pathways indicated should be considered as integral parts of this system. "Supra-cortical motor" pathway carries the impulses to precentral gyrus that result in voluntary movement. "Memory mechanism" pathways render the records of past experience available.

Figure 2. The centrencephalic hypothesis of Wilder Penfield and Herbert Jasper.

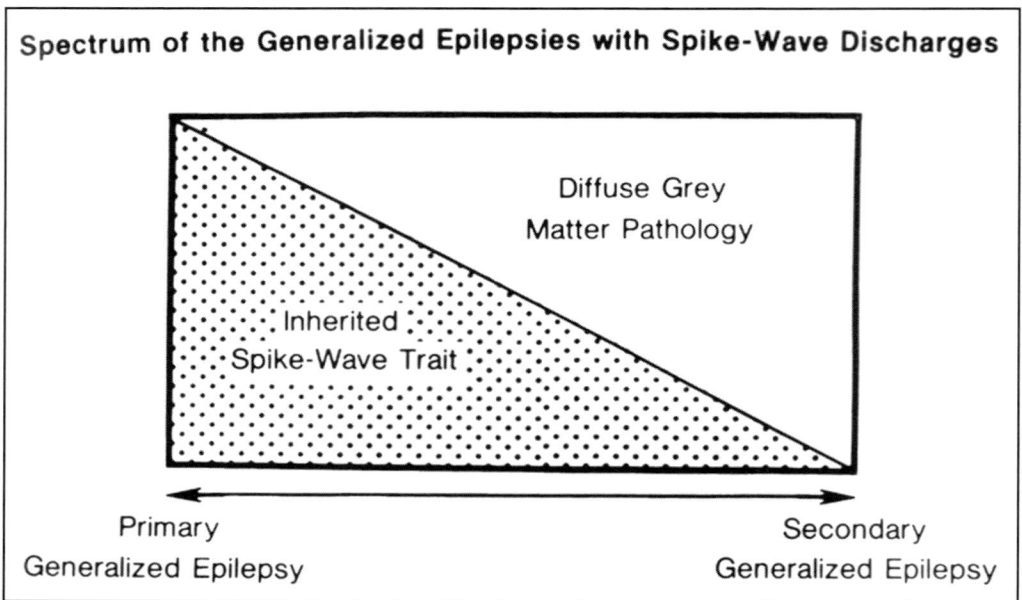

Figure 3. The continuum between genetic and acquired components in the primary and secondary generalized epilepsies (modified from Gloor with permission).

Focal changes in idiopathic epilepsy may contribute to difficulties in seizure control and certainly asymmetries demonstrated by imaging are probably significant in this sense as well. The effectiveness of antiepileptic medications is not based only on recognition of the epileptic syndrome that patients being treated have, but also in many instances on the lack of responsiveness of these patients to the usually most effective drugs, in which presumably focal accentuation and focalization play an important role.

The recognition of sensitivity of many epileptic syndromes to drugs like valproate and conversely the tendency of drugs like carbamazepine, gabapentin, or gamma vinyl gaba, to bring out patterns, usually associated with the generalized manifestations of diffuse epilepsies, is another aspect that highlights the difference between the primarily diffuse and the primarily focal epileptic disorders.

The role of focal lesions leading to diffuse or generalized epileptic discharges such as the mesial frontal lesions described by Tukel and Jasper, provoking generalized spike and wave, suggests that focal abnormalities can indeed activate, what from an EEG point of view, appears to be a diffuse process (Tükel and Jasper, 1952). This is the concept of secondary generalization as distinct from secondary generalized epilepsy. However, attempts to prove focal origin and consider the possibility of surgical treatment in patients with diffuse spike and wave by means of the intracarotid amytal metrazol test, or the Lombroso Erba test (Lombroso and Erba, 1969), have not been fruitful and have now largely been abandoned in the light of progress in epileptology.

This volume brings together recent contributions and developments in our understanding of the systems and networks underlying the different mechanisms of the epilepsies in which diffuse or generalized features predominate.

References

Andermann F, Kobayashi E, Andermann E. Genetic focal epilepsies: state of the art and paths to the future. *Epilepsia* 2005; 46 (Suppl 10): 61-7.

Arruda F, Cendes F, Andermann F, Dubeau F, Villemure JG, Jones-Gotman M, Poulin N, Arnold DA, Olivier A. Mesial atrophy and outcome after amygdalohippocampectomy or temporal lobe removal. *Ann Neurol* 1996; 40: 446-50.

Berkovic S, Andermann F, Carpenter S, Andermann E, Wolfe LS. Progressive myoclonus epilepsies: specific causes and diagnosis. *N Engl J Med* 1986; 135: 296-305.

Bernasconi A, Martinez V, Rosa-Neto P, D'Agostino D, Bernasconi N, Berkovic S, MacKay M, Harvey AS, Palmini A, Da Costa JC, Paglioli E, Kim HI, Connolly M, Olivier A, Dubeau F, Andermann E, Guerrini R, Whisler W, De Toledo-Morrell L, Morrell F, Andermann F. Surgical resection for intractable epilepsy in "double cortex" syndrome yields inadequate results. *Epilepsia* 2001; 42 (9): 1124-9.

Blumenfeld H, Westerveld M, Ostroff RB, *et al*. Selective frontal, parietal, and temporal networks in generalized seizures. *Neuroimage* 2003; 19: 1556-66.

Chugani HT, Shields WD, Shewmon DA, Olson DM, Phelps ME, Peacock WJ. Infantile spasm: I. PET identifies focal cortical dysgenesis in cryptogenic cases for surgical treatment. *Ann Neurol* 1900; 27: 406-13.

Devinsky O, Gershengorn J, Brown E, Perrine K, Vazquez B, Luciano D. Frontal functions in juvenile myoclonic epilepsy. *Neuropsychiatry Neuropsychol Behav Neurol* 1997; 10: 243-6.

Doose H, Gerken H, Leonhardt R, Voltzke E, Colz C. Centrencephalic myoclonic-astatic petit-mal. *Neuropediatrics* 1970; 2: 59-78.

Ferlazzo E, Zifkin BG, Andermann E, Andermann F. Cortical triggers in generalized reflex seizures and epilepsies. *Brain* 2005; 128 (4): 700-10.

Friedmann M. Über die nicht epileptischen Absencen oder kurzen narkoleptischen Anfälle. *Deutsche Ztschr Nervenh* 1906; 30: 462-91.

Gastaut H, Roger J, Soulayrol R, *et al*. Childhood epileptic encephalopathy with diffuse slow spike-waves (otherwise known as "petit mal variant") or Lennox syndrome. *Epilepsia* 1966; 7: 139-79.

Janz D. Pitfalls in the diagnosis of grand mal on awakening. In: Wolf P, ed. *Epileptic Seizures and Syndromes* London: John Libbey, 1994: 213-20.

Gibbs FA, Davis H, Lennox WG. The electroencephalogram in epilepsy and in conditions of impaired consciousness. *Arch Neurol Psychiatry* 1935; 34: 1133-48.

Gloor P. Generalized cortico-reticular epilepsies. Some considerations on the pathophysiology of generalized bilaterally synchronous spike and wave discharge. *Epilepsia* 1968; 9: 249-63.

Gloor P. Generalized epilepsy with spike-and-wave discharge: a reinterpretation of its electrographic and clinical manifestations. *Epilepsia* 1979; 20: 571-88.

Lennox WG, Davis JP. Clinical correlates of the fast and the slow spike-wave electroencephalogram. *Pediatrics* 1950; 5: 626-44.

Lombroso CT, Erba G. A test separating secondary from primary bilateral synchrony in epileptic subjects. [Journal Article] *Epilepsia* 1969; 3: 415-6.

Meencke HJ. Neuron density in the molecular layer of the frontal cortex in primary generalized epilepsy. *Epilepsia* 1985; 26: 450-4.

Penfield W, Jasper H. *Epilepsy and the Functional Anatomy of the Human Brain*. London: J & A Churchill, 1954.

Savic I, Lekvall A, Greitz D, Helms G. MR spectroscopy shows reduced frontal lobe concentrations of N-acetyl aspartate in patients with juvenile myoclonic epilepsy. *Epilepsia* 2000; 41: 290-6.

Simister RJ, McLean MA, Barker GJ, Duncan JS. Proton MRS reveals frontal lobe metabolite abnormalities in idiopathic generalized epilepsy. *Neurology* 2003a; 44: 550-8.

Tükel K, Jasper H. The electroencephalogram in parasagittal lesions. *Electroencephalogr Clin Neurophysiol* 1952; 4: 481-94.

Walsh FM. The brain-stem conceived as the highest level of function in the nervous system; with particular reference to the automatic apparatus of Carpenter (1850) and to the centrencephalic integrating system of Penfield. *Brain* 1957; 80 (4): 510-39.

Section II :
Tonic seizures and brainstem systems

From brainstem to forebrain in generalized animal models of seizures and epilepsies

Phillip C. Jobe[1], Ronald A. Browning[2]

[1] Department of Biomedical and Therapeutic Sciences,
The University of Illinois College of Medicine at Peoria, Peoria, Illinois
[2] Department of Physiology, Southern Illinois University School of Medicine, Carbondale, Illinois, USA

Arguments supporting a major role of the subcortical brain in seizure generation and maintenance have been advanced by outstanding academic figures of recent and somewhat more distant history (Gastaut, 1987; Fromm, 1987). Other prominent investigators have emphasized the cardinal role of the cerebral cortex (Aicardi, 1986b). Still others have advanced the primacy of "rostral" structures, while acknowledging that tonic seizures may be mediated by the brainstem (Engel, 1989). Within this milieu of ideas, consensus definitions have been recently developed by the International League Against Epilepsy and the International Bureau for Epilepsy: the "Cerebral cortex is the primary element in the generation of epileptic seizures, but it is not the only one. In some circumstances, epileptic seizures can originate in thalamocortical interactive systems or in the brainstem" (Fisher et al., 2005).

Normal mammals as well as many, if not all, of their counterparts with epilepsy are characterized by two sets of convulsive seizure circuitry: the forebrain seizure circuitry; and the brainstem seizure circuitry. As will be demonstrated in subsequent sections of this monograph, partial seizures in humans with epilepsy (Engel, Jr. and Schwartzkroin, 2006) correspond with seizures known to be driven by the forebrain seizure circuitry (Jobe et al., 1999). Moreover, GTCSs coincide with episodes known to be driven by the brainstem seizure circuitry (Jobe and Browning, 2006). Partial seizures evolving to secondarily generalized tonic/clonic seizures correspond to forebrain seizures that secondarily evoke brainstem seizures (Coffey et al., 1996).

This chapter describes the reciprocal functional relationship between the forebrain and brainstem seizure circuitry. Concepts regarding the secondary ignition of one seizure circuitry by the other are also included with an emphasis on partial seizures that activate tonic/clonic seizures.

■ Seizure types *versus* seizure circuitry of the forebrain and brainstem

Table I summarizes seizure types that occur within the seizure circuitry of the forebrain and of the brainstem. The seizure-free, normal brain is depicted in Row 1. In a unilateral focal forebrain seizure, brain activity within non-focal areas may also be altered, with many of the consequences becoming evident at a later point in time. These alterations may include kindling of non-focal areas. In a seizure determined by the forebrain circuitry and generalized throughout the musculature of the body, an electrographic seizure occurs throughout the rostral but not the brainstem circuitry. The resulting behaviors are those that have commonly been attributed to partial seizures or limbic/cortical seizures in the clinical literature and as forebrain seizures in the integrative basic sciences literature.

Electrographic seizures localized to the brainstem may be rarely detected and reported in the clinical literature. On the other hand, such seizures have been well documented in studies of audiogenic seizures in GEPRs. Accordingly, a sound stimulus produces a seizure within the inferior colliculus before the onset of a GTCS within the brainstem seizure circuitry (Faingold and Randall, 1995).

A brainstem seizure generalized throughout the relevant circuitry of the caudal brain may occur in the absence of a seizure within the forebrain. As will be illustrated subsequently, seizures of this distribution have been detected in GEPRs. The conditions required for detection of such seizures may never be fulfilled in human studies. The behavioral and electrographic characteristics of a seizure fully generalized throughout the rostral and caudal seizure circuitry of the brain are largely determined by the seizure within the brainstem circuitry. Whether the forebrain is exhibiting a brainstem-determined seizure makes little difference in the convulsion that is driven by the brainstem seizure. Some evidence supports the concept that a simultaneous brainstem-determined seizure in the rostral and caudal brain will activate the spinal cord more rapidly than will a brainstem seizure restricted to the caudal circuitry. This difference may determine whether the convulsion is preceded in some mammals by a running episode.

■ Generalized tonic-clonic seizures

Generalized tonic-clonic seizures (GTCSs) in mammals are behaviorally, electrographically and neuroanatomically distinct from partial seizures. Evidence supports the concept that GTCSs in humans are closely mimicked by brainstem seizures in other mammals. Although the electrographic signature of GTCSs can be detected in cortical recordings both in human and subhuman species, the neuroanatomical determinants of these seizures are largely contained within the brainstem.

Table I. Relationship between seizures in rostral and caudal brain and behaviors.

Condition	Brain Activity	Exemplification of Behavioral Consequences
Seizure-free, Normal brain		Typical mammalian behaviors.
Unilateral focal forebrain seizure		Brain activity & behaviors altered in a manner consonant with the motor and sensory functions localized to the part of the brain with the focal seizure.
Generalized forebrain seizure		Immobility, muscle tone sufficient to maintain posture, facial, neck, and bilateral forelimb clonus; head & trunk turning, alteration of postural tone with gradual slumping to floor.
Focal brainstem seizure		Running, high amplitude clonus, loss of righting posture, tonic dorsiflexion of neck & trunk with tonic flexion of the shoulder, hip, elbow, & knee joints (Class 1-3 brainstem seizure).
Generalized brainstem seizure		Running, righting posture lost, tonic dorsiflexion of neck & trunk with tonic flexion of thoracic & pelvic limbs. Conversion into tonic ventriflexion of neck & trunk & tonic extension of forelimbs & continued tonic flexion of pelvic limbs.
Generalized brainstem seizure with invasion of the forebrain		Massive limb thrusts, righting posture lost, tonic rigidity throughout body with superimposition of very low amplitude clonus. Amplitude of clonus increases as tonus subsides.

Key to symbols and colors			
Brain Part		Symbol/Function	
Forebrain			
Brainstem		Normal Function	
Spinal Cord			Seizure
Variable locus			

(Symbols: Forebrain = blue; Brainstem = green; Spinal Cord = yellow; Normal Function shown in natural colors; Seizure shown in red; Non-seizure responses to seizures in other brain parts shown in mauve/pink.)

The electroencephalographic and behavioral manifestations of GTCSs in humans and GEPR-10s are compared in *table II*. All seizure components of GTCSs including those of initiation, continuation and termination in humans with epilepsy are closely approximated by GTCSs in GEPR-10s. Also, GTCSs in the epileptic *Papio papio* correspond closely to those in the humans and GEPR-10s.

GTCSs are known to occur both in epileptic and in non-epileptic mammals. However, in non-epileptic individuals, these episodes do not occur spontaneously, nor do they occur in response to environmental stimuli; rather, they occur in response to electrical stimulation, or a convulsant drug. Moreover, analogous behavioral events

Table II. Sequential Events of GTCSs in Humans & GEPR-10s.

Temporal Event	Electroencephalogram (EEG)		Behavior	
	Human	GEPR-10	Human	GEPR-10
1	Polyspikes		Sudden onset, massive myoclonus	
2	Electrodecremental interval		Extreme tonic rigidity of skeletal muscles	
3	High amplitude spike/wave complexes, temporally increasing in duration & amplitude		Partial relaxation & recurrence of rigidity	
4			Clonus superimposed on dominant tonic rigidity	
5	Marked postictal amplitude reduction		Muscular flaccidity	

[a] GEPR-10s (Moraes et al., 2005a; Moraes et al., 2005b; Jobe et al., 1995; Naritoku et al., 1992; Ludvig and Moshe, 1989).
[b] Humans with epilepsy (Engel, 1989; Gastaut and Broughton, 1972).

are also characteristic of non-paralyzed humans undergoing maximal seizures in response to electroshock or pentylenetetrazol (Goodman and Gilman, 1941; Toman et al., 1947). In humans and other mammals, the dose of the convulsant stimulus required to produce GTCSs in these non-epileptic mammals is substantially above that required for epileptic subjects (Jobe and Browning, 2006; Jobe and Weber, 2005; Cure et al., 1948).

The concept that brainstem seizure circuitry drives the behaviors of generalized tonic/clonic seizures is supported by investigations of neurologically normal mammals and of mammals with epilepsy. For example, electrical stimulation of the reticular core of the brainstem produces GTCSs that are self-sustained and that occur even after the removal of the forebrain (Burnham, 1987). Another verification of concept arises from behavioral studies after complete precollicular transection of the brain. In the first of these studies, non-epileptic rats exhibit the behaviors of GTCSs in response to maximal electroshock despite the absence of intact neuronal connections of the brainstem to the forebrain (Browning and Nelson, 1986). A companion experiment demonstrates that pentylenetetrazol-induced GTCSs in non-epileptic rats also occur under these conditions. In epileptic animals, both GEPR-3s and GEPR-9s exhibit behavioral concomitants of sound-induced GTCSs despite the transections (Browning et al., 1999; Moraes et al., 2005b). Under these conditions, GEPR-3s and GEPR-9s respectively exhibit class 3 and Class 9 seizures as defined by Jobe and colleagues (Moraes et al., 2005b). These observations support the concept that the spectrum of seizures so defined is of brainstem origin.

EEG recordings from intact GEPRs provide additional evidence for brainstem circuitry as the origin of GTCSs. Relatively early in the development of the GEPR strains, major EEG components of the typical GTCSs in the cerebral cortex were missing during the behavioral manifestations of the first GTCS in previously seizure naïve subjects (Naritoku et al., 1992). For example, high amplitude spikes were absent immediately before the onset of tonic rigidity, as were clearly developed spike/wave complexes during the characteristic interval of clonus superimposed on predominant tonus (see *Table II* for sequential events of GTCSs in GEPR-10s). With seizure repetition at daily intervals, these EEG components became evident in the cerebral cortex.

A temporal analysis of the EEG undertaken in the year 1993 demonstrated that in GEPR-9s, which had experienced three GTCS in the weeks preceding the experimental recording, the initial high amplitude spikes characteristic of GTCSs occurred first in the reticular formation of the brainstem and subsequently in the cerebral cortex (Jobe et al., 1999). Experiments undertaken in the late 1990s, after the GEPR-9 colony had undergone further development with brother/sister inbreeding for seizure predisposition, revealed that the temporal differences between the initial EEG spikes in the different parts of the brain in any given seizure were no longer detectable with the type of technology used in the earlier investigation. Nevertheless, new approaches were developed for determination of the anatomical direction of voltage alterations in the field potential EEG (Moraes et al., 2005a; Moraes et al., 2005b). The results support the hypothesis that the different components of the spike and wave complexes in the GTCSs arise from different anatomical influences, the spikes stemming from the midbrain/hindbrain and the waves from the midbrain/forebrain. In transected GEPRs, the spikes occur in the brainstem in rapid succession without intervening waves. After a delay of approximately 4 seconds, spikes of sharply reduced amplitude begin to appear in the cerebral cortex. With this particular finding, we suggest that volume transmission may play a role in communication between the caudal and rostral brain despite transection. The absence of the wave component of the spike/wave complexes in the brainstem of transected animals suggests that neuronal connections are important for the occurrence of this feature.

The behaviors driven by brainstem seizures are ultimately determined within the spinal cord (Esplin and Freston, 1960; Esplin, 1959; Vernadakis, 1962; Jobe, 1987). Evidence supports the concept that a seizure within the brainstem invades the spinal cord with neuronal frequencies that are sufficient to initiate a seizure within this most caudal part of the CNS. Seizures of different severities within the brainstem appear to deliver differing numbers of impulses per unit time to the proximal cord. A maximal behavioral response (Class 9 or 10 brainstem seizure) occurs when a relatively large number of seizure derived impulses per unit time invade the cord and ignite a seizure therein. These seizures have the capacity to continue in the absence of additional seizure driven impulses from the brain. Activation of behaviorally specific circuitry within the brain is not required to produce the various behaviors driven by brainstem seizures. The complete behavioral repertoire appears to be "hard wired" within the spinal cord. All of the behaviors from class 1 through 10 brainstem seizures are determined within the cord. All of the components of brainstem seizures are produced even when the brain is completely bypassed so that high frequency impulses are delivered directly to the proximal cord in mammals wherein the brain is severed from the cord at the atlanto-occipital junction (Jobe, 1987).

The reticular formation, periaqueductal gray of the midbrain, superior and inferior colliculi, the superior lateral parabrachial area, and the cerebellum participate in the generation of high frequency impulses that produce GTCSs within the spinal cord (Gale, 1992; Browning, 1994; Ryu et al., 1997; Yan et al., 1998; Patel, 1988; Chakravarty and Faingold, 1999; Faingold et al., 1985; Faingold et al., 1988a; Faingold, 1999; Feng et al., 2001; Faingold et al., 1988b; Faingold, 1999; Clough et al., 1997; Eells et al., 1998). In the milder form of brainstem seizures that occur in GEPR-3s, the amygdala has also been implicated in the seizure circuit (Raisinghani and Faingold, 2003).

Areas of the reticular core have been investigated *via* electrical stimulation, mechanical lesions and microinfusions of non-epileptic cats, rabbits and rats and of epileptic rats (GEPRs) (Kreindler et al., 1958; Bergmann et al., 1963; Burnham, 1987). During electrical stimulations of the brainstem, GTCSs occur in animals with or without precollicular transections. Moreover, GTCSs can be evoked independently from every level of the reticular core; and the tonic components of these seizures in GEPRs are attenuated by bilateral mechanical lesions of the pontine reticular formation, or by more specific damage to the reticularis pontis oralis or reticularis pontis caudalis (Browning et al., 1985). In contrast, these pontine lesions do not affect facial and forelimb clonus (forebrain seizures) (Browning et al., 1981b). The reticular core is further implicated in GTCS by the demonstration that anticonvulsant effects occur in response to infusion of an excitant amino acid antagonist into the reticularis pontis caudalis or the mesencephalic reticular formation (Millan et al., 1988).

Other brainstem structures have been evaluated with analogous approaches. A reduction in cerebellar efferent activity inhibits GTCSs and facilitates forebrain seizures (Raines and Anderson, 1976; Browning et al., 1981a, b; Dow, 1965; Dow et al., 1962). The inferior colliculus appears to play two roles in brainstem seizures: one focal; the others generalized. The localized seizure role occurs in the mechanisms of sound-induced seizures. The generalized role probably occurs regardless of the stimulus that provokes the brainstem seizure. In GEPR-9s the inferior colliculus undergoes transition to a localized seizure in response to sound stimulation (Chakravarty and Faingold, 1996; Faingold, 2004). This limited response has been detected *via* microwire technology (unit recording). Almost immediately after the onset of a sound stimulus in a GEPR-9, the excessive firing within the inferior colliculus triggers a GTCS within the reticular formation of the brainstem, which tertiarily evolves to include the inferior colliculus *per se* (Jobe et al., 1999). These generalized brainstem events have been detected *via* field potential recordings. In recent measurements, the components of the brainstem seizure circuitry are activated pervasively in such rapid succession that the separation of early and late electrographic field potential components can no longer be made *via* traditional field potential recordings (Moraes et al., 2005a; Moraes et al., 2005b). In earlier generations in development of the GEPR-9 strain, a four component process was evident in the evolution of an audiogenic seizure. First, the inferior colliculus developed a sound-induced focal seizure, which then ignited a second component: a tonic/clonic seizure throughout the brainstem reticular formation. The third and fourth components became evident as the tonic/clonic seizure in the reticular formation ignited an electrographically similar event in the inferior colliculus and probably other structures in the brainstem, and subsequently in the cerebral cortex and spinal cord.

The role of the superior colliculus in GTCSs is a topic of previous reviews (Browning, 1994; Gale, 1992; Gale, 1993; Gale, 1992; Faingold, 1999). Activation of the superior colliculus can be achieved by microinjections of GABA agonists into the pars reticulata of the substantia nigra, which disinhibits the superior colliculus. Such treatments suppresses brainstem seizures induced by maximal electroshock (Gale et al., 1993; Depaulis et al., 1990; Dean and Gale, 1989; Redgrave et al., 1992a). Moreover, the superior colliculus has been shown to be involved in the propagation and ignition of the brainstem seizures induced by sound in GEPRs and Wistar rats (Faingold and Randall, 1999; Faingold, 1999; Merrill et al., 2003). Lesions (Merrill et al., 2003) of the superior colliculus or microinjections of glutamate antagonists (Faingold and Casebeer, 1999) have been shown to suppress markedly the severity of sound induced seizures in GEPRs. Moreover, the superior colliculus has been identified as a site of action for norepinephrine in its seizure suppressant effects on GTCS in GEPR-9s (Jobe et al., 1994; Yan et al., 1998). Thus, the superior colliculus is a participant in the brainstem seizure. One problem with this idea is that infusion of GABA antagonists into the superior colliculus has been shown to reduce the severity of brainstem seizures induced by maximal electroshock. A recent study in our laboratory suggests that the inhibition of maximal electroshock induced seizure may not be due to the direct activation of the superior colliculus, but rather to the post-ictal depression that follows the class 1 brainstem seizure that typically results from the infusion of biculline into the superior colliculus (Merrill et al., 2003).

We use the term "generalized brainstem seizure" to convey five major concepts: (1) the bilateral and major components of the brainstem seizure circuitry are exhibiting a seizure; (2) the resulting behaviors are occurring in response to a spinal cord seizure activated by the intense neuronal activity of the brainstem circuitry; (3) any accompanying seizure in the cerebral cortex is driven by the brainstem seizure; and (4) the signature characteristics of the field potential EEG are determined by an interaction between the brainstem and the forebrain. Accordingly, the field potential spikes arise within the brainstem. The waves of the spike/wave complexes may be caused by inhibitory influences of the forebrain which may retard the rate of neuronal spiking within the brainstem (Moraes et al.; 2005b).

■ Forebrain (Limbic/Cortical) Seizures

Forebrain seizures do not occur in neurologically normal, non-epileptic mammals, at least partially because the naturally occurring anticonvulsant properties of the brain are sufficient preventatives. In epileptic subjects such as the *Papio papio*, spontaneous seizures infrequently occur in as much as endogenous anticonvulsant influences provide insufficient protection against seizure initiating events (Jobe and Browning, 2006).

Behaviorally and electrographically, forebrain and brainstem seizures differ sharply even within the same strain and species. In contrast, partial seizures correspond closely across species from humans to mice and rats (Jobe et al., 1999; Jobe and Browning, 2006). Behavioral similarities are illustrated in *table III*.

Whereas intact rats exhibit pentylenetetrazol- or electroshock-induced behaviors commonly associated with human partial seizures *(Table III)*, animals with complete precollicular transections do not (Browning and Nelson, 1986; Browning, 1994). These findings support the hypothesis that the circuitry for partial seizures in mammals resides rostral to the midbrain. Additional evidence for this concept is provided by investigations with kindling paradigms for induction of partial seizure status epilepticus. Data from electrographic and/or 2-deoxyglucose autoradiographic methodology, indicate that partial seizure status epilepticus terminates rostral to or upon reaching the level of the substantia nigra (Thompson and Galosy, 1983; Handforth and

Treiman, 1995b; Handforth and Treiman, 1995a; Handforth and Treiman, 1994; Handforth and Ackermann, 1993; Handforth and Ackermann, 1992; Handforth and Ackermann, 1988b). Accordingly, with the exception of the substantia nigra, generalized forebrain seizures do not appear to increase 2-deoxyglucose uptake in the brainstem as they do in the forebrain (Handforth and Ackermann, 1988a; Browning, 1994; Morimoto et al., 2004). However, the absence of a caudal seizure does not imply the absence of impulse transmission. Rather, the behaviorally determinant neuronal impulses initiated by the seizure continue caudally so that the coherency of the descending neuronal impulses is preserved and delivered to the skeletal muscles in the absence of a seizure in the brainstem (Thompson and Galosy, 1983; Handforth and Treiman, 1995b; Handforth and Treiman, 1994; Handforth and Treiman, 1995b; Handforth and Treiman, 1995a; Handforth and Ackermann, 1993; Handforth and Ackermann, 1992; Handforth and Ackermann, 1988b).

Forebrain seizure behaviors differ sharply from those determined by the brainstem circuitry. The onset of a GTCS (class 10 brainstem convulsion) in GEPRs and in humans occurs with sudden and dramatic myoclonic thrusts in all extremities. In contrast, forebrain seizures involving the limbic nuclei in humans, *Papio papio*, GEPRs and other mammals often begin with behavioral arrest (immobility), evolving into palpebral clonus and spasm, mandibular clonus, grimacing, head bobbing, scratching, and alternating and synchronous thoracic limb clonus. Thus, from the outset, the clonus of brainstem seizures is pervasively evident throughout the musculoskeletal system, whereas in forebrain seizures early movements are "localized" and subtle. Much of the clonus in forebrain seizures occurs with the maintenance of righting posture, whereas, with the exception of coordinate clonus, brainstem clonus occurs with sudden loss of posture. In cases of forebrain seizures wherein postural impairment occurs, the onset is often gradual, and subjects slump to the floor. Finally, the clonus of brainstem convulsions is initially superimposed on a dominant and extreme tonic rigidity, with clonus of increasing amplitude progressively displacing rigidity. In contrast, forebrain clonus occurs in the absence of severe rigidity.

The behaviors of many forebrain seizures are driven by circuitry within and between limbic and olfactory structures (Browning, 1994; Gale, 1992; Handforth and Ackermann, 1988a; Lothman et al., 1981; Lothman and Collins, 1981; McIntyre et al., 1991; Turski et al., 1984; Patel, 1988; Collins et al., 1983b; Collins et al., 1983a; Handforth and Ackermann, 1988a; Handforth and Ackermann, 1988b). In some instances, the seizure extends caudally to the substantia nigra and the superior colliculus, and rostrally to the cerebral cortex. Within this large part of the brain, seizures may encompass the hippocampus, amygdala, septum, piriform cortex, perirhinal cortex, prepiriform cortex (area tempestas), nucleus accumbens, olfactory bulb, entorhinal cortex, dentate gyrus and the subiculum. Extralimbic participants in the forebrain seizure circuitry may include the neocortex, caudate-putamen, entopeduncular nucleus, thalamus (mediodorsal), substantia innominata, habenula, substantia nigra and superior colliculus. In some cases, specific components of the forebrain (*e.g.*, cerebral cortex) may drive motor behaviors without involvement of limbic structures.

The role of brainstem structures in forebrain seizures has been a topic of several important studies. For example, the effect of the superior colliculus on forebrain seizures appears to be mediated through the nigro-collicular pathway and therefore is believed to be involved in the mechanism by which the substantia nigra inhibits seizures (Depaulis et al., 1990; Depaulis, 1992; Deransart et al., 1998; Nail-Boucherie et al., 2005; Merrill et al., 2003; Merrill et al., 2000; Browning, 1994; Dean and Gale, 1989; Gale, 1986). Other closely related studies describe additional details and components of the caudal/rostral interactions in the mechanisms of forebrain seizures (both convulsive and non-convulsive) (Redgrave et al., 1988; Dean and Gale, 1989; Redgrave et al., 1992b; Nail-Boucherie et al., 2005; Depaulis et al., 1990; Gale et al., 1993; Depaulis et al., 1990; Dean and Gale, 1989; Redgrave et al., 1992a; Depaulis et al., 1994).

■ Forebrain seizures of limited distribution progress to greater neuroanatomical representation within the rostral circuitry

As frequently employed, the term "focal" (or perhaps "localization related") implies that a seizure or the beginning of a seizure is located unilaterally in a small part of the brain (Treiman and Treiman, 2001). The behavioral consequences of these unilateral focal events depend partly on the neuroanatomical location of the seizure. Progression beyond a unilateral focus is common in humans and other mammals. For example, unilateral focal forebrain seizures are known to activate seizures in contralateral areas (Engel, 1989). Clinically, such seizure evolution is exemplified by a simple partial seizure onset followed by impairment of consciousness, a condition often designated as complex partial seizure. But this limited progression is only one of several types that may occur within the forebrain seizure circuitry. Bilateral forebrain seizures within a limited part of the forebrain seizure circuitry may become rostrally pervasive. Kindling data from rodents and other mammals indicates that this type of evolution underlies the bilateral facial and forelimb clonus, which progresses to include rearing, turning of the trunk, alterations of postural tone and slumping to the floor ("falling").

Partly to avoid ambiguity, we find it useful to apply the term "generalized seizure" both to the forebrain and brainstem seizure circuitry. We use the term "generalized forebrain seizure" to signify that the major components of the forebrain seizure circuitry are exhibiting a forebrain-determined seizure, and that the skeletal muscles are pervasively active bilaterally in the behavioral expression of the seizure *(Table III)*.

According to our usage, motor commands of a generalized forebrain seizure need only be transmitted through the brainstem to cause the associated behaviors of such a seizure. It is not essential that the brainstem exhibit field potential evidence of a seizure in order to transmit the neuronal impulses that it receives from the forebrain.

A fascinating point has arisen with regard to kindling seizure progression. In our view, all common classes (1-5) of kindling correspond to human partial seizures. However, some investigators suggest that GTCSs rather than partial seizures are modeled by

Table III. Correspondence of motor behaviors of complex partial seizures in humans and of forebrain seizures in epileptic baboons, GEPRs and other rats.

Body Region	Humans[a]	Papio papio[b]	GEPRs & other rats[c]
Whole body	Arrest with motionless stare	Arrest of behavior	Immobility
Face	Palpebral & other facial clonus	Facial clonus, jaw clonus, grimacing	Palpebral clonus & spasm, jaw clonus, mouth opening
Thoracic limbs	Picking at clothes, scratching, rubbing of hands, boxing, flailing, & hand elevation as head turns	Clonus	Scratching, forelimb clonus; occasional shoulder flexion & head turning
Trunk & Legs	Lateral incurvation, head flexion or turning, sitting up, alteration of postural tone with gradual slumping to floor the floor	Sitting up or rearing, slumping to floor	Rearing; turning of trunk, alteration of postural tone & gradual slumping to floor ("falling")

[a] Humans (Jobe and Browning, 2006; Aicardi, 1986a; Aicardi, 1986c; Engel, 1989).
[b] *Papio papio* (Jobe and Browning, 2006).
[c] Rats (Savage *et al.*, 1986a; Savage *et al.*, 1986b; Coffey *et al.*, 1996; Racine, 1972).

bilateral class 3 through class 5 kindled seizures (Sutula and Ockuly, 2006). We agree with the idea that neuroanatomical seizure generalization within the forebrain occurs as part of kindling progression from class 1 through class 5 seizures. We do not agree, however, that the transition from class 3 to class 5 seizures represents a conversion from a partial seizure to a GTCS.

According to our line of thought, the transition beyond class 2 seizures occurs in response to neuroanatomical and pathophysiologic seizure progression within the forebrain circuitry, including an extension to the substantia nigra. Our hypothesis is supported by several factors. First, behaviors of classes 1 through 5 – not merely classes 1 through 3 – closely resemble behaviors of human partial seizures. *Table III* illustrates the similarities of these behavioral seizure types in GEPRs, other rats, *Papio papio*, and humans with epilepsy. Second, the behaviors of classes 4 and 5 kindled seizures have negligible similarities to human GTCSs *(Tables I and II)*. Third, the field potential EEG morphologies of kindled or partial seizures are markedly dissimilar to those of GTCSs. The dissimilarity is evident whether the determinations are made in rats or other mammals including humans with epilepsy. For example, the EEG morphology of a GTCS in a GEPR-10 or in a human with epilepsy is characterized by initial high amplitude spikes followed immediately by a sudden onset electrodecremental interval. Behaviorally, the initial spikes and the electrodecremental interval are accompanied respectively by massive myoclonic thrusts of the extremities and extreme tonic rigidity with complete loss of righting posture. Classes 1 through 5 kindled seizures are not linked to such behavioral or electrographic events.

◼ Forebrain seizures ignite brainstem seizures in epileptic mammals

In the practice of medicine, partial seizures have long been known to undergo conversion to tonic/clonic seizures (Engel, 1989; Gastaut and Broughton, 1972). The data presented in previous sections of this manuscript support the hypothesis that this transition in humans occurs when a partial seizure within the forebrain seizure circuitry activates a GTCSs within the brainstem seizure circuitry. Also, transition from forebrain to brainstem seizures has been observed in mice treated with chemoconvulsants (Samoriski et al., 1997; Samoriski and Applegate, 1997). Several years ago, we anticipated that a forebrain seizure fully generalized within the rostral circuitry would be more likely to activate a brainstem seizure than would a localized forebrain seizure. Nevertheless, the medical literature suggests that humans with partial seizure epilepsy may undergo secondary transition at any point along the continuum of seizure progression within the forebrain (Engel, 1989). For example, GTCSs occur either in response to simple or complex partial seizures, diagnostic seizure subtypes that are usually unilateral and bilateral, respectively.

Studies in GEPR-9s and GEPR-10s underscore the validity of the principle that forebrain seizures of any degree of kindling progression have a potential to activate brainstem seizures in epileptic subjects (Coffey et al., 1996). In these investigations, brainstem seizure behaviors occurred in a fraction of the experimental subjects in response to forebrain seizures initiated by electrical kindling stimuli delivered to the amygdala in GEPR-9s. Seventy-one percent of the experimental GEPR-9s exhibited secondary class 1 through 9 brainstem seizures at least once during the course of the kindling process. This same percentage of responders was obtained from subjects selected as naïve to sound-induced seizures versus GEPR-9s with a history of audiogenic seizure experiences. None of the non-epileptic control subjects exhibited secondary GTCSs during the course of kindling stimuli. This failure of forebrain-induced brainstem seizures with non-epileptic control rats reinforces the idea that limbic stimulation of nonepileptic animals does not elicit brainstem seizures except, perhaps, under extreme experimental conditions. In an earlier study that employed = 550 kindling stimulations per rat (Pinel and Rovner, 1978b; Pinel and Rovner, 1978a), the animals ultimately responded with episodes that according to the brainstem seizure ranking scale (Jobe and Dailey, 2000) appear to have represented minimal expressions of brainstem circuitry activation. Accordingly, during the advanced stages of stimulation, the rats exhibited running episodes with or without terminal intervals wherein the animals reared and supported themselves against a wall of the test chamber.

Thus, GEPR-9s appear to have an innate mechanism for forebrain to brainstem seizure transition, and this process is not dependent on kindling progression. In contrast, such a mechanism does not appear to exist in non-epileptic control subjects, at least not until the animal has been exposed to an extreme number of kindling stimuli, and even at this late time, the brainstem circuitry remains highly seizure resistant so as to exhibit the least severe of brainstem seizure episodes. The almost complete absence of brainstem seizure activation in response to seizures in limbic nuclei in normal, non-epileptic, kindled rats supports the hypothesis that mechanisms for the rostral to caudal seizure transition reside specifically within genetically epileptic mammals.

■ Brainstem seizures ignite forebrain-determined seizures in mammals with epilepsy

Repeated sound-induced brainstem seizures lead to ignition of forebrain-determined seizures (*i.e.*, limbic motor seizure). These rostrally determined events follow or replace brainstem seizures. In some paradigms the forebrain-determined seizure behavior is not observed until the subjects have experienced 10 – 40 sound-induced brainstem seizures. The ignition of forebrain seizures using this procedure has been referred to as "audiogenic kindling". This phenomenon was first described by Marescaux and colleagues using a Wistar strain of audiogenic seizure susceptible rats (Marescaux *et al.*, 1987; Vergnes *et al.*, 1987), but has now been demonstrated by several laboratories using other audiogenic seizure susceptible rodent models (*e.g.* GEPRs, KM rats and WAG/Rij rats) (Naritoku *et al.*, 1992; Garcia-Cairasco *et al.*, 1994; Naritoku *et al.*, 1992; Kiesmann *et al.*, 1988; Hirsch *et al.*, 1992; Garcia-Cairasco *et al.*, 1996; Merrill *et al.*, 2005; Vinogradova *et al.*, 2005).

Ignition of a forebrain-determined seizure by a brainstem seizure occurs as a consequence of propagation of seizure discharge from the inferior colliculus to the amygdala by way of the medical geniculate nucleus in the thalamus. This anatomical pathway is involved in the classical conditioning of emotional reactions to auditory tones when paired with aversive stimuli (Bordi and LeDoux, 1994; McCown *et al.*, 1987). Several lines of evidence indicate that the brainstem seizure can ignite the forebrain seizure *via* this particular pathway. Repeated daily electrical stimulation of the inferior colliculus has been shown to produce forebrain seizures which follow an initial brainstem seizure (McCown *et al.*, 1987; Hirsch *et al.*, 1993). The forebrain seizures resulting from audiogenic kindling can be blocked by microinjecting lidocaine or GABA agonists into the medial geniculate body or the amygdala (Hirsch *et al.*, 1997; Feng *et al.*, 2001). Moreover, the basolateral amygdala and subsequently other limbic structures are activated in audiogenic kindling but not by a single sound-induced seizure (Hirsch *et al.*, 1997; Simler *et al.*, 1999). This is typically followed by activation of other limbic structures that have been shown to be involved in limbic motor seizures (Simler *et al.*, 1999; Hirsch *et al.*, 1997; Pereira, V *et al.*, 1997; Raisinghani and Faingold, 2005a; Raisinghani and Faingold, 2005b).

Thus the amygdala may undergo plastic changes similar to those occurring during electrical kindling of the amygdala, but in this case the daily stimulus to the amygdala is triggered by the inferior colliculus in response to sound stimulation (Feng and Faingold, 2002). Indeed, the initial plastic changes appear to occur in the inferior colliculus since repetitive sound induced seizures in GEPR-9s were shown to cause elevated neuronal firing in this structure (N'Gouemo and Faingold, 1996). Such seizures facilitate electrical kindling of the hippocampus (Hirsch *et al.*, 1992) and cause mossy fiber sprouting in the hippocampus (Garcia-Cairasco *et al.*, 1996). Moreover, increases in COX-2 gene expression are associated with the activation of the forebrain seizure network following repeated electrical stimulation of the inferior colliculus (McCown *et al.*, 1997).

Examination of the audiogenic kindling paradigm in GEPRs has provided further evidence of the separation of the forebrain and brainstem seizure circuitry, but also a greater understanding of how these two convulsive seizure networks interact and influence one another. Indeed, it is clear that the brainstem seizure controls convulsive behavior irrespective of seizure discharge in the forebrain. This phenomenon has been observed by several investigators (Kreindler *et al.*, 1958; Jobe *et al.*, 1999; Moraes *et al.*, 2005b; Browning *et al.*, 1990).

Evidence suggests that the severity of brainstem seizures may act as a determinant of whether forebrain-determined seizures are ignited by seizures in the caudal circuitry. Two additional experiments in the domain of "audiogenic kindling" have been undertaken on this subject in GEPR-3s and GEPR-9s. In one, sound-induced brainstem seizures were evoked once daily for up to 24 days (Merrill *et al.*, 2005). In the other, three brainstem seizures were induced each day (Garcia-Cairasco *et al.*, 1994). For the present narrative, we are distinguishing between the paradigms used in these studies with the terms *close-interval* and *very close-interval* seizure repetition. In both experiments, untreated GEPR-3s developed typical forebrain seizure behaviors which occurred as anticonvulsant effects against brainstem seizures became progressively evident in response to the repetition paradigms. However, differences between the experiments became evident in GEPR-9s. In the close-interval study, untreated GEPR-9s did not exhibit forebrain seizure behaviors, whereas in the very close-interval paradigm such behaviors became readily evident. We suggest that two mechanisms are operative in the transition from brainstem- to forebrain-determined seizure activity. First, severe brainstem-determined seizures have a limited capacity to protect against forebrain-determined seizures. As a result, forebrain-determined seizures do not become evident in the short-interval paradigm. Second, we suggest that brainstem seizures kindle components of the forebrain. The appearance of forebrain-determined seizures in the very-short interval study provides evidence for this hypothesis. We suggest that with the large number of brainstem seizures in the very short interval study, forebrain kindling was sufficient to overcome anticonvulsant effects exerted on this circuitry by severe brainstem seizures.

The anticonvulsant effect of severe brainstem-determined seizures on the forebrain was explored further with the close-interval paradigm in GEPR-9s pretreated with low-dose phenytoin or lesions of the superior colliculus (Merrill *et al.*, 2005). Both protocols selectively reduced brainstem seizure severity. Moreover, both gave rise to the appearance of forebrain-determined seizure behaviors. In an experiment with GEPR-3s, serotonin was depleted with 5,7-dihydroxytryptamine to increase brainstem seizure severity above that of the phenotypical class 3 episodes. As anticipated, the increase in brainstem seizure severity was associated with a reduction in the incidence of forebrain seizure behavior.

Another factor may influence the occurrence of forebrain-determined seizures in response to brainstem-determined seizures: the duration of the brainstem-determined seizure. Essentially all recordings show that brainstem seizure repetition increases the duration of the set of spike-wave complexes that occurs following the electrodecremental interval in class 9 brainstem seizures (Merrill *et al.*, 2005; Moraes *et al.*, 2005a). Thus, the interval between the initial high amplitude spikes and spike/wave complexes increases dramatically with repetition, as does the interval between the initial spikes and the onset of forebrain-determined seizures. Perhaps, the anticonvulsant properties of the brainstem-determined seizure arise from the initial high amplitude activity at the beginning of the brainstem seizure and dissipate during the long interval of post-electrodecremental spike/wave activity that is developed *via* brainstem seizure repetition.

The cortical EEG of class 9 and 10 brainstem-determined seizures in GEPR-9s corresponds very closely to the morphology of EEGs recorded from the caudal circuitry in fully generalized brainstem-determined seizures (Jobe et al., 1995; Moraes et al., 2005a; Moraes et al., 2005b; Jobe et al., 1995; Jobe et al., 1999). At the termination of caudally-determined seizures, spike/wave complexes devolve into the postictal stage. However, with the secondary onset of a forebrain-determined seizure, the cortical seizure EEG appears to change morphology, with different events occurring in association with different classes of forebrain-determined seizure. Quantitative analyses of the cortical EEGs before, during and after the transition to forebrain-determined seizure activity may reveal characteristic distinctiveness in the tonic/clonic spike/wave complexes driven by brainstem-determined seizures *versus* the secondary clonic behaviors characteristic of forebrain circuitry. Future studies may determine the mechanism by which a brainstem seizure acts to preclude and to initiate the expression of the forebrain-determined seizure.

■ Summary and conclusions

Two major sets of seizure circuitry characterize normal mammalian brain and probably most brains with epilepsy. These are the seizure circuitry of the forebrain and of the brainstem. Localized seizures may occur in either set of circuitry. Focal seizures within the forebrain circuitry are well known clinically and experimentally. These may remain localized or may invade additional components of the circuitry in which they reside. The different degrees of generalization within the rostral circuitry are associated with expansion of behavioral repertoires. These are described in the "Racine" seizure classification system, which in its totality we have applied to partial seizures in the various mammalian species, including humans and other primates.

In contrast, to progression within the forebrain circuitry *per se*, seizures within the rostral brain may ignite seizures within the brainstem circuitry. Accordingly, patients with localized or generalized forebrain seizures may experience secondary ignition of a brainstem seizure. This transition across these major sets of seizure circuitry can probably be viewed clinically as a partial seizure secondarily generalized to tonic/clonic seizures. In contrast, seizures within the forebrain circuitry do not mimic GTCSs. Rather, the behavioral and electrophysiological characteristics of GTCSs appear to mimic those of brainstem seizures. Ultimately, the behaviors driven by brainstem seizures are determined by the magnitude of another seizure that is secondarily ignited within the spinal cord. A behavioral rating scale for mammalian brainstem seizures has arisen from studies of sound-induced seizures. The scale of "Jobe and colleagues" is now known to be applicable to brainstem seizures induced by several different stimuli, including those induced by chemoconvulsants and electroshock, as well as those ignited by forebrain seizures in GEPRs.

In contrast to seizures exported from the rostral to caudal circuitry, several mammals are known to undergo transition from brainstem seizure to forebrain seizure. For example, many GEPR-3s will express secondary forebrain-determined seizures if previously exposed to close-interval repetition of sound-induced brainstem seizures. However, these rostrally determined seizures do not occur during the course of a brainstem seizure. Rather, termination of brainstem seizures in mammals already exposed to brainstem seizure repetition is associated with the ignition of forebrain-determined seizures. Different mechanisms may be operative in determining the possibility of secondary forebrain seizures. Brainstem seizure-induced kindling of the forebrain seizure circuitry may play a prominent role in this process. Also, brainstem seizures of short duration do not appear to ignite forebrain-determined seizures. Since preliminary evidence suggests that long duration brainstem seizures are more likely to ignite forebrain-determined seizures, the time between the initial high amplitude EEG events of a brainstem seizure and the onset of the postictal period may also play a role. Forebrain seizure ignition appears to be associated with long intervals preceding the onset of postictal events.

Although focal brainstem seizures may be obscure clinically, studies in other mammals suggest that seizures determined by the brainstem circuitry may also be focal, partially or fully generalized within the brainstem. Alternatively, brainstem-determined seizures may be fully generalized throughout the entire brain. Nevertheless, behaviors driven by the brainstem circuitry are largely determined within the caudal CNS. Indeed, invasion of the forebrain by the brainstem-determined seizure is not an essential biological underpinning of the resulting convulsive behaviors.

References

Aicardi J. Epilepsies characterized by simple partial seizures. In: *Epilepsy in Children*. New York: Raven Press, 1986a: 112-39.

Aicardi J. Epilepsy: Overview and definitions. In: *Epilepsy in Children*. New York: Raven Press, 1986b.

Aicardi J. Epilepsies with affective-psychic manifestations and complex partial seizures. In: *Epilepsy in Children*. New York: Raven Press, 1986c: 140-75.

Bergmann F, Costin A, Gutman J. A low threshold convulsive area in the rabbit's mesencephalon. *Electroencephalogr Clin Neurophysiol* 1963; 15: 683-90.

Bordi F, LeDoux JE. Response properties of single units in areas of rat auditory thalamus that project to the amygdala. I. Acoustic discharge patterns and frequency receptive fields. *Exp Brain Res* 1994; 98: 261-74.

Browning RA. Anatomy of generalized convulsive seizures. In: Malafosse A, Genton P, Hirsch E, Marescaux C, Broglin D, Bernasconi R, eds. *Idiopathic Generalized Epilepsies*. London, England: John Libbey & Company, Ltd., 1994: 399-413.

Browning RA, Nelson DK. Modification of electroshock and pentylenetetrazol seizure patterns in rats after precollicular transections. *Exp Neurol* 1986; 93: 546-56.

Browning RA, Nelson DK, Mogharreban N, Jobe PC, Laird HE. Effect of midbrain and pontine tegmental lesions on audiogenic seizures in genetically epilepsy-prone rats. *Epilepsia* 1985; 26: 175-83.

Browning RA, Simonton RL. Antagonism of experimentally induced tonic seizures following a lesion in the midbrain tegmentum. *Epilepsia* 1981a; 22: 595-601.

Browning RA, Turner FJ, Simonton RL, Bundman MC. Effect of midbrain and pontine tegmental lesions on the maximal electroshock seizure pattern in rats. *Epilepsia* 1981; 22: 583-94.

Browning RA, Wang C, Lanker ML, Jobe PC. Electroshock- and pentylenetetrazol-induced seizures in genetically epilepsy-prone rats (GEPRs): differences in threshold and pattern. *Epilepsy Res* 1990; 6: 1-11.

Browning RA, Wang C, Nelson DK, Jobe PC. Effect of precollicular transection on audiogenic seizures in genetically epilepsy-prone rats. *Exp Neurol* 1999; 155: 295-301.

Burnham WM. Electrical stimulation studies: Generalized convulsions triggered from the brain-stem. In: Fromm GH, Faingold CL, Browning RA, Burnham WM, eds. *Epilepsy and the Reticular Formation: The Role of the Reticular Core in Convulsive Seizures*. New York: Alan R. Liss, 1987: 25-38.

Chakravarty DN, Faingold CL. Differential roles in the neuronal network for audiogenic seizures are observed among the inferior colliculus subnuclei and the amygdala. *Exp Neurol* 1999; 157: 135-41.

Chakravarty DN, Faingold CL. Increased responsiveness and failure of habituation in neurons of the external nucleus of inferior colliculus associated with audiogenic seizures of the genetically epilepsy-prone rat. *Exp Neurol* 1996; 141: 280-6.

Clough RW, Eells JB, Browning RA, Jobe PC. Seizures and proto-oncogene expression of Fos in the brain of adult genetically epilepsy-prone rats. *Exp Neurol* 1997; 146: 341-53.

Coffey LL, Reith ME, Chen NH, Mishra PK, Jobe PC. Amygdala kindling of forebrain seizures and the occurrence of brainstem seizures in genetically epilepsy-prone rats. *Epilepsia* 1996; 37: 188-97.

Collins RC, Olney JW, Lothman EW. Metabolic and pathological consequences of focal seizures. *Res Publ Assoc Res Nerv Ment Dis* 1983a; 61: 87-107.

Collins RC, Tearse RG, Lothman EW. Functional anatomy of limbic seizures: focal discharges from medial entorhinal cortex in rat. *Brain Res* 1983b; 280: 25-40.

Cure D, Rasmussen T, Jasper H. Activation of seizures and electroencephalographic disturbances in epileptic and in control subjects with "metrazol". *Arch Neurol Psychiatr* 1948; 59: 691-717.

Dean P, Gale K. Anticonvulsant action of GABA receptor blockade in the nigrotectal target region. *Brain Res* 1989; 477: 391-5.

Depaulis A. The inhibitory control of the substantia nigra over generalized non-convulsive seizures in the rat. *J Neural Transm Suppl* 1992; 35: 125-39.

Depaulis A, Liu Z, Vergnes M, Marescaux C, Micheletti G, Warter JM. Suppression of spontaneous generalized non-convulsive seizures in the rat by microinjection of GABA antagonists into the superior colliculus. *Epilepsy Res* ????: 5: 192-8.

Depaulis A, Vergnes M, Marescaux C. Endogenous control of epilepsy: the nigral inhibitory system. *Prog Neurobiol* 1994; 42: 33-52.

Deransart C, Vercueil L, Marescaux C, Depaulis A. The role of basal ganglia in the control of generalized absence seizures. *Epilepsy Res* 1998; 32: 213-23.

Dow RS. Extrinsic regulatory mechanisms of seizure activity. *Epilepsia* 1965; 13: 122-40.

Dow RS, Fernandez-Guardiola A, Manni E. The influence of the cerebellum on experimental epilepsy. *Electroencephalogr Clin Neurophysiol* 1962; 14: 383-98.

Eells JB, F.A.U., Clough RW, F.A.U., Browning R.A. Expression of Fos in the superior lateral subdivision of the lateral parabrachial (LPBsl) area after generalized tonic seizures in rats. *Brain Res Bull* 1998; 47: 155-61.

Engel J. Epileptic seizures. In: Engel J, F.A., ed. *Seizures and Epilepsy*. Philadelphia: Davis Company, 1989: 137-78.

Engel J, Jr, Schwartzkroin PA. What should be Modeled? In: Pitkanen A, Schwartkroin PA, Moshe SL, eds. *Models of Seizures and Epilepsy*. New York: Elsevier Academic Press, 2006: 1-14.

Esplin DW. Spinal cord convulsions. *Arch Neurol* 1959; 1: 485-90.

Esplin DW, Freston JW. Physiological and pharmacological analysis of spinal cord convulsions. *J Pharmacol Exp Ther* 1960; 130: 68-80.

Faingold C, Casebeer D. Modulation of the audiogenic seizure network by noradrenergic and glutamatergic receptors of the deep layers of superior colliculus. *Brain Res* 1999; 821: 392-9.

Faingold CL. Neuronal networks in the genetically epilepsy-prone rat. *Adv Neurol* 1999; 79: 311-21.

Faingold CL. Emergent properties of CNS neuronal networks as targets for pharmacology: application to anticonvulsant drug action. *Prog Neurobiol* 2004; 72: 55-85.

Faingold CL, Copley CA, Boersma CA. Effects of microinjection of a new excitant amino acid (EAA) antagonist, CPP, into inferior colliculus (IC) and amygdala (AMG) on audiogenic siezures (AGS) in the genetically epilepsy-prone rat (GEPR). *FASEB J* 1988a; 2: A1067.

Faingold CL, Hoffmann WE, Caspary DM. Comparative effects of convulsant drugs on the sensory responses of neurons in the amygdala and brainstem reticular formation. *Neuropharmacology* 1985; 24: 1221-30.

Faingold CL, Millan MH, Boersma CA, Meldrum BS. Excitant amino acids and audiogenic seizures in the genetically epilepsy-prone rat. I. Afferent seizure initiation pathway. *Exp Neurol* 1988b; 99: 678-86.

Faingold CL, Randall ME. Neurons in the deep layers of superior colliculus play a critical role in the neuronal network for audiogenic seizures: mechanisms for production of wild running behavior. *Brain Res* 1999; 815: 250-8.

Faingold CL, Randall ME. Pontine reticular formation neurons exhibit a premature and precipitous increase in acoustic responses prior to audiogenic seizures in genetically epilepsy-prone rats. *Brain Res* 1995; 704: 218-26.

Feng HJ, Faingold CL. Synaptic plasticity in the pathway from the medial geniculate body to the lateral amygdala is induced by seizure repetition. *Brain Res* 2002; 946: 198-205.

Feng HJ, Naritoku DK, Randall ME, Faingold CL. Modulation of audiogenically kindled seizures by gamma-aminobutyric acid-related mechanisms in the amygdala. *Exp Neurol* 2001; 172: 477-81.

Fisher RS, van Emde BW, Blume W, Elger C, Genton P, Lee P, Engel J, Jr. Epileptic seizures and epilepsy: definitions proposed by the International League Against Epilepsy (ILAE) and the International Bureau for Epilepsy (IBE). *Epilepsia* 2005; 46: 470-2.

Fromm GH. The brain-stem and convulsions: Historical overview. In: Fromm GH, Faingold CL, Browning RA, Burnham WM, eds. *Epilepsy and the Reticular Formation: The Role of Reticular Core in Convulsive Seizures*. New York: Alan R. Liss, 1987: 1-8.

Gale K. Focal trigger zones and pathways of propagation in seizure generation. In: Schwartzkroin PA, ed. *Epilepsy: Models, Mechanisms, and Concepts*. Cambridge: Cambridge University Press, 1993: 48-93.

Gale K. Role of the substantia nigra in GABA-mediated anticonvulsant actions. *Adv Neurol* 1986; 44: 343-64.

Gale K. Subcortical structures and pathways involved in convulsive seizure generation. *J Clin Neurophysiol* 1992; 9: 264-77.

Gale K, Pazos A, Maggio R, Japikse K, Pritchard P. Blockade of GABA receptors in superior colliculus protects against focally evoked limbic motor seizures. *Brain Res* 1993; 603: 279-83.

Garcia-Cairasco N, Terra VC, Mishra PK, Dailey JW, Jobe PC. Neuroethology of brainstem-induced forebrain seizure kindling in genetically epilepsy-prone rats (GEPRs). Society for Neuroscience Abstracts 20[1], 406. 1994.

Garcia-Cairasco N, Wakamatsu H, Oliveira JA, Gomes EL, Del Bel EA, Mello LE. Neuroethological and morphological (Neo-Timm staining) correlates of limbic recruitment during the development of audiogenic kindling in seizure susceptible Wistar rats. *Epilepsy Res* 1996; 26: 177-92.

Gastaut H. Forward. In: Fromm GH, Faingold CL, Browning RA, Burnham WM, Liss AR, eds. *Epilepsy and the Reticular Formation: The Role of the Reticular Core in Convulsive Seizures*. New York, 1987: 11-2.

Gastaut H, Broughton RJ. *Epileptic seizures; clinical and electrographic features, diagnosis and treatment*. Thomas: Springfield, IL, 1972.

Goodman L, Gilman A. Metrazol, coramine and camphor. In: *The Pharmacological Basis of Therapeutics*. New York: MacMillan, 1941: 267-73.

Handforth A, Ackermann RF. Functional [14C]2-deoxyglucose mapping of progressive states of status epilepticus induced by amygdala stimulation in rat. *Brain Res* 1988b; 460: 94-102.

Handforth A, Ackermann RF. Hierarchy of seizure states in the electrogenic limbic status epilepticus model: behavioral and electrographic observations of initial states and temporal progression. *Epilepsia* 1992; 33: 589-600.

Handforth A, Ackermann RF. Electrogenic status epilepticus induced from numerous limbic sites. *Epilepsy Res* 1993; 15: 21-6.

Handforth A, Ackermann RF. Electrically induced limbic status and kindled seizures. In: Meldrum BS, Ferrendelli JA, Wieser HG, eds. *Anatomy of Epileptogenesis*. London-Paris: John Libbey & Company Ltd., 1988a: 71-87.

Handforth A, Treiman DM. A new, non-pharmacologic model of convulsive status epilepticus induced by electrical stimulation: behavioral/electroencephalographic observations and response to phenytoin and phenobarbital. *Epilepsy Res* 1994; 19: 15-25.

Handforth A, Treiman DM. Functional mapping of the early stages of status epilepticus: a 14C-2-deoxyglucose study in the lithium-pilocarpine model in rat. *Neuroscience* 1995a; 64: 1057-73.

Handforth A, Treiman DM. Functional mapping of the late stages of status epilepticus in the lithium-pilocarpine model in rat: a 14C-2-deoxyglucose study. *Neuroscience* 1995b; 64: 1075-89.

Hirsch E, Danober L, Simler S, Pereira DV, Maton B, Nehlig A, Marescaux C, Vergnes M. The amygdala is critical for seizure propagation from brainstem to forebrain. *Neuroscience* 1997; 77: 975-84.

Hirsch E, Maton B, Vergnes M, Depaulis A, Marescaux C. Reciprocal positive transfer between kindling of audiogenic seizures and electrical kindling of inferior colliculus. *Epilepsy Res* 1993; 15: 133-9.

Hirsch E, Maton B, Vergnes M, Depaulis A, Marescaux C. Positive transfer of audiogenic kindling to electrical hippocampal kindling in rats. *Epilepsy Res* 1992; 11: 159-66.

Jobe PC. Spinal seizures induced by electrical stimulation. In: *Epilepsy and the Reticular Formation: The Role of the Reticular Core in Convulsive Seizures*. Alan R. Liss, Inc., 1987: 81-91.

Jobe PC, Browning RA. Mammalian models of genetic epilepsy characterized by sensory-evoked seizures and generalized seizure susceptibility. In: Pitkanen A, Schwartzkroin PA, Moshe SL, eds. *Models of Seizures and Epilepsy*. Amsterdam: Academic Press, 2006: 261-71.

Jobe PC, Dailey JW. Genetically epilepsy-prone rats (GEPRs) in drug research. *CNS Drug Rev* 2000; 6: 241-60.

Jobe PC, Mishra PK, Adams-Curtis LE, Deoskar VU, Ko KH, Browning RA, Dailey JW. The genetically epilepsy-prone rat (GEPR). *Ital J Neurol Sci* 1995; 16: 91-9.

Jobe PC, Mishra PK, Browning RA, Wang C, Adams-Curtis LE, Ko KH, Dailey JW. Noradrenergic abnormalities in the genetically epilepsy-prone rat. *Brain Res Bull* 1994; 35: 493-504.

Jobe PC, Mishra PK, Dailey JW, Ko KH, Reith MEA. Genetic predisposition to partial (focal) seizures and to generalized tonic/clonic seizures: Interactions between seizure circuitry of the forebrain and brainstem. In: Berkovic SF, Genton P, Hirsch E, Picard F, eds. *Genetics of Focal Epilepsies*. Avignon, France: John Libbey & Company, Ltd., 1999: 251-60.

Jobe PC, Weber RW. Affective disorder and epilepsy comorbidity in the genetically epilepsy prone-rat (GEPR). In: Gilliam F, Kanner AM, Sheline YI, eds. *Depression and Brain Dysfunction*. London: Taylor & Francis Medical Books, 2005.

Kiesmann M, Marescaux C, Vergnes M, Micheletti G, Depaulis A, Warter JM. Audiogenic seizures in Wistar rats before and after repeated auditory stimuli: clinical, pharmacological, and electroencephalographic studies. *J Neural Transm* 1988; 72: 235-44.

Kreindler A, Zuckermann E, Steriade M, Chimion J. Electroclinical features of convulsions induced by stimulation of brain-stem. *J Neurophysiol* 1958; 21: 430-6.

Lothman EW, Collins RC. Kainic acid induced limbic seizures: metabolic, behavioral, electroencephalographic and neuropathological correlates. *Brain Res* 1981; 218: 299-318.

Lothman EW, Collins RC, Ferrendelli JA. Kainic acid-induced limbic seizures: electrophysiologic studies. *Neurology* 1981; 31: 806-12.

Ludvig N, Moshe SL. Different behavioral and electrographic effects of acoustic stimulation and dibutyryl cyclic AMP injection into the inferior colliculus in normal and in genetically epilepsy-prone rats. *Epilepsy Res* 1989; 3: 185-90.

Marescaux C, Vergnes M, Kiesmann M, Depaulis A, Micheletti G, Warter JM. Kindling of audiogenic seizures in Wistar rats: an EEG study. *Exp Neurol* 1987; 97: 160-8.

McCown TJ, Greenwood RS, Breese GR. Inferior colliculus interactions with limbic seizure activity. *Epilepsia* 1987; 28: 234-41.

McCown TJ, Knapp DJ, Crews FT. Inferior collicular seizure generalization produces site-selective cortical induction of cyclooxygenase 2 (COX-2). *Brain Res* 1997; 767: 370-4.

McIntyre DC, Don JC, Edson N. Distribution of 14C 2-deoxyglucose after various forms and durations of status epilepticus induced by stimulation of a kindled amygdala focus in rats. *Epilepsy Res* 1991; 10: 119-33.

Merrill MA, Clough RW, Dailey JW, Jobe PC, Browning RA. The effect of serotonin (5-HT) in the deep layers of the superior colliculus (DLSC) and intercollicular nucleus (ICN) on audiogenic seizures (AGS) in the genetically epilepsy-prone rat (GEPR). Society for Neuroscience Abstracts 26[1], 1010. 2000.

Merrill MA, Clough RW, Jobe PC, Browning RA. Brainstem seizure severity regulates forebrain seizure expression in the audiogenic kindling model. *Epilepsia* 2005; 46: 1380-8.

Merrill MA, Clough RW, Jobe PC, Browning RA. Role of the superior colliculus and the intercollicular nucleus in the brainstem seizure circuitry of the genetically epilepsy-prone rat. *Epilepsia* 2003; 44: 305-14.

Millan MH, Meldrum BS, Boersma CA, Faingold CL. Excitant amino acids and audiogenic seizures in the genetically epilepsy-prone rat. II. Efferent seizure propagating pathway. *Exp Neurol* 1988; 99: 687-98.

Moraes MFD, Chavali M, Mishra PK, Jobe PC, Garcia-Cairasco N. A comprehensive electrographic and behavioral analysis of generalized tonic-clonic seizures of GEPR-9s. *Brain Res* 2005a; 1033: 1-12.

Moraes MFD, Mishra PK, Jobe PC, Garcia-Cairasco N. An electrographic analysis of the synchronous discharge patterns of GEPR-9s generalized seizures. *Brain Res* 2005b; 1046: 1-9.

Morimoto K, Fahnestock M, Racine RJ. Kindling and status epilepticus models of epilepsy: rewiring the brain. *Prog Neurobiol* 2004; 73: 1-60.

N'Gouemo P, Faingold CL. Repetitive audiogenic seizures cause an increased acoustic response in inferior colliculus neurons and additional convulsive behaviors in the genetically-epilepsy prone rat. *Brain Res* 1996; 710: 92-6.

Nail-Boucherie K, Le Pham BT, Gobaille S, Maitre M, Aunis D, Depaulis A. Evidence for a role of the parafascicular nucleus of the thalamus in the control of epileptic seizures by the superior colliculus. *Epilepsia* 2005; 46: 141-5.

Naritoku DK, Mecozzi LB, Aiello MT, Faingold CL. Repetition of audiogenic seizures in genetically epilepsy-prone rats induces cortical epileptiform activity and additional seizure behaviors. *Exp Neurol* 1992; 115: 317-24.

Patel S. Chemically induced limbic seizures in rodents. In: Meldrum BS, Ferrendelli JA, Wieser HG, eds. *Current Problems In Epilepsy: Anatomy of Epileptogenesis*. London: John Libbey, 1988: 89-106.

Pereira DV, Vergnes M, Boyet S, Marescaux C, Nehlig A. Forebrain metabolic activation induced by the repetition of audiogenic seizures in Wistar rats. *Brain Res* 1997; 762: 114-20.

Pinel JP, Rovner LI. Electrode placement and kindling-induced experimental epilepsy. *Exp Neurol* 1978b; 58: 335-46.

Pinel JP, Rovner LI. Experimental epileptogenesis: kindling-induced epilepsy in rats. *Exp Neurol* 1978a; 58: 190-202.

Racine RJ. Modification of seizure activity by electrical stimulation: II. motor seizure. *Electroencephalogr Clin Neurophysiol* 1972; 32: 281-94.

Raines A, Anderson RJ. Effects of acute cerebellectomy on maximal electroshock seizures and anticonvulsant efficacy of diazepam in the rat. *Epilepsia* 1976; 17: 177-82.

Raisinghani M, Faingold CL. Evidence for the perirhinal cortex as a requisite component in the seizure network following seizure repetition in an inherited form of generalized clonic seizures. *Brain Res* 2005a; 1048: 193-201.

Raisinghani M, Faingold CL. Neurons in the amygdala play an important role in the neuronal network mediating a clonic form of audiogenic seizures both before and after audiogenic kindling. *Brain Res* 2005b; 1032: 131-40.

Raisinghani MF, Faingold CL. Identification of the requisite brain sites in the neuronal network subserving generalized clonic audiogenic seizures. *Brain Res* 2003; 967: 113-22.

Redgrave P, Dean P, Simkins M. Intratectal glutamate suppresses pentylenetetrazole-induced spike-and-wave discharges. *Eur J Pharmacol* 1988; 158: 283-7.

Redgrave P, Marrow LP, Dean P. Anticonvulsant role of nigrotectal projection in the maximal electroshock model of epilepsy-II. Pathways from substantia nigra pars lateralis and adjacent peripenduncular area to the dorsal midbrain. *Neuroscience* 1992a; 46: 391-406.

Redgrave P, Simkins M, Overton P, Dean P. Anticonvulsant role of nigrotectal projection in the maximal electroshock model of epilepsy-I. Mapping of dorsal midbrain with bicuculline. *Neuroscience* 1992b; 46: 379-90.

Ryu JR, Steenbergen JL, Mishra PK, Clough RW, Dailey JW, Ko KH, Jobe PC. Culture of locus ceruleus (LC) and superior colliculus (SC): cells characterization of noradrenergic (NA) system. Society for Neuroscience Abstracts 23, 2420. 1997.

Samoriski GM, Applegate CD. Repeated generalized seizures induce time-dependent changes in the behavioral seizure response independent of continued seizure induction. *J Neurosci* 1997; 17: 5581-90.

Samoriski GM, Piekut DT, Applegate CD. Differential spatial patterns of Fos induction following generalized clonic and generalized tonic seizures. *Exp Neurol* 1997; 143: 255-68.

Savage DD, Reigel CE, Jobe PC. Angular bundle kindling is accelerated in rats with a genetic predisposition to acoustic stimulus-induced seizures. *Brain Res* 1986a; 376: 412-5.

Savage DD, Reigel CE, Jobe PC. The development of kindled seizures is accelerated in the genetically epilepsy-prone rat. *Life Sci* 1986b; 39: 879-86.

Simler S, Vergnes M, Marescaux C. Spatial and temporal relationships between C-Fos expression and kindling of audiogenic seizures in Wistar rats. *Exp Neurol* 1999; 157: 106-19.

Sutula TP, Ockuly J. Kindling, spontaneous seizures, and the consequences of epilepsy: More than a model. In: Pitkanen A, Moshe SL, Schwartzkroin PA, eds. *Models of Seizures and Epilepsy*. Amsterdam: Elsevier Academic Press, 2003: 395-406.

Thompson ME, Galosy RA. Electrical brain activity and cardiovascular function during amygdaloid kindling in the dog. *Exp Neurol* 1983; 82: 505-20.

Toman JEP, Loewe S, Goodman L. Physiology and therapy of convulsive disorders. *Arch Neurol and Psychiatr* 1947; 58: 312-24.

Treiman LJ, Treiman DM. Genetic aspects of epilepsy. In: Wyllie E, ed. *The Treatment of Epilepsy: Principles & Practice*. Philadelphia: Lippincott, Williams & Wilkins, 2001: 115-30.

Turski WA, Cavalheiro EA, Bortolotto ZA, Mello LM, Schwarz M, Turski L. Seizures produced by pilocarpine in mice: a behavioral, electroencephalographic and morphological analysis. *Brain Res* 1984; 321: 237-53.

Vergnes M, Kiesmann M, Marescaux C, Depaulis A, Micheletti G, Warter JM. Kindling of audiogenic seizures in the rat. *Int J Neurosci* 1987; 36: 167-76.

Vernadakis A. Spinal cord convulsions in developing rats. *Science* 1962; 137: 532.

Vinogradova LV, Kuznetsova GD, Shatskova AB, Van Rijn CM. Vigabatrin in low doses selectively suppresses the clonic component of audiogenically kindled seizures in rats. *Epilepsia* 2005; 46: 800-10.

Yan QS, Dailey JW, Steenbergen JL, Jobe PC. Anticonvulsant effect of enhancement of noradrenergic transmission in the superior colliculus in genetically epilepsy-prone rats (GEPRs) – A microinjection study. *Brain Res* 1998; 780: 199-209.

Systems and network in tonic seizures and epilepsies in humans

Warren T. Blume

*London Health Sciences Centre – University Campus, Epilepsy Unit,
University of Western Ontario, London, Ontario, Canada*

According to the Oxford Dictionary, "generalised" means "including or affecting or applicable to all or most parts or cases or things" (Concise Oxford Dictionary, 1982). Applying this definition to epilepsy designates epileptic conditions that begin without specific warning, whose motor manifestations are usually symmetrically bilateral, in which awareness is usually impaired or lost and which terminate without focal postictal manifestations. When generalized epilepsy begins in early childhood, a common manifestation is tonic seizures.

■ Tonic seizures: semiology

The comprehensive description of tonic seizures by Gastaut and Broughton (1972) remains the standard. They delineated three types: axial, axorhizomelic, and global.

Axial

Neck muscles contract with flexion or extension, eyelids and eyebrows elevate, eyes deviate upwards, and jaws and lips contract tonically. Respiratory excursion attenuates from contraction of sternocleidomastoid, scalene and then thoracic muscles. The consequent forced expiration across a glottis in spasm produces a cry.

Axorhizomelic

In addition to axial features, proximal limb muscles contract: shoulders elevate; arms abduct; elbows flex or extend; hips, knees flex or more commonly extend and legs may abduct or adduct.

Global

To axial and axorhizomelic features are added: elevation of arms in front of the face and clenching of fists. Legs may be triply flexed or extended. These diffuse flexion motor features comprise an emprosthotonic posture.

Autonomic features may prominently appear: mydriasis, tachycardia, hypertension, tachypnea, apnea, flushing and cyanosis; lacrimal, salivary and tracheobronchial hypersecretion; sweating and urinary incontinence.

Tonic seizures may begin abruptly or gradually. They may end with a brief clonic phase that is much shorter than that of a generalised tonic-clonic attack.

Bisynchronous slow spike-waves are the most common interictal correlate of generalised tonic seizures. Fast rhythmic waves, termed also "the epileptic recruiting rhythm" accompany tonic seizures and may also appear interictally (Blume, 1999). Both EEG phenomena reflect excess cortical excitability as described below.

■ Clinical syndromes with tonic seizures

Infantile Encephalopathy with Suppression-burst Pattern (Ohtahara Syndrome)

These unfortunate children have several hundred per day of tonic seizures in flexion lasting a few to 10 seconds occurring during wakefulness or in sleep and therefore represent epileptic spasms in this respect (Ohtahara, 1992; Aicardi, 1994). Diffuse cortical dysgenesis and neonatal asphyxia are the principal two etiologies. Their EEGs consist of bursts of spikes, sharp-waves and slow-waves lasting 1-5 seconds alternating with periods of electrical attenuation, *i.e.* "suppression". These bursts may appear asymmetrically or symmetrically, synchronously or asynchronously but the individual spikes and waves are never bilaterally synchronous either during wakefulness or sleep. Such "suppression-bursts" occur during wakefulness or sleep and therefore are distinguished from hypsarrhythmia, which has similar bursts only in non-REM sleep. The ictal phase is manifested by diffuse desynchronisation and sequences of low voltage fast activity and therefore resemble somewhat that of epileptic spasms. The burst-suppression pattern may progress to hypsarrhythmia *via* a gradual increase in voltage of the suppression phase which first appears in the awake state. A second outcome is progression to focal spikes.

These infants, manifesting evidence of severe cerebral dysfunction, may progress to the West Syndrome at about age 4 months; but all become handicapped or die.

Epileptic Spasms

Epileptic spasms consist of 2-10 seconds tonic events usually flexing the trunk and abducting the extended arms at the shoulders.

Hypsarrhythmia is the most remarkable but not the only EEG pattern associated with epileptic (infantile) spasms. It appears in 40-70% of cases (Aicardi, 1994), but is the most characteristic interictal EEG pattern seen with epileptic spasms. According to Jeavons and Bower (Jeaons, 1974) about two-thirds of first EEGs done for epileptic spasms contain hypsarrhythmia; other EEG abnormalities occur in 30% while only 2% of first EEGs are normal. All subsequent EEGs of these 2% are abnormal. Be alert to the possibility of pyridoxine dependency or deficiency in this condition.

During the spasm, a widely synchronous single spike is followed by diffuse attenuation upon which may be superimposed high frequency low amplitude rhythmic waves (Blume, 1999).

The Lennox-Gastaut Syndrome

This syndrome consists of an intractable generalised seizure disorder of childhood onset consisting of multiple seizure types including tonic, atonic, and atypical absence attacks. Some patients may have tonic or non-convulsive status epilepticus. EEG criteria include bilaterally synchronous slow spike-waves and 10-20 Hz epileptic recruiting rhythm, the latter appearing principally in sleep. According to Genton *et al.* (2000) both the slow spike-waves and the paroxysmal 10-20 Hz activity must be present in the same recording in any given patient to satisfy the diagnosis of the syndrome. Therefore, a sleep recording should be carried out in any patient suspected of having the Lennox-Gastaut Syndrome (LGS) in whom the 10-20 Hz activity does not appear in the awake state. To document EEG-clinical correlations, particularly subtle attacks, polygraph recordings are often valuable. These would include: EEG, video, axial and deltoid EMG, and monitors of respiration and ocular movements. Adolescents who have had the LGS may continue to have atypical absence, generalised tonic-clonic seizures and atonic seizures. Although their EEGs retain slow spike-waves, rapid rhythms and tonic seizures become rare to absent.

■ Mechanisms of generalised seizures: clinical data

A close association exists between bisynchronous epileptiform discharges and generalised seizure disorders. Jasper and Kershman (1941) correlated clinical seizure manifestations with interictal EEG abnormalities: bilaterally synchronous spike-wave discharges occurred in 84% of their patients with absences and in 48% of patients with generalised tonic-clonic seizures. Bilaterally synchronous epileptiform paroxysms occurred in all 90 children with myoclonic epilepsy studied by Aicardi and Chevrie (1971). Conversely, 80% of patients with bisynchronous paroxysms had generalised seizures in the Jasper and Kershman series (1941). 98% of children with bilaterally synchronous slow spike-waves have generalised seizures which are most commonly tonic (Blume, 1973; Markand, 1977).

Spike-waves, the most common bisynchronous epileptiform discharge, consist of one or more electronegative spikes within a positive trough followed by a broad negative wave (Weir, 1965). Bilaterally synchronous spike-waves are usually maximally expressed over the frontal regions (Gibbs, 1936). Sequential field plots of evolving spike-wave discharges confirm this location over the frontal lobes corresponding principally to the premotor and prefrontal cortices (Lemieux, 1986). Bancaud *et al.* (1965) and Goldring (1972), recording from implanted electrodes in humans, found that generalised motor seizures originated principally from the frontal cortex and that subcortical structures became involved secondarily.

Gloor et al. (1968) correlated EEG features in patients with diffuse encephalopathies with their histopathological abnormalities. Patients with both cortical and subcortical grey matter disorders developed bisynchronous bursts, either as slow spike-waves, sharp waves or delta. Such abnormalities rarely appeared among those whose lesions involved only the cortical grey matter.

■ EEGs and tonic seizures

Slow Spike-Waves (SSWs)

The slow spike-wave is the principal interictal correlate of tonic seizures. These are spike-waves with a repetition rate between 1 and 2 Hz and a total duration of each complex from 450 to 600 milliseconds (Gastaut, 1966). The epileptiform component may be either a spike or a sharp wave. The complexes are usually bilaterally synchronous and symmetrical but they may be principally expressed in, or confined to, the anterior or the posterior head regions. Morphology, amplitude and repetition rate may vary between and within SSW bursts; shifting asymmetries may occur. Hyperventilation has little effect on these discharges and photic stimulation has none. Sleep increases their abundance. During sleep, polyspike waves, generalised polyspikes, and 10-20 Hz rhythmic waves or even electrodecremental events (sudden attenuation for 1-2 seconds) may appear. Sleep spindles and V-waves may be absent (Blume, 1999). The maximum incidence of such discharges occurs between 1 and 5 years (Blume, 1973) but SSWs may be mixed with hypsarrhythmia at the younger part of this range and with 3 Hz spike-waves at the later part. In contrast to recordings with 3 Hz spike-wave discharges, the interparoxysmal recording is usually abnormally slow. This phenomenon usually occupies a greater portion of the awake recording than generalised spike-wave complexes. No clinical alteration may be discerned in such patients at the onset of a burst of slow spike-waves in contradistinction to 3 Hz spike-wave discharges in which a closer EEG-clinical correlation occurs. However, in other instances "atypical absence" may coincide with SSWs.

Seizures occur in about 98% of patients with slow spike-waves; the most common are tonic seizures followed by atypical absence attacks. Atonic, myoclonic, and tonic-clonic seizures are also seen (Markand, 1977; Gastaut, 1966; Chevrie, 1972; Blume, 1973). Unfortunately, the majority of patients have more than one type of seizure and have daily attacks that are usually difficult to control. Tonic seizures are most often accompanied by diffuse electrodecremental events, fast rhythmic waves, or polyspikes (Markand, 1977; Gastaut, 1972; Chevrie, 1972; Blume, 1973). Atypical absence may be detected at the onset of slow spike-waves or may accompany any of the patterns of tonic seizures. Myoclonic attacks occur in association with high voltage bisynchronous spikes.

Fast Rhythmic Waves and Sequential Polyspikes

These are bursts of sinusoidal waves at 8-30 Hz with a widespread or generalised distribution (Blume, 1999). They may appear subtly and occasionally may be difficult to distinguish from ongoing beta activity (Blume, 1999). The usual clinical accompaniment is tonic seizures when hypsarrhythmia or slow spike-waves appear in the recording. When spike-wave complexes appear in the same recording, the usual clinical accompaniment is absence.

Basic mechanisms

Participating structures

Clinical data of tonic seizures implicate the cortex, thalamus, and brainstem originating motor tracts. Mechanisms relevant to these components comprise this section.

The neuronal aggregates participating in the spike-wave phenomenon include: cortico-thalamic neurones and their axons (excitatory), thalamo-cortical relay cells (TCR) and their axons (excitatory), adjacent cortical and thalamic GABAergic interneurones (inhibitory), and thalamic reticular nucleus neurones (inhibitory). Thalamocortical neurones extend glutamergic excitatory connections to the cortical pyramidal neurones, principally in cortical layers III-IV and V-VI but they also excite adjacent inhibitory interneurones and thalamic reticular neurons. Projection back to the thalamus derives from cortical layer VI (Blumenfeld, 2005) to excite thalamo-cortical cells (excitatory), thalamic interneurones (inhibitory) and thalamic reticular neurones (inhibitory) (Lothman, 1993; Blumenfeld, 2000). Recurrent cortical inhibition also occurs. Although inhibitory interneurones exist throughout the cortex and thalamus, the thalamic reticular nucleus is virtually exclusively composed of GABAergic inhibitory interneurons, underpinning its major role in sleep spindle and spike-wave generation and regulation. As stated, the thalamic reticular nucleus receives excitatory axon collaterals from both thalamocortical and corticothalamic neurons and sends inhibitory GABAergic connections to the thalamic relay neurones. Additionally, inhibitory GABAergic connections and gap junctions exist between the thalamic reticular nucleus neurones (Blumenfeld, 2005).

Cortical Participation

The feline generalised penicillin epilepsy FGPE model (Prince, 1969) disclosed several properties of bisynchronous spike-wave discharges. Bilateral participation of both the thalamus and cortex are required for development of the spike-wave complex. Parenteral penicillin injection produced epileptiform activity in the cortex before subcortical regions (Fisher, 1977; Gloor, 1990). Moreover, Fisher and Prince (Fisher, 1977) produced spike-wave discharges by bilateral cortical penicillin application but thalamic application did not elicit spike-waves. However, inactivation of the thalamus by potassium chloride can abolish spike-wave discharges (Avoli, 1981). In fact, removal of cortex or the thalamus or their interconnections in the FGPE model will abolish spike-waves (Avoli, 1982; Avoli, 1981; Pellegrini, 1979). Therefore no locus in the cortex or the thalamus can be considered an origin of spike-waves. Instead, this phenomenon and its associated epilepsies, should be considered as abnormalities of a system(s).

Micro-electrode recordings reveal that the negative spikes of spike-wave complexes are associated with depolarising potentials resembling excitatory post-synaptic potentials (EPSPs) in upper cortical layers while positive troughs are linked with excitation in lower cortical layers (Fisher, 1977; Kostopoulos, 1982). Kostopoulos *et al.* (Fisher, 1977) found the peak incidence of cortical action potential firing to coincide with the junction of the spike and positive trough of the spike-wave complex. Similarly, Elger and Speckmann (1983) found that corticofugal potentials correlate with electronegative discharges in deeper cortical layers. Although the latter work was performed in the primary motor cortex, its finding combined with the field distribution of spike-wave discharges may lead one to postulate that the junction of the electronegative spike and positive trough is that point in the spike-wave complex that correlates with corticofugal discharges from the premotor and prefrontal areas. In contrast, cortical action potential firing virtually ceases during the wave (Avoli, 1982). This oscillatory pattern of alteration between a high incidence of action potential discharge (spike and trough) and longer periods of near neuronal silence (wave) was found in both cortex and the thalamus. This oscillation corresponds to the intracellular correlates of spike-waves as alternating sequences of depolarising and hyperpolarising potentials (Pumain, 1992; Avanzini, 1999). Further mechanisms underlying these sequences are discussed below.

Thalamic Participation

As the thalamic neuronal aggregates creating sleep spindles play a crucial role in this oscillation, the relationships of its relevant components are significant.

The "non-specific" thalamic nuclei, a rostral portion of the ascending reticular activating system, comprise the intralaminar nuclei, the midline nuclei, and the reticular thalamic nucleus (Brodal, 1981). Midline and intralaminar nuclei, which receive reticulothalamic connections from the reticular formation of the brain stem, project onto the thalamic reticular nucleus. Neurones of these nuclei resemble those of the reticular formation of the brain stem and their richly branching axons enter neighbouring "non-specific" and "specific" thalamic nuclei (Brodal, 1981). These latter are relay nuclei.

Single shock stimulation of these "non-specific" nuclei trigger widely distributed "spindle bursts" in the cortex (Dempsey, 1942). Dempsey and M3n (1942) found that repeated stimulation of these nuclei, at rates close to those of spontaneous cortical rhythms, would produce long latency, monophasic, surface negative, widely distributed association cortex responses. They termed this phenomenon the "recruiting rhythm" as the response increased in amplitude with successive stimuli (1942). This contrasts to stimulation of "specific" thalamic sensory relay nuclei that produces a short latency, diphasic "augmenting" response, restricted to the relevant projection area (Brazier, 1968). By blocking local cortical $GABA_A$ inhibition, bilateral application of penicillin over the cerebral cortex transformed the stimulation-induced thalamocortical response from a spindle or recruiting rhythm to spike-wave discharges (Gloor, 1979; Gloor, 1977). Spike-waves in the penicillin model could only be elicited by stimulation of those thalamic nuclei ("non-specific") that elicited the recruiting rhythm or spindles before penicillin. However, no spike-waves occurred when penicillin was injected into the thalamus.

Thalamic relay cells and thalamic reticular neurones each possess a unique type of calcium channel, so-called "T" channels, which are typically closed at resting membrane potentials (Avanzini, 1999; Lothman, 1993). T-type calcium channels are activated by first *hyperpolarizing* this type of cell through gabaergic interneurone innervation. Such hyperpolarisation "de-inactivates" T-type calcium channels. De-inactivation allows calcium to enter the thalamic relay cell whenever any afferent input slightly depolarises the neurone. This calcium current allows thalamic relay neurones to possess, in normals, two distinct responses to stimuli depending upon the resting membrane potential and corresponding to level of awareness. The "relay mode", predominant during wakefulness, occurs at intracellular membrane potentials positive to –60mV (depolarised): action potential rates of 1-200 Hz occur corresponding to stimulus intensity. Intracellular membrane potentials more negative than –60mV (hyperpolarised) convert the "relay mode" to a "burst firing" mode. In this mode, characteristic of sleep but occurring in wakefulness, 300-500 Hz bursts of action potentials occur, only weakly related to input strength (Huguenard, 1995). The "relay mode" provides an accurate reconstruction of the afferent stimulus while the "burst firing" mode indicates that something has changed in the environment (Sherman, 2001). The mechanism of generalised spike-wave and seizure generation appears to represent an accentuation of this normally-occurring "burst firing mode". In the Genetic Absence Epilepsy Rat of Strasbourg (GAERS) model, reticular thalamic nucleus lesions abolish spike and wave discharges (Avanzini, 1999). The selective inhibition of such "T" calcium channels by the anti-absence drugs ethosuximide and valproic acid supports the essential role of such channels in spike-wave generation (Coulter, 1989; Kelly, 1990).

Cortical-Thalamic Interaction

Recall that the same thalamocortical network that generated spindle waves could switch to spike-wave activity in the feline generalised penicillin epilepsy model. Spindle waves are generated through a reciprocal interaction between excitatory thalamocortical cells and inhibitory gabaergic thalamic reticular neurones and depend upon fast (100-150 msec) $GABA_A$ receptor-mediated IPSPs in the thalamocortical cells, setting the oscillation frequency at about 6-14 Hz. Blocking $GABA_A$ receptors in the thalamocortical relay cells can convert spindles to 3-4 Hz activity (Blumenfeld, 2000). Blumenfeld and McCormick (2000) and Kim et al. (1997) found in the ferret that brief bursts of action potentials in thalamic reticular cells produces fast (100-150 msec) IPSPs in thalamocortical cells mediated by $GABA_A$ receptors. However, more sustained bursts in thalamoreticular cells elicits, in addition to $GABA_A$ IPSPs, slow (approximately 300 msec) $GABA_B$ receptor-mediated IPSPs in thalamocortical cells.

Blumenfeld and McCormick (2000) thus demonstrated that increased firing in the corticothalamic pathway can actually transform the thalamoreticular cell discharge from brief to sustained bursts thereby effecting conversion to $GABA_B$ IPSPs. A possible decrease in thalamic $GABA_A$ receptors in the GAERS absence model may contribute to this conversion to the $GABA_B$ mechanism. The slow metabotropic IPSPs are particularly effective in removing inactivation of the low threshold calcium current and therefore in generating large delayed rebound bursts of action potentials that initiate the next cycle of the oscillation (Sherman, 2001). Gap junctions between thalamic reticular neurones may also aid in generating low frequency synchronous activity in the thalamus, thus spindles and spike-waves.

Given the foregoing, it follows that the slower rate of "slow spike-waves" (1-2 Hz in humans) of the Lennox-Gastaut syndrome and its medical intractability both reflect even greater cortical excitability than is present in most epilepsy syndromes associated with spike-waves (Blume, 2001). Fast rhythmic waves, a signature of the

Lennox-Gastaut syndrome, also likely reflect heightened cortical excitability as they may relate to "ripples" *i.e.* ultra-fast oscillations produced by fast rhythmic-bursting neurones, those cortical neurones having the highest propensity to develop seizures (Blume, 2001; Timofeev, 2004).

Tonic Seizure Mechanisms

Most investigations have centred on the pathophysiology of epileptic spasms with which tonic seizures share many features (Egli, 1985; Ikeno, 1985). These attacks involve the excitatory portions of the pontomedullary reticular system as disclosed by PET studies that show an increase in brainstem glucose metabolism in over 50% of children with spasms (Chugani, 1992). However, several lines of investigation indicate a neocortical origin or at least a dominant role in their genesis. Clinically focal cortical EEG spikes may immediately precede and accompany spasms (Dulac, 1999). NMDA excitatory synapses are over-represented in the cortex of immature rats (Represa, 1989) and GABAergic synapses are transiently depolarising (Ben Ari, 1990). These features of immature cortex may underlie the onset of tonic seizures in early years. Intracerebral propagation is enhanced in the immature brain (Berbel, 1988). Systemically administered NMDA produces emprosthotonic seizures in developing rats, reproducing the fully developed tonic seizure position described above (Mares, 1992).

Several lines of evidence indicate that corticotrophin-releasing hormone (CRH) is an excitatory neurotransmitter independently involved in producing epileptic spasms and other generalised epilepsy manifestations, acting independently from NMDA (Rho, 2004; Baram, 1993; Wang, 2001; Brunson, 2001). One study showed higher cortical CRH levels in children with generalised epilepsies than in controls (Wang, 2001).

These data support earlier subdural recordings in humans whose findings are consistent with frontal cortical origin for tonic seizures (Fisher, 1987). They are also consistent with the anatomical-physiological relationships described earlier.

■ Determinants of Generalised Seizure Type

Manifestations of generalised seizures depend principally upon 1) the region of epileptogenesis, 2) the maturity of the brain at seizure onset and currently, and 3) the physiological state of the system at any point.

Cortical Region

Motor seizures and their electrographic correlates in generalised epilepsy represent epileptic discharges in the frontal association cortex, the thalamic reticular system and the brain stem.

Studies in the Rhesus monkey and the cat found that cortical projections to the pontine and medullary tegmental fields arise principally from area 6, the rostral part of area 4, the prefrontal cortex and the supplementary motor area (Catsman-Berrevoets, 1979; Keizer, 1984; Kuypers, 1981; Newman, 1989). The premotor cortex sends its most prominent corticofugal projections to the medullary reticular formation (Catsman-Berrevoets, 1979). These corticoreticular fibres terminate at or near the regions from which the reticulospinal tract originates. Mechanisms in the forebrain appear to be crucial for triggering facial and forelimb clonic convulsions (Browning, 1985). Site of neocortical involvement may also affect generalised seizure phenomena. Thus, Marcus *et al.* (1968), using bilateral acute epileptogenic foci in the cerebral cortex of monkeys, correlated seizure type with epileptic focus localisation. Anterior foci gave absence whereas progressively more posterior foci gave increasing motor components from myoclonic events to generalised tonic-clonic seizures.

Ontogenesis

The principal expression of generalised seizures appears to evolve with age. Chevrie and Aicardi (1972), studying childhood epileptic encephalopathy with slow spike-waves, found that tonic seizures began at a mean age of 16.6 months whereas atypical absences began at 32 months, myoclonic attacks at 39 months, and clonic or tonic-clonic seizures as 42 months.

Physiological State

Modifications of pathophysiology in a component of generalised seizures may convert one seizure type to another: an absence or myoclonic seizure may evolve to a generalised tonic-clonic event. This transition from an absence attack to a generalised tonic-clonic seizure has been associated with a progressive decrease in recurrent $GABA_A$ inhibition in the cortex (Avoli, 1990). In several models of seizure activity, cortical extracellular potassium levels rise (Lux, 1986). This rise causes a shift of the chloride equilibrium potential in a positive (depolarising) direction thus decreasing the hyperpolarising effect of $GABA_A$ activity. A higher extracelllar potassium level also decreases the normally hyperpolarising outward potassium current from $GABA_B$ receptor activation (Avoli, 1990).

■ Motor seizure pathways

A specific and complete pathophysiology of ictal motor epileptic events remains to be delineated. Progress to date has centred upon the reticulospinal system emanating from the mesencephalon, pons and medulla. Other brainstem-originating descending motor tracts unlikely contribute measurably to tonic seizures. The rubrospinal tract extends throughout the spinal cord (Brodal, 1981) but its progressively smaller size in higher primates may limit its role in tonic seizures. The vestibulospinal tract lacks cortical afferents. The tectospinal tract terminates in the cervical spinal cord; its only motor afferents arise from the frontal eye fields (Brodal, 1998). Deriving a cogent concept of the intricate brainstem mechanisms producing tonic seizures from literature to date is impeded by distinct methodological differences and the intricate anatomy of the brain stem reticular formation.

Cortical projections to the brainstem reticular formation emanate principally from areas that give origin to the pyramidal tract (Brodal, 1998). These corticofugal tracts project principally to the nucleus reticularis pontis caudalis and the caudal part of the NR pontis oralis in the pons and to the NR gigantocellularis in the medulla. The reticulospinal tracts originate from these pontine and medullary origins.

Magoun and Rhines (Rhines, 1946) first showed that electrical stimulation of the medullary reticular formation inhibited spinal reflexes in the anaesthetised cat whereas excitatory effects were distributed far more widely throughout the brain stem. Subsequent studies have disclosed that the most powerful excitatory influences on spinal motor neurones likely originate from the lower pons and rostral medulla corresponding to the NR pontis caudalis pars beta in the caudal pons and to the NR gigantocellularis in the rostral medulla (Newman, 1995). Inhibitory effects derive from the NR gigantocellularis in the medulla. However, this nucleus receives rostrally-originating afferents, especially the dorsorostral pons (Mori, 1995). Moreover, diagrams of brainstem slices disclose a close juxtaposition of areas exerting excitatory and inhibitory effects on spinal motor neurones (Newman, 1995).

Jimenez et al. (2000) studied the location and extent of feline brain stem "convulsive" area(s) using focal microinjections of Penicillin, a $GABA_A$ receptor blocker. The mesencephalic tegmentum was the only brainstem area in which seizures were induced. Seizure type depended upon penicillin dose and not stereotactic coordinates, suggesting direction or amount of spread of its physiological effect may determine the type of seizure produced. This group (Velasco, 1990) also perfused discrete feline brainstem regions with Pentylenetetrazol (PTZ), a GABA antagonist. Rostral mesencephalic reticular formation perfusion evoked myoclonic seizures; more caudal mesencephalic perfusion evoked tonic-clonic seizures; pontine PTZ administration produced diffuse hypotonia (their *Figure 26.4*). This latter effect likely resulted from stimulation of the nucleus reticularis pontis oralis that projects to the medullary N.R. gigantocellularis which is an origin of the reticulospinal tract (Mori, 1995) (see further). Instead of myoclonic and tonic-clonic seizures, electrical stimulation of the mesencephalon evoked tonic seizures (Kreindler, 1958). Similarly midbrain teqmental lesions blocked the hindlimb tonic extensor component of maximal electroshock seizures (Browning, 1981). However, the reticulospinal tract, considered the principal conveyor of tonic seizures, originates from the pons and medulla which are also the termini of cortico reticular fibres (Brodal, 1998). This discrepancy may relate to the extensive vertical descending and ascending connections in the brainstem reticular system.

The pontine-originating reticulospinal tracts facilitate axial and limb extension while the medullary originating reticulospinal tract inhibits axial extensors and promotes flexors (Mori, 1995; Brooks, 1986). However electrical stimulation and glutamate stimulation of the pontomedullary and pontine reticular formation, respectively, each elicited ipsilateral forelimb flexion and contralateral forelimb extension(through spinal cord commissural fibres) in the monkey and cat respectively (Davidson, 2006; Shimamura, 1990). This indicates that the reticulospinal tract may convey either extensor or flexor motor effect. The pattern and origin of afferent input as well as activity of other descending tracts may determine whether output will be flexor or extensor.

The extensor and the flexor phenomena of tonic seizures each resembles extensor and flexor synergy, described by Foerster in 1936 and detailed by Brodal (1981), in patients with lesions involving the primary motor area or the posterior limb of the internal capsule. Extensor synergy consists of arm adduction at the shoulder with elbow and wrist extension and leg adduction at the hip, extension at the knee, and plantar flexion of the ankle and toes. Flexor synergy consists of elevation and abduction of the arm at the shoulder, flexion at the elbow, wrist and fingers and leg abduction and flexion at the hip, and flexion at the knee and dorsiflexion of the foot and toes (Brodal, 1981). The hemiparetic or monoparetic patient with a restricted lesion, can perform either one of these movements voluntarily, indicating their cortical involvement. Such synergies may appear simultaneously in supplementary motor seizures, with a *tendency* for extensor postures to appear contralaterally to side of seizure origin and flexion to appear ipsilaterally (Bleasel, 1996). Kotagal and colleagues (2000) found a remarkably asymmetrical arm posture during secondarily generalised tonic-clonic seizures, the extended arm almost always contralateral to seizure onset and the flexed arm ipsilateral. This suggests that an ictal extensor synergy may reflect a more severe tonic seizure than a flexor synergy in a mature nervous system.

Ajmone Marsan and Ralston (1957) described fundamentally two phases of pentylenetetrazol-induced generalised tonic-clonic seizures: the first phase exhibits predominantly flexor synergy and the second principally extensor synergy. However, their sequential descriptions do not match Foerster's synergies in all respects. This sequence may reflect a progressively intense cortically-originating bilateral seizure discharge.

Substantial clinical and experimental evidence has been presented to indicate a principally frontal cortical origin of tonic seizures whose mechanism apparently does not involve the primary motor system. Corticofoqual discharges descend to the pontomedullary component of the brain stem to induce the pontine-originating reticulospinal system to excite axial and proximal limb musculature at multiple levels.

Delineation of specific descending pathways for each motor seizure phenomenon has yet to be achieved. Overlapping excitatory and inhibitory zones and multiple interconnections among brainstem nuclei underlie this difficulty (Newman, 1995).

Conclusions

Tonic seizures involve the malignant cooperation of almost the entire neuraxis: at least the cortex, thalamus, brain stem and spinal cord. Evaluation of the patient requires careful documentation of seizure semiology and polygraph EEG recording. Basic science will hopefully continue to focus upon interaction of these involved systems.

References

Aicardi J. *Epilepsy in Children*. Second Edition. New York: Raven Press, 1994: 21-5.

Aicardi J, Chevrie JJ. Myoclonic epilepsies of childhood. *Neuropaediatrie* 1971; 3: 177-90.

Ajmone Marsan C, Ralston BL. *The epileptic seizure*. Springfield Illinois. CC Thomas. 1957: 104-7.

Avanzini G, de Curtis M, Pape HC, Spreafico R. Intrinsic properties of reticular thalamic neurons relevant to genetically determined spike-wave generation. *Adv Neurol* 1999; 79: 297-309.

Avoli M, Gloor P. Interaction of cortex and thalamus in spike and wave discharges of feline generalized penicillin epilepsy. *Exp Neurol* 1982; 76: 196-217.

Avoli M, Gloor P. The effects of transient functional depression of the thalamus on spindles and on bilateral synchronous epileptic discharges of feline generalized penicillin epilepsy. *Epilepsia* 1981; 22: 443-52.

Avoli M, Gloor P, Kostopoulos G. Focal and generalized epileptiform activity in the cortex: in search of differences in synaptic mechanisms, ionic movements, and long-lasting changes in neuronal excitability. In: Avoli M, Gloor P, Kostopoulos G, et al., eds. *Generalized Epilepsy Neurobiological Approaches*. Massachusetts: Birkhauser Boston, Inc., 1990: 213-31.

Bancaud J, Talairach J, Bonis A, et al. *La Stéréo-électroencéphalographie dans l'épilepsie*. Paris: Masson 1965.

Baram, T. Z. "Pathophysiology of massive infantile spasms: perspective on the putative role of the brain adrenal axis." *Ann Neurol* 1993; 33.3: 231-36.

Ben Ari, Y, et al. "GABAergic mechanisms in the CA3 hippocampal region during early postnatal life." *Prog Brain Res* 1990; 83: 313-21.

Berbel P, Innocenti GM. "The development of the corpus callosum in cats: a light- and electron-microscopic study." *J Comp Neurol* 1988; 276.1: 132-56.

Bleasel AF, Morris HH. Supplementary sensorimotor area epilepsy in adults. In: Luders Ho, ed. *Advances in Neurology*. Vol. 70: Suppplementary Sensorimotor area. Philadelphia Lippincott-Raven, 1996: 271-84.

Blume WT. "Pathogenesis of Lennox-Gastaut syndrome: considerations and hypotheses." *Epileptic Disord* 2001; 3.4: 183-96.

Blume WT, Kaibara M. Abnormal electroencephalogram; epileptiform potentials. In: *Atlas of Pediatric Electroencephalography*. Second Edition. Philadelphia: Lippincott-Raven, 1999: 155.

Blume WT, Kaibara M. Abnormal electroencephalogram: epileptiform potentials. In: *Atlas of Pediatric Electroencephalography*. Second Edition. 2 edn. Philadelphia: Lippincott-Raven, 1999: 156-7.

Blume WT, Kaibara M. *Atlas of Pediatric Electroencephalography*. Second Edition. Philadelphia: Lippincott-Raven, 1999: 221-4.

Blume WT, Kaibara M. *Atlas of Pediatric Electroencephalography*. Second Edition. Philadelphia: Lippincott-Raven, 1999: 231-3.

Blume WT, David RB, Gomez MR. Generalized sharp and slow wave complexes. Associated clinical features and long-term follow-up. *Brain* 1973; 96: 289-306.

Blumenfeld, H. "Cellular and network mechanisms of spike-wave seizures." *Epilepsia* 2005; 46 (suppl 9): 21-33.

Blumenfeld H, McCormick DA. Corticothalamic inputs control the pattern of activity generated in thalamocortical networks. *J Neuroscience* 2000; 20: 5153-62.

Brazier MAB. *Neurological Anatomy in Relation to Clinical Medicine*. Third Edition. London: Pitman Medical Publishing Co. Ltd., 1968: 260.

Brodal A. *Neurological Anatomy in Relation to Clinical Recidive*. Third Edition. New York: Oxford University Press, 1981: 99.

Brodal P. Central motor pathways. In: Brodal P. *The Central Nervous System*. Oxford: Oxford University Press, 1998: 339-70.

Brooks VB. *The Neural Basis of Motor Control*. New York: Oxford University Press, 1986; 82-110.

Brooks VB. *The Neural Basis of Motor Control*. New York: Oxford University Press, 1986; 151-9.

Browing RA, Turner FJ, Simonson R, et al. Effect of Midbrain and Pontine Tegmental Lesions on the Maximal Electroshock Seizure Pattern in Rats. *Epilepsia* 1981; 22: 583-94.

Browning R, Nelson D. Variation in threshold and pattern of electroshock-induced seizures in rats depending on site of stimulation. *Life Sci* 1985; 37: 2205-11.

Brunson, KL, Eghbal-Ahmadi M, Baram TZ. "How do the many etiologies of West syndrome lead to excitability and seizures? The corticotropin releasing hormone excess hypothesis." *Brain Dev* 2001; 23: 533-8.

Catsman-Berrevoets CE, Kuypers HGJM. Cells of origin of cortical projections to dorsal column nuclei, spinal cord and bulbar medial reticular formation in the rhesus monkey. *Neurosci Lett* 1976; 3: 245-52.

Chevrie JJ, Aicardi J. Childhood epileptic encephalopathy with slow spike-wave. A statistical study of 80 cases. *Epilepsia* 1972; 13: 259-71.

Chugani HT, et al. Infantile spasms: II. Lenticular nuclei and brain stem activation on positron emission tomography. *Ann Neurol* 1992; 31.2: 212-9.

Concise Oxford Dictionary. 7th ed. 1982.

Coulter DA, Huguenard JR, Prince DA. Characterization of ethosuximide reduction of low-threshold calcium current in thalamic neurons. *Ann Neurol* 1989; 25: 582-93.

Davidson AG, Buford JA. Bilateral actions of the reticulospinal tract on arm and shoulder muscles in the monkey: stimulus triggered averaging. *Exp Brain Res* 2006; 28 (Epub ahead of reprint).

Dempsey EW, Morison RS. Production of rhythmically recurrent cortical potentials after localised thalamic stimulation. *Amer J Physiol* 1942; 135: 293-300.

Dulac OJ, et al. *Infantile Spasms: A Physiological Hypothesis*. Nehlig A, et al. London: Libbey, 1999: 93-102.

Egli M, Mothersill I, O'Kane M, O'Kane F. The axial spasm--the predominant type of drop seizure in patients with secondary generalized epilepsy. *Epilepsia* 1985; 26: 401-15.

Elger CE, Speckmann EJ. Vertical inhibition in motor cortical epileptic foci and its consequences for descending neuronal activity to the spinal cord. In: Speckmann EJ, Elger CE, eds. *Epilepsy and Motor System*. Baltimore, MD: Urban & Schwarzenberg, 1983: 152-60.

Fisher RS, Niedermeyer E. "Depth EEG studies in the Lennox-Gastaut syndrome." *Clin Electroencephalogr* 1987; 18.4: 191-200.

Fisher RS, Prince DA. Spike-wave rhythms in cat cortex induced by parenteral penicillin. I. Electroencephalographic features. *Electroencephalogr Clin Neurophysiol* 1977; 42: 608-24.

Fisher RS, Prince DA. Spike-wave rhythms in cat cortex induced by parenteral penicillin. II. Cellular features. *Electroencephalogr Clin Neurophysiol* 1977; 42: 625-39.

Gastaut H, Broughton R. *Epileptic Seizures. Clinical and Electrographic Features, Diagnosis and Treatment*. In: Springfield, Ill.: Charles C. Thomas, 1972: 37-47.

Gastaut H, Roger J, Soulayrol R, et al. Childhood epileptic encephalopathy with diffuse slow spike-waves (otherwise known as "petit mal variant") or Lennox Syndrome. *Epilepsia* 1966; 7: 139-79.

Genton P, Guerrini R, Dravet C. The Lennox-Gastaut syndrome. In: Meinardi H, ed. Handbook of Clinical Neurology, Vol. 73 (29): *The Epilepsies, Part II*. Amsterdam: Elsevier, 2000: 211-22.

Gibbs FA, Lennox WG, Gibbs EL. The electroencephalogram in diagnosis and localization of epileptic seizures. *Arch Neurol Psychiatry* 1936; 36: 1225-35.

Gloor P. Generalized epilepsy with spike-and-wave discharge: a reinterpretation of its electrographic and clinical manifestations. The 1977 William G. Lennox Lecture, American Epilepsy Society. *Epilepsia* 1979; 20: 571-88.

Gloor P, Avoli M, Kostopoulos G. Thalamocortical relationships in generalized epilepsy with bilaterally synchronous spike-and-wave discharge. In: Avoli M, Gloor P, Kostopoulos G, et al. eds. *Generalized Epilepsy: Neurobiological Approaches*. Massachusetts: Birkhauser Boston, Inc., 1990: 190-212.

Gloor P, Kalabay O, Giard N. The electroencephalogram in diffuse encephalopathies: electroencephalographic correlates of grey and white matter lesions. *Brain* 1968; 91: 779-802.

Gloor P, Quesney LF, Zumstein H. Pathophysiology of generalized penicillin epilepsy in the cat: the role of cortical and subcortical structures. II. Topical application of penicillin to the cerebral cortex and to subcortical structures. *Electroencephalogr Clin Neurophysiol* 1977; 43: 79-94.

Goldring S. The role of prefrontal cortex in grand mal convulsion. *Arch Neurol* 1972; 26: 109-19.

Huguenard JR, McCormick DA, Coulter D. Thalamocortical interactions. In: Gutnick MJ, Mody I, eds. The Cortical Neuron. New York: Oxford University Press, 1995: 156-73.

Ikeno T, et al. An analytic study of epileptic falls. *Epilepsia* 1985; 26.6: 612-21.

Jasper H, Kershman J. Electroencephalographic classification of the epilepsies. *Arch Neurol Psychiatry* 1941; 45: 903-43.

Jeavons PM, Bower BD. Infantile spasms. In: Vinken PJ, Bruyn GW, eds. *Handbook of Clinical Neurology*, Vol. 15: The Epilepsies. New York: American Elsevier, 1974: 219-34.

Jimenez, F, et al. Seizures induced by penicillin microinjections in the mesencephalic tegmentum. *Epilepsy Res* 2000; 38.1: 33-44.

Keizer K, Kuypers HGJM. Distribution of corticospinal neurons with collaterals to lower brain stem reticular formation in cat. *Exp Brain Res* 1984; 54: 107-20.

Kelly KM, Gross RA, Macdonald RL. Valproic acid selectively reduces the low-threshold (T) calcium current in rat nodose neurons. *Neurosci Lett* 1990; 116: 233-8.

Kim U, Sanchez-Vives MV, McCormick DA. Functional dynamics of GABAergic inhibition in the thalamus. *Science* 1997; 278: 130-4.

Kostopoulos G, Avoli M, Pellegrini A, Gloor P. Laminar analysis of spindles and of spikes of the spike and wave discharge of feline generalized penicillin epilepsy. *Electroencephalogr Clin Neurophysiol* 1982; 53: 1-13.

Kostopoulos G, Gloor P, Pellegrini A, Gotman J. A study of the transition from spindles to spike and wave discharge in feline generalised penicillin epilepsy: microphysiological features. *Exp Neurol* 1981; 73: 55-77.

Kotagal P, Bleasel A, Geller E, et al. Lateralixzing value of assymetric tonic limb posturing observed in secondarily qenneralized tonic-clonic seizures. *Epilepsia* 2000; 41: 457-62.

Kreindler A, Zuckermann E, Steriade M, Chiminion D. Electroclinical features of convulsions induced by stimulation of the brain stem. *J Neurophysiol* 1958; 2 (5): 430-6.

Kuypers HGJM. Anatomy of the descending pathways. In: Brookhart JM, Mountcastle VB, Brooks VB, et al. eds. *Handbook of Physiology*. Section 1: The Nervous System. Vol. II. Bethesda, Maryland: American Physiological Society, 1981: 597-666.

Lemieux JF, Blume WT. Topographical evolution of spike-wave complexes. *Brain Res* 1986; 373: 275-87.

Lothman EW. The neurobiology of epileptiform discharges. *American Journal of EEG Technology* 1993; 33: 93-112.

Lux HD, Heinemann U, Dietzel I. Ionic changes and alterations in the size of the extracellular space during epileptic activity. *Adv Neurol* 1986; 44: 619-39.

Magoun HW, Rhines R. An Inhibitory Mechanism in the Bulbar Reticular Formation. *J Neurophysiol* 1946; 9: 165-71.

Marcus EM, Watson CW, Simon SA. An experimental model of some varieties of petit mal epilepsy. Electrical-behavioral correlations of acute bilateral epileptogenic foci in cerebral cortex. *Epilepsia* 1968; 9: 233-48.

Mares P, Velisek L. N-methyl-D-aspartate (NMDA)-induced seizures in developing rats. *Brain ResDev Brain Res* 1992; 65.2: 185-9.

Markand ON. Slow spike-wave activity in EEG and associated clinical features: often called "Lennox" or "Lennox-Gastaut" syndrome. *Neurology* 1977; 27: 746-57.

Mori S, et al. Neuroanatomical and neurophysiological bases of postural control. *Adv Neurol* 1995; 67: 289-303.

Newman DB. "Anatomy and neurotransmitters of brainstem motor systems." *Adv Neurol* 1995; 67: 219-44.

Newman DB, Hilleary SK, Ginsberg CY. Nuclear terminations of corticoreticular fiber systems in rats. *Brain Behav Evol* 1989; 34: 223-64.

Ohtahara S, Ohtsuka Y, Yamatogi Y, Oka E, Inoue H. Early infantile epileptic encephalopathy with suppression-bursts. In: Roger J, Bureau M, Dravet C, et al. eds. *Epileptic Syndromes in Infancy, Childhood and Adolescence*, Second Edition. London: John Libbey, 1992: 25-34.

Pellegrini A, Musgrave J, and Gloor P. "Role of afferent input of subcortical origin in the genesis of bilaterally synchronous epileptic discharges of feline generalized penicillin epilepsy." *Exp Neurol* 1979; 64.1: 155-73.

Prince DA, Farrell D. "Centrencephalic" spike-wave discharges following parenteral penicillin injection in the cat. *Neurology* 1969; 19: 309-10.

Pumain R, Louvel J, Gastard M, Kurcewicz I, Vergnes M. Responses to N-methyl-D-aspartate are enhanced in rats with petit mal- like seizures. *J Neural Transm Suppl* 1992; 35: 97-108.

Represa A, Tremblay E, Ben Ari Y. "Transient increase of NMDA-binding sites in human hippocampus during development." *Neurosci Lett* 1989; 99.1-2: 61-6.

Rhines R, Magoun HW. Brain Stem Facilitation of Cortical Motor response. *J Neurophysiol* 1946; 9: 219.

Rho J. M. "Basic science behind the catastrophic epilepsies." *Epilepsia* 2004; 45 (suppl 5): 5-11.

Sherman SM. Tonic and burst firing: dual modes of thalamocortical relay. *Trends Neurosci* 2001; 24: 122-6.

Shimamura M, Fuwa T and Tanaka I. Crossed forelimb extension produced in thalamic cats by injection of putative transmitter substances into the paraleminiscal pontine reticular formation. *Brain Res* 1990; 524 (2): 282-90.

Timofeev I, Steriade M. Neocortical Seizures: Iniation, Development and Cessation. *Neuroscience* 2004; 123 (2): 299-336.

Velasco F, Velasco M. Mesencephalic structures and tonic-clonic generalized seizures. In: Avoli M, Gloor P, Kostopoulos G, *et al.* eds. *Generalized Epilepsy*. Boston: Birkhauser Boston, Inc., 1990: 368-84.

Wang W, Dow KE, Fraser DD. "Elevated corticotropin releasing hormone/corticotropin releasing hormone-R1 expression in postmortem brain obtained from children with generalized epilepsy." *Ann Neurol* 2001; 50.3: 404-9.

Weir B. The morphology of the spike-wave complex. *Electroencephalogr Clin Neurophysiol* 1965; 19: 284-90.

Comments from participants

Ajay Gupta

*Section of Pediatric Epilepsy, Cleveland Clinic Foundation
Cleveland OH, USA*

The premise that brainstem could be a primary generator or is primarily involved in the network for generating seizures is not usually seen in clinical practice in humans. A variety of congenital disorders, sporadic or familial (with or without a known causative gene), are now known that result in primary brainstem and hind brain malformations (Gleeson, 2004). Seizures are not reported as a symptom in any of these congenital disorders of brainstem. Moebius syndrome, Joubert syndrome, ARIMA syndrome, and Senior-Löken syndrome are some examples of congenital disorders of upper and lower brainstem malformations. These syndromes present with a variety of clinical features including cranial nerve palsies, hyptonia, oculomotor impairment, tremors, mental retardation, and oro-facial dysmorphism. However, seizures have not been reported in these congenital disorders of brainstem and hindbrain. Brain MRI findings in these syndromes comprise of upper and lower brainstem malformations with absence of brainstem nuclei, thinning of brainstem, mal-position of long tracts, molar tooth sign, and hypoplastic cerebellar vermis (Gleeson, 2004). If congenital lesions are considered to be paralytic (non-epileptogenic) rather than irritative (epileptogenic) type of lesions, then one can look at other examples of acquired conditions like brainstem glioma, which is a common solid brain tumor in children that usually presents with ataxia and multiple cranial palsies. Seizures are not reported in children with brainstem glioma (Rutka, 2004). Even in adults, central nervous system disorders like ischemic stroke that can purely affect brain stem usually do not results in seizures.

References

1. Gleeson JG, Keeler L, Parisi MA, Marsh SE, Chance, PF, Glass, IA, Graham Jr, JM, Maria, BL, Barkovich, AJ, Dobyns, WB. Molar tooth sign of the midbrain-hindbrain junction: occurrence in multiple distinct syndromes. *Am J Med Genet* 2004; 125 (2): 125-34.
2. Rutka JT, Kuo JS. Pediatric surgical neuro-oncology: Current best care practices and stratergies. *Journal of Neuro-Oncology* 2004; 69 (1): 139-50.

Comments from participants

Pavel Mareš

Institute of Physiology, Academy of Sciences of the Czech Republic, Prague

▪ Generalized seizures in rodents – only two patterns?

Forebrain (clonic seizures involving head and forelimb muscles) and brainstem (generalized tonic-clonic) seizures represent basic types of convulsive seizures in rodents. In addition, nonconvulsive seizures can be elicited by convulsant drugs with an affinity to limbic structures, the two well known examples are kainic acid or pilocarpine. Nonconvulsive partial seizures characterized by presence of epileptic automatisms (*e.g.* wet dog shakes, scratching) are induced by low doses of these drugs (Nadler 1981; Turski 1983; Kršek 2001). Increasing the doses of either kainic acid or pilocarpine results in a transition into the pattern of forebrain seizures what may be taken as a sign of generalization. Similar situation is with electrical stimulation of limbic structures (amygdala, hippocampus, entorhinal cortex) – low stimulation intensities lead to an appearance of automatisms and repetition of these stimulations or a marked increase in intensity of stimulation current results in a transition into typical forebrain seizures (McIntyre, 2006). Models of generalized seizures of the absence type are characterized by minute clonic seizures – movements of vibrissae, nose or ears (Depaulis, 2006).

At least immature laboratory rats can exhibit also another type of generalized convulsive seizures – emprosthotonic, flexion seizures. This type of seizures can be elicited during the first three postnatal weeks by agonists of N-methyl-D-aspartate type of receptors for excitatory amino acids (NMDA – [Mareš, 1997]; homocysteic acid – [Mareš, 1997]). Increasing the dose of these drugs never led to an appearance of forebrain seizures; as a rule, generalized clonic-tonic (*i.e.* in contrast to the typical brainstem seizures the sequence of the two phases is reversed) seizures were observed. Structure responsible for generation of emprosthotonic seizures is not yet known.

Localization of a generator of forebrain seizures is undisputable (Browning, 1985). We confirmed their conclusions in 18-day-old rats with intercollicular transsection of the brainstem. Intact animals of this age can generate both types of seizures; pentylenetetrazol administration in rats with transsection led only to an appearance of generalized tonic-clonic seizures (Mareš and Schickerová – data on file). On the other hand, generalized tonic-clonic seizures must not be generated only by the brainstem. Vernadakis (1962) demonstrated a possibility to induce this type of seizures by electrical stimulation of isolated spinal cord in newborn rats. We examined this possibility in the same age group as the effects of intercollicular transsection. A complete transverse section of the thoracic spinal cord was made at a level of Th 11-12 and when the spinal shock faded out different doses of pentylenetetrazol were administered. Tonic-clonic seizures were observed on forelimbs after doses of pentylenetetrazol identical with those effective in intact controls. Hindlimbs exhibited the same pattern only after higher doses of pentylenetetrazol (Figure 1). It can be concluded that under conditions of intact central nervous system spinal cord machinery serves only as a "final comon path" subdue to higher levels of the central nervous system but if released from this influence it is able to generate basic pattern of generalized tonic-clonic seizures.

Message to be taken is that rodent nervous system is able to generate more than the two basic types of seizures and therefore we can model different types of human seizures.

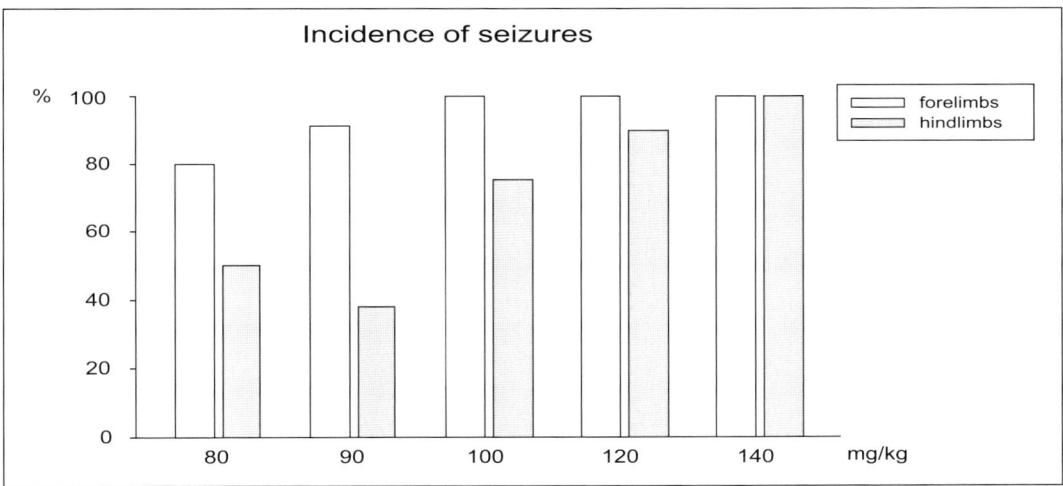

Figure 1. Incidence of generalized tonic-clonic seizures in rats with spinal cord transsection at the level of Th 11-12. White columns – seizures of forelimbs; cross-hatched columns – seizures of hindlimbs. Abscissa – doses of pentylenetetrazol; ordinate – percentage of rats exhibiting seizures.

References

1. Nadler JV. Kainic acid as a tool for the study of temporal lobe epilepsy. Life Sci 1981; 29: 2031-42.
2. Turski WA, Cavalheiro EA, Schwarz M, Czuczwar SJ, Kleinrok Z, Turski L. Limbic seizures produced by pilocarpine in rats: A behavioural, electroencephalographic and neuropathological study. Behav Bran Res 1983; 9: 315-35.
3. Kršek P, Mikulecká A, Druga R, Hliňák Z, Kubová H, Mareš P. An animal model of nonconvulsive status epilepticus: a contribution to clinical controversies. Epilepsia 2001; 42: 171-80.
4. McIntyre DC. The kindling phenomenon. In: Pitkänen A, Schwartzkroin PA, Moshé SL. Models of Seizures and Epilepsy. Amsterdam: Elsevier, 2006: 351-63.

5. Depaulis A, van Luijtelaar G. Genetic models of absence epilepsy in the rat. In: Pitkänen A, Schwartzkroin PA, Moshé SL. *Models of Seizures and Epilepsy*. Amsterdam: Elsevier, 2006: 233-48.
6. Mareš P, Velíšek L. N-Methyl-D-aspartate (NMDA)-induced seizures in developing rats. *Dev Brain Res* 1992; 65: 185-9.
7. Mareš P, Folbergrová J, Langmeier M, Haugvicová R, Kubová H. Convulsant action of D,L-homocysteic acid and its stereoisomers in immature rats. *Epilepsia* 1997; 38: 767-76.
8. Browning RA, Nelson DK. Variation of threshold and pattern of electroshock-induced seizures depending on site of stimulation. *Life Sci* 1985; 37: 2205-11.
9. Vernadakis A. Spinal cord convulsions in developing rats. *Science* 1962; 137: 532 only.

Section III:
Absence seizures and cortico-thalamic systems

Propagation and dynamic processing of cortical paroxysms in the basal ganglia networks during absence seizures

Jeanne T. Paz, Pierre-Olivier Polack, Seán J. Slaght*,
Jean-Michel Deniau, Séverine Mahon, Stéphane Charpier

Institut National de la Santé et de la Recherche Médicale U667, Collège de France, Paris. Université Pierre-et-Marie-Curie, Paris, France
* North Middlesex University Hospital, Sterling way, London, UK.

■ New emerging concepts on the physiopathology of absence seizures

Absence epilepsy is classically described as an idiopathic, non-convulsive, generalized epilepsy of multifactorial origin. Typical absence seizures consist of a sudden, mild or severe, impairment of consciousness concomitant with the abrupt occurrence of bilateral synchronous 3-Hz spike-and-wave discharges (SWDs) in the electroencephalogram (EEG) over wide cortical areas (Panayiotopoulos, 1997; Crunelli and Leresche, 2002). Electrophysiological recordings in patients (Williams, 1953) and in various animal models of absence epilepsy (Danober *et al.*, 1998; Crunelli and Leresche, 2002; Timofeev and Steriade, 2004) indicate that SWDs are the surface reflections of synchronized oscillations in thalamo-cortical networks. As described from *in vivo* intracellular recordings in GAERS (Genetic Absence Epilepsy Rats from Strasbourg), a well-established genetic model of absence epilepsy, and in the cat under ketamine-xylazine, corticothalamic neurons exhibit during SWD rhythmic suprathreshold depolarizations leading to a repetitive bursting in the inhibitory thalamic reticular neurons which, in turn, produce steady and phasic synaptic inhibitions in thalamocortical cells (Pinault *et al.*, 1998; Charpier *et al.*, 1999; Slaght *et al.*, 2002; Timofeev and Steriade, 2004). The relative contributions of neocortex and thalamus in the generation of SWDs have been the matter of intense debate among clinicians and experimental neurophysiologists and the endogenous mechanisms controlling the duration and the termination of the corticothalamic paroxysms remain to be fully characterized (see for review Timofeev and Steriade, 2004 and Meeren *et al.*, 2005).

Recent *in vivo* electrophysiological and pharmacological investigations in GAERS and WAG/Rij rats, another genetic model of absence epilepsy (Coenen and van Luijtelaar, 2003) close to GAERS, provided important new insights into the mechanisms of initiation and modulation of SWDs. Indeed, a number of converging data strongly suggest that SWDs are initiated in a restricted region of the cerebral cortex (Meeren et al., 2002; Meeren et al., 2005; Manning et al., 2004) and are dynamically controlled by the basal ganglia (BG) networks *via* their feed-back pathway to the cerebral cortex (Deransart et al., 1998, 2002; Slaght et al., 2004; Paz et al., 2005) (*Figure 1*).

The spatiotemporal properties of cortical and thalamic SWDs in WAG/Rij rats, examined by means of the advanced signal analysis method of nonlinear association analysis, clearly indicate a consistent focus within the facial region of the somatosensory cortex (Meeren et al., 2002; Meeren et al., 2005). In this new

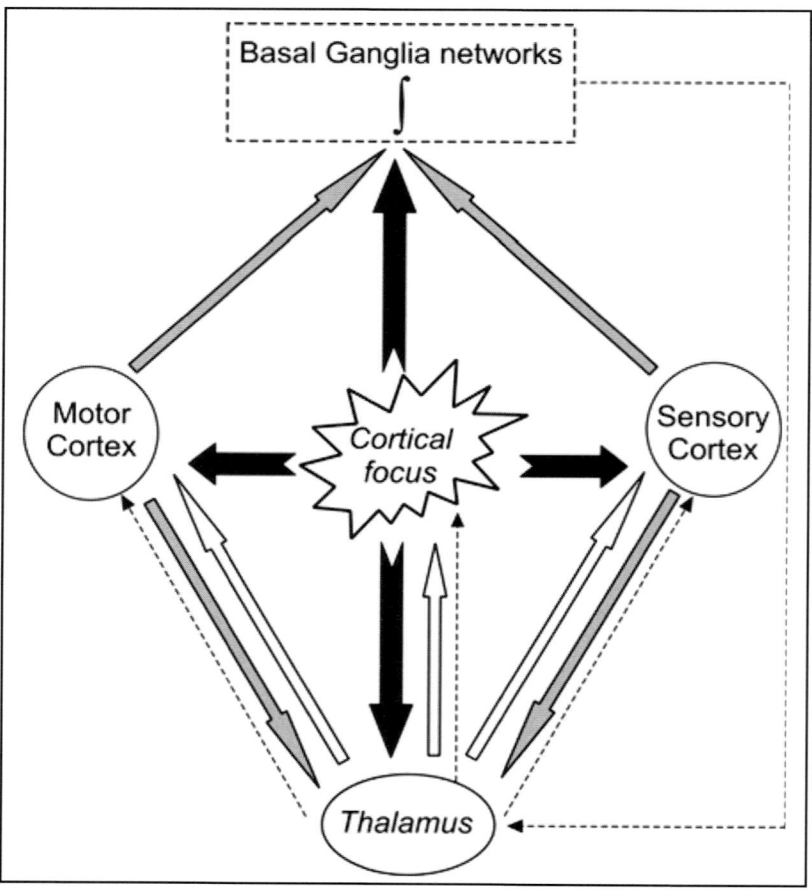

Figure 1. Generation and remote control of absence seizures: a new conceptual framework.
Seizure activity is initiated in a cortical focus and rapidly generalizes over the cortex. Cortical spike-and-wave discharges, which are promoted by synchronized oscillations in the cortico-thalamic loops, also propagate to the basal ganglia nuclei which, in turn, can modulate the cortical paroxysms *via* their thalamic projections.

conceptual scheme, paroxysmal activity is rapidly generalized from this cortical focus, then maintained and amplified through coherent oscillations within the corticothalamic loops. Consistent with this finding, local injection of ethosuximide, a first choice anti-absence drug, into the facial somatosensory cortex of GAERS specifically suppresses SWDs (Manning *et al.*, 2004). Recent EEG and intracellular investigations performed in GAERS further support the hypothesis that a cortical focus is a dominant factor in initiating the paroxysmal activities during absence seizures *(unpublished data)*. We found that EEG spikes in the motor cortex are systematically lagged behind those recorded from a limited region of the somatosensory cortex *(Figure 2A-C)* consistent with the cortical focus found in WAG/Rij rats.

The temporal delay measured between the somatosensory and motor surface paroxysms is on average of 3 ms *(Figure 2B)*, a value that can reach ~15 ms during the peak cortical synchronization *(Figure 2C)*. The apparent leading role of the somatosensory cortex neurons in the generation of generalized SWDs in GAERS is associated with an elevated cellular excitability manifested as a relatively high firing rate during interictal and seizure activities *(Figure 2D)* compared to that observed in motor cortex neurons in the same animal *(Figure 2E)*. The assumption that somatosensory cortex acts as the primary driving source of SWDs is also supported by the fact that neuronal discharges in this cortical region mostly precede those of motor cortex neurons *(Figure 2E, inset)*.

As stated above, it is very likely that a specific region of the cerebral cortex plays a leading role in the induction of generalized SWDs whereas the thalamic networks operate as a "resonant" device amplifying and sustaining the epileptic discharges (Timofeev and Steriade, 2004; Meeren *et al.*, 2005). It is also expected that cortical paroxysms can propagate, *via* active corticofugal neurons, to subcortical nuclei, which could affect through feed-back pathways the propensity of cortical networks to generate SWDs. Support for the existence of such a remote control system for absence seizures came from recent studies in GAERS suggesting that a modulation of activity in BG circuits could affect the occurrence of SWDs (Depaulis *et al.*, 1988; Depaulis *et al.*, 1989; Danober *et al.*, 1998; Deransart *et al.*, 1998, 2000, 2001; Deransart and Depaulis, 2002). In the following sections of this chapter, we will first describe the anatomo-functional organization of the BG and the pharmacological manipulations of these circuits leading to the modulation of cortical seizures in GAERS. Then, we will summarize our recent data showing how cortical paroxysms are propagated and dynamically processed, at cellular and network levels, by the BG. Finally, we will discuss the cellular and networks mechanisms by which these subcortical nuclei can positively or negatively modulate absence seizures.

■ Basal ganglia circuits: functional anatomy and control of absence seizures

The BG are connected to the cerebral cortex through multi-synaptic loop circuits. As illustrated in *Figure 3A*, the cerebral cortex provides a main source of afferents to the striatum and the subthalamic nucleus (STN), the two major input structures of

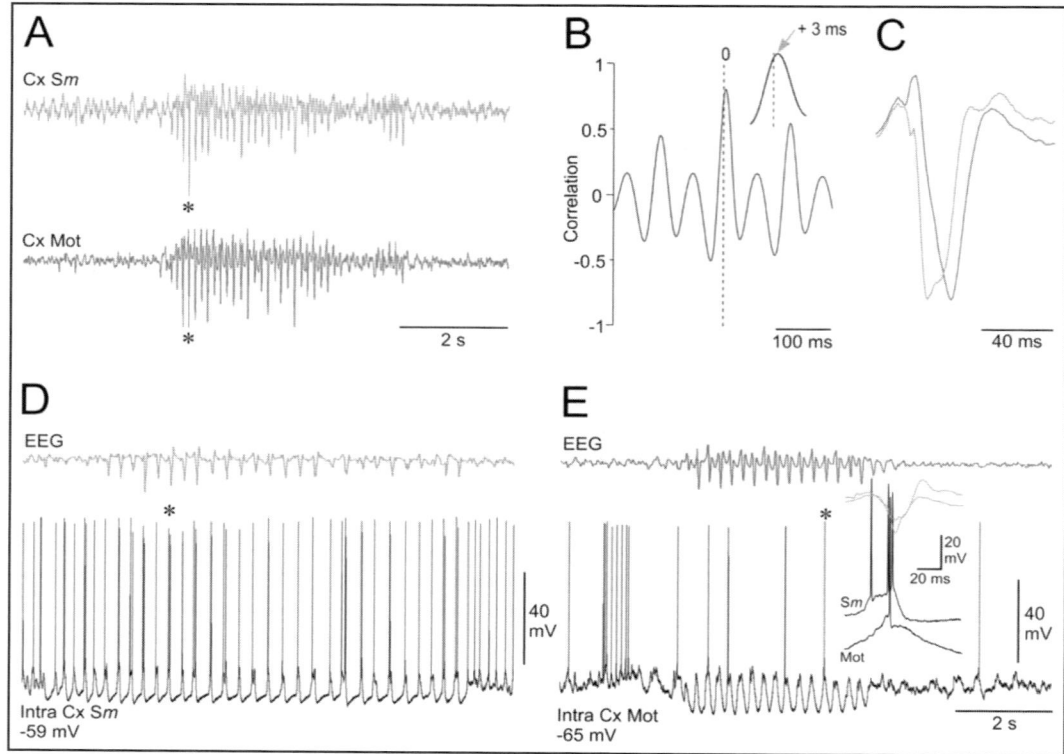

Figure 2. Increased excitability of cortical neurons located in the presumed cortical focus of GAERS. (A) Simultaneous EEG recordings from the motor (Mot) and somatosensory (Sm) cortices showing the abrupt occurrence of a SWD activity. (B) The cross-correlogram between the EEG seizure activities shown in (A) indicates a strong temporal coherence between the two oscillatory signals, with a temporal delay of about +3ms in the motor paroxysms with respect to the somatosensory activity *(Inset)*. (C) Superimposition of the EEG spikes indicated by the asterisks in (A), showing a clear-cut delay in the electrical paroxysms of the motor cortex compared to the somatosensory region. (D, E) Simultaneous recordings of the intracellular activity of somatosensory (D) and motor (E) cortical neurons (bottom traces) and of the corresponding EEGs (top traces). The occurrence of a SWD in the EEG is accompanied in both somatosensory and motor cortical neurons by rhythmic depolarizations, which are superimposed on a tonic membrane hyperpolarization. Note the high rate and the strong periodicity of firing in the somatosensory cortical neuron. The *inset* in (E) depicts the superimposition of cellular depolarizations (bottom traces) indicated by the asterisks in (D) and (E), with respect to the peak negativity of the EEG spike simultaneously recorded from the somatosensory cortex (top traces). Recordings in (D) and (E) are from the same GAERS.

the basal ganglia. In turn, the BG output nuclei, the substantia nigra pars reticulata (SNR) and the internal segment of the globus pallidus (GPi) innervate a diversity of thalamic and brain stem nuclei through which they can influence cortical electrogenesis. In rodents, specie in which the control exerted by the BG onto paroxysmal cortical discharges has been mostly documented, the thalamic projections of the BG extends throughout the entirety of the ventral medial nucleus, the lateral and ventral parts of the medial dorsal nucleus, the intralaminar nuclei: parafascicular, central medial, paracentral and restricted parts of the ventral anterior/ventral lateral complex and the lateral dorsal nucleus (Gerfen et al., 1982; Deniau and Chevalier, 1992; Deniau and Thierry, 1997; Groenewegen and Berendse, 1994; Sakai et al., 1998). Through these thalamic nuclei, the BG are in a position to influence a large portion of the frontal cortex including the prelimbic and orbital prefrontal areas, the anterior cingulate and the sensory-motor areas. In addition, the BG also innervate the intermediate and deep layers of the superior colliculus and the pedunculo-pontine nucleus from which arise major projections to the ventral medial and intralaminar thalamic nuclei (Chevalier and Deniau, 1984; Sugimoto and Hattori, 1984; Grofova and Zhou, 1998; Krout et al., 2001). Via the ascending projections of these brain stem structures, the BG might influence widespread areas of the cerebral cortex. Such a set of connections indicates that the BG are tightly related to regions of the frontal cortex playing a leading role in the induction of generalized SWDs and are in position to control the propagation of the cortical paroxysmal discharges via the BG-thalamo-cortical loop circuits.

Based on anatomical and electrophysiological observations, a conceptual model of BG and their relationships to the cerebral cortex has been proposed (Albin et al., 1989; Smith et al., 1998). In this model, cortical information is transmitted from the input to the output structures of the BG via three main pathways: a direct striato-nigral pathway (pathway 2 in Figure 3A), a direct subthalamo-nigral pathway (also defined as the hyperdirect pathway due to its fast conduction velocity; pathway 1 in Figure 3A) and an indirect striato-pallido-subthalamo-nigral pathway (pathway 3 in Figure 3A).

Because the striatal projection neurons are GABAergic and the STN neurons are glutamatergic, the trans-striatal and trans-subthalamic pathways exert opposite effects, respectively inhibitory and excitatory, on the BG output neurons. In accordance with this model, electrical stimulation of the cerebral cortex induces in BG output neurons a sequence of synaptic events consisting of an inhibition preceded or not by an early excitation and followed or not by a late excitatory event (Figure 3B). The inhibitory event results from the activation of the direct striato-nigral neurons; the early excitation results from the activation of the hyperdirect subthalamo-nigral pathway and the late excitation of the indirect pathway (Kita, 1994; Maurice et al., 1999; Kolomiets et al., 2003). In this indirect pathway the inhibition of the GABAergic pallido-subthalamic neurons by the cortically evoked striatal discharge leads to a disinhibition of the STN cells. Because the BG output neurons are tonically active and GABAergic, their inhibition by the direct striatal pathway leads to a disinhibition of the BG targets in thalamus and brain stem. Conversely, the trans-STN circuits (hyperdirect and indirect) reinforce the inhibitory influence that BG exerts on their targets. Interestingly, a pharmacological manipulation of synaptic transmission at different levels of these circuits modulates the occurrence of absence seizures, stressing the role of the BG as a remote system control of seizure induction and/or propagation (Deransart and Depaulis, 2002). Briefly, decreasing the activity of SNR cells by a local injection of GABA, by activating the direct striato-nigral pathway or by reducing the activity of the STN decreases the occurrence of seizures. Conversely, increasing the discharge of SNR cells by stimulating the glutamatergic subthalamo-nigral pathway favours the occurrence of seizures.

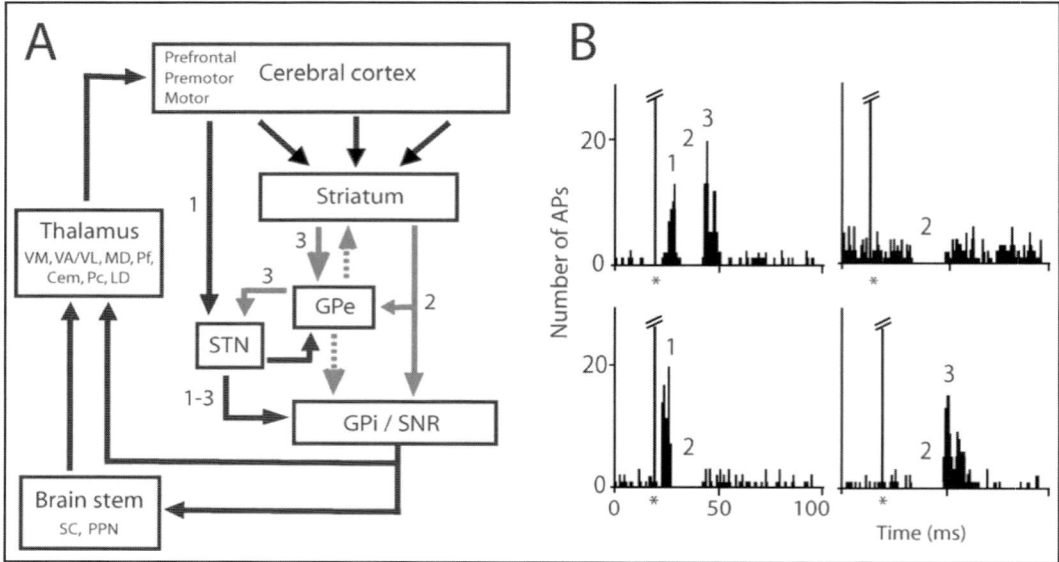

Figure 3. Functional organization of circuits connecting the basal ganglia and the cerebral cortex. (A) Schematic representation of fibre connections of the basal ganglia nuclei with the cerebral cortex. For clarity, the thalamic connections to the striatum and the STN have been omitted. Glutamatergic excitatory pathways are indicated in black and the GABAergic inhibitory pathways in grey. Abbreviations: Cem, centralis medialis thalamic nucleus; GPe, external segment of the globus pallidus; GPi, internal segment of the globus pallidus; LD, lateral dorsal thalamic nucleus; MD, medial dorsal thalamic nucleus; Pc, paracentral thalamic nucleus; Pf, parafascicular thalamic nucleus; PPN, pedunculo pontine nucleus; SC, superior colliculus; SNR, substantia nigra pars reticulata; STN, subthalamic nucleus; VA/VL, ventral anterior/ventral lateral thalamic nuclear complex; VM, ventral medial thalamic nucleus. (B) Peristimulus time histograms illustrating typical electrophysiological effects induced in the substantia nigra pars reticulata by stimulation of the motor cortex. Numbers refer to the pathway implicated (see A). Stars below the histograms indicate the time of stimulation. APs, action potentials.

Although the three pathways model of the BG provided important conceptual advance, it is unlikely to disclose the functional role of BG in the pathophysiology of seizures. Indeed, a seizure is characterized by the development of synchronized oscillations in the cortical network. The way cortical oscillatory activities are transmitted in the BG network depends on dynamic properties that cannot be approached by a simple hierarchical network model in which a steady state change of activity at a given level of the BG is readily transmitted positively or negatively to the next level in a simple cascade of events (Bar Gad and Bergman, 2001). The dynamic properties of the BG network result from complex interactions between the specific membrane properties of the neurons in each of the BG nuclei, the local intranuclear neuronal interactions and the mutual synaptic interactions between the BG nuclei that are highly interconnected. Finally, the impact of the cortically-driven oscillatory behaviour of the BG on the thalamo-cortical oscillators might favour or interfere with the propagation of the SWD in the thalamo-cortical circuits, depending on the relative phase and frequency of discharges in the BG output neurons and thalamus.

Corticostriatal neurons *vs* corticosubthalamic neurons: an unfair contest

As mentioned above, excitatory cortical information propagate to BG *via* two distinct corticofugal pathways, the corticostriatal (CStr) neurons, mainly projecting to the striatal GABAergic output neurons (Kincaid et al., 1998) and interneurons (Ramanathan et al., 2002), and the corticosubthalamic (CSth) neurons exciting the glutamatergic projection neurons of STN (Maurice et al., 1998; Bevan et al., 2002). By performing *in vivo* intracellular recordings of GAERS CStr and CSth neurons located in the motor cortex, we determined how epileptic activities propagate from the cortex to the striatum and the STN (Slaght et al., 2004; Paz et al., 2005; Paz et al., 2005). The comparison of electrophysiological properties of both types of cortical output neurons indicates a dramatic imbalance between the two pathways, including a relatively high axonal conduction velocity, intrinsic excitability and synaptic activity in CSth neurons compared to that observed in CStr neurons.

Corticostriatal *(Figure 4A1)* and CSth neurons *(Figure 4B1)* can be identified by their antidromic activation following electrical stimulation of their respective targets. The measured antidromic latencies in CStr (3-9 ms) and CSth (1-3 ms) neurons indicate a higher axonal conduction velocity in CSth neurons (~ 7 m.s^{-1} *vs* $\sim .5$ m.s^{-1} in CStr axons) (Kitai and Deniau, 1981; Mahon et al., 2001; Slaght et al., 2004; Paz et al., 2005) and thus suggest a faster propagation of cortical epileptic discharges to the STN. Although the mean interictal membrane potentials measured in CStr and CSth neurons are remarkably similar ($\sim$-61 mV in both neuronal types), their membrane excitabilities noticeably differ as attested to by the voltage changes induced in both cell populations in response to intracellular injection of square current pulses of the same intensity *(Figure 4A2, B2)*. In CStr neurons, the firing pattern evoked by intracellular injection of +1 nA-current pulse is characteristic of "regular-spiking" neocortical neurons (Connors and Gutnick, 1990; Steriade, 2004) with a mean rate of discharge of 20 Hz *(Figure 4A2)*. In contrast, CSth neurons can exhibit, in response to the same current pulse *(Figure 4B2)*, the firing mode of either "regular spiking" or "intrinsic bursting" neocortical neurons (Connors and Gutnick, 1990; Steriade, 2004) and reach a maximal firing rate of 100 Hz (Paz et al., 2005). Moreover, in most CSth neurons (Paz et al., 2005), large-amplitude hyperpolarizing current pulses induce a depolarizing sag of membrane potential *(Figure 4C, top, red record)* likely due to a hyperpolarization-activated inward cationic current (I_h) (Gutnick and Crill, 1995), and a post-inhibitory rebound of depolarization *(Figure 4C, bottom, red record)* possibly provoked by the slow kinetics of I_h and/or by a low voltage-activated Ca^{2+} current (I_T) (Gutnick and Crill, 1995). Such active membrane properties, promoting rebound depolarizations and repetitive discharge, could not be revealed in the recorded CStr neurons *(Figure 4C, black records)* (Slaght et al., 2004).

Corticostriatal (*Figure 4D*) and CSth (*Figure 4E*) neurons exhibit during SWD rhythmic depolarizations, in phase with the EEG spikes, superimposed on a tonic hyperpolarization lasting for the entire surface paroxysm (Slaght et al., 2004; Paz et al., 2005). In both types of neurons, the sustained membrane hyperpolarization probably results from a process of disfacilitation, leading to a passive return to the resting membrane potential due to a transient interruption in the tonic excitatory synaptic drive (Charpier et al., 1999). It is also very likely that the cortical membrane oscillations associated with seizure activity mainly reflect rhythmic synaptic potentials since their amplitude is increased during membrane hyperpolarization whereas their frequency is not altered by DC-induced changes in membrane potential (Charpier et al., 1999; Slaght et al., 2004; Paz et al., 2005). It is possible that these synaptic potentials represent a mixture of glutamatergic and GABAergic events since the membrane potential reached during the hyperpolarizing envelope is close or below the equilibrium potential of chloride in cortical neurons (Gulledge and Stuart, 2003). The firing rate of CSth neurons, during spontaneous interictal activity and SWD, is significantly elevated compared to that observed in CStr cells in the same conditions (*Figure 4F*) (Slaght et al., 2004; Paz et al., 2005). This imbalance in the output activity of CSth and CStr neurons might result, at least in part, from the relatively high membrane excitability in CSth cells (see above) and/or from exacerbated excitatory synaptic events in this cell population.

The measurement of the timing of individual action potentials in CStr and CSth neurons, relative to the peak negativity of the corresponding spike component in the EEG (*Figure 4G*, inset), allows a quantitative assessment of temporal relationships between the firing of these two cell populations. Whereas the latencies of discharge in CSth neurons exhibit a broad bimodal distribution, with two principal values at −38 ms and −10 ms (*Figure 4G*, red curve), CStr action potentials show a single narrow distribution centred around −20 ms (*Figure 4G*, black curve).

The experimental findings reviewed here demonstrate that cortical paroxysms associated with absence seizures are effectively propagated to basal ganglia. They also reveal an important functional imbalance between CStr and CSth neurons during SWD, with epileptic activities propagating earlier, faster and with a higher rate of neuronal firing in the corticosubthalamic pathway.

Figure 4. Differential membrane excitability and firing pattern of GAERS corticostriatal and corticosubthalamic neurons. (A1, B1) Corticostriatal (CStr, A1) and corticosubthalamic (CSth, B1) neurons were identified by their antidromic activation after electrical stimulation of the contralateral striatum (Stim. Str) and the ipsilateral STN (Stim. STN), respectively. As shown by the superimposed traces in (A1), the activation of the CStr neuron, using a threshold stimulus, was obtained in the absence of any underlying synaptic potential. The superimposed records in (B1) show a collision of an antidromic spike with a spontaneous orthodromic action potential (asterisk). (A2, B2) Voltage responses (top traces) of CStr (A2) and CSth (B2) neurons to intracellular injection of negative and positive square current pulses (bottom traces). Note the elevated current-induced firing rate in the CSth neuron compared to that evoked in the CStr cell by the same current pulse. (C) Enlargement, from the records shown in A2 and B2, of the CStr and CSth neurons responses at the onset (top traces) and

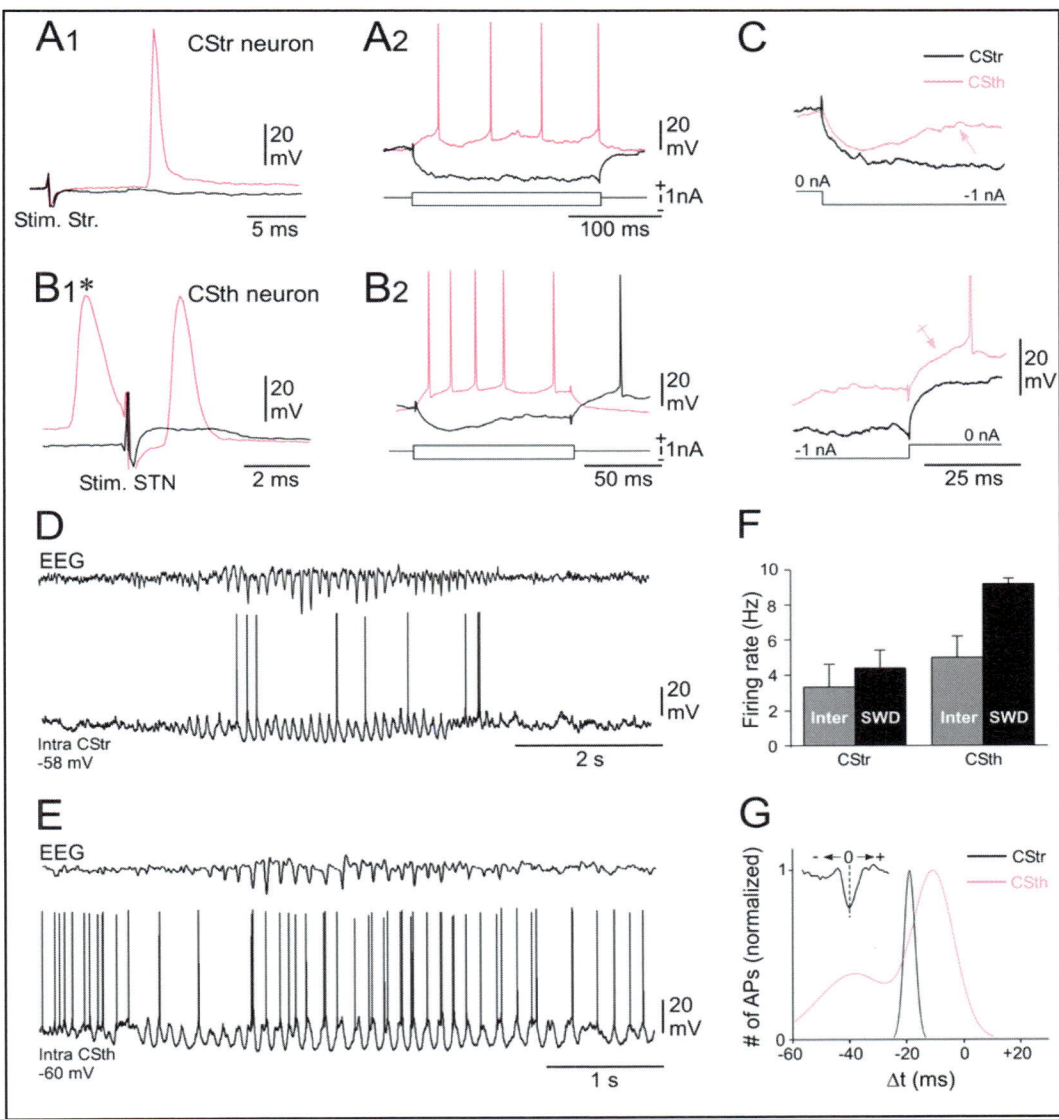

the termination (bottom traces) of the square negative current pulse. Note the presence in the CSth neuron, and the lack in the CStr neuron, of a hyperpolarization-activated membrane depolarization (arrow) and of a post-anodal break depolarization (crossed arrow). The action potential is truncated. (D, E) Simultaneous recordings of the intracellular activity of CStr (D) and CSth (E) neurons (bottom traces) and of the corresponding EEG (top traces) during seizure activity. (F) Pooled histogram (n > 4 cells) showing the increase in the firing rate of both types of cortical neurons during SWD compared to the interictal activity (Inter). (G) Superimposition of the firing probability densities of CStr and CSth neurons during SWD. The timing of action potentials in both neuronal populations is measured with respect to the peak negativity of the corresponding EEG waves, which is used as the zero time reference *(Inset)*. (A1), (D) and (F) are modified from Slaght et al., 2004. (B1,2), (E) and (G) are modified from Paz et al., 2005.

▪ Striatal output neurons are knocked-down during absence seizures

A large number of converging corticostriatal inputs impinge on GABAergic striatal output neurons (Kincaid *et al.*, 1998; Zheng and Wilson, 2002). Thus, it was expected that the synchronized rhythmic discharges in CStr neurons during SWDs (see above) produce a powerful ongoing excitation leading to repetitive firing in striatal output neurons (Mahon *et al.*, 2001). Surprisingly, we found that these neurons are silenced during seizures. This collapse in the output activity of striatal neurons is not due to an alteration in their membrane excitability but rather results from a feed-forward synaptic inhibition originating from the powerful activation of GABAergic striatal interneurons (Slaght *et al.*, 2004: Paz *et al.*, 2005).

The intrinsic excitability of striatal output neurons in epileptic rats is not altered as compared to that of non-epileptic animals (Slaght *et al.*, 2004). As exemplified by the striatonigral cell shown in *Figure 5A*, the striatal output neurons, recorded in GAERS, exhibit their classical electrical membrane properties (Wilson, 1995; Mahon *et al.*, 2001, 2003, 2004), including a highly polarized resting membrane potential (~-80 mV), a relatively low apparent input resistance and the distinctive slow ramp-like membrane depolarization in response to a suprathreshold current pulse *(Figure 5B)*.

Both extra- and intracellular recordings *(Figure 5C)* reveal that action potential discharge in striatal output neurons, which occurs irregularly and with a low frequency during interictal periods, is transiently interrupted during SWDs (Slaght *et al.*, 2004). This lack of firing is associated with a tonic hyperpolarization and subthreshold rhythmic synaptic depolarizations are superimposed on it *(Figure 5C)*. In most striatal output neurons, a rebound of synaptic depolarization, which can generate spike discharge, is observed at the end of the SWD *(Figure 5C, inset)*. The inability of seizure-associated striatal synaptic depolarizations to reach action potential threshold is due to an increase in membrane conductance. This is evidenced by the decrease in current-evoked firing, and the concomitant reduction of the underlying membrane depolarization, during the SWD-associated membrane depolarizations *(Figure 5D)*. The fact that striatal subthreshold oscillations are converted into large-amplitude suprathreshold rhythmic depolarizations after intracellular injection of chloride *(Figure 5E)*, demonstrates the presence of a powerful chloride-dependent conductance and strongly suggests that the shunting inhibition observed during SWD results from $GABA_A$-mediated synaptic activity. This hypothesis is corroborated by the rhythmic bursting, during SWDs, of GABAergic striatal interneurons *(Figure 5F)*, which are known to produce a robust chloride-dependent inhibition able to block the generation of action potentials in striatal output neurons (Plenz and Kitai, 1998; Koos and Tepper, 1999).

The experimental results described above, showing that cortical excitation of striatal output neurons during epileptic discharges is dampened by the activation of striatal inhibitory interneurons, suggest that the propagation of cortical paroxysms through the corticostriatal pathway during absence seizures transiently decreases the striatal-mediated synaptic inhibition of basal ganglia output nuclei.

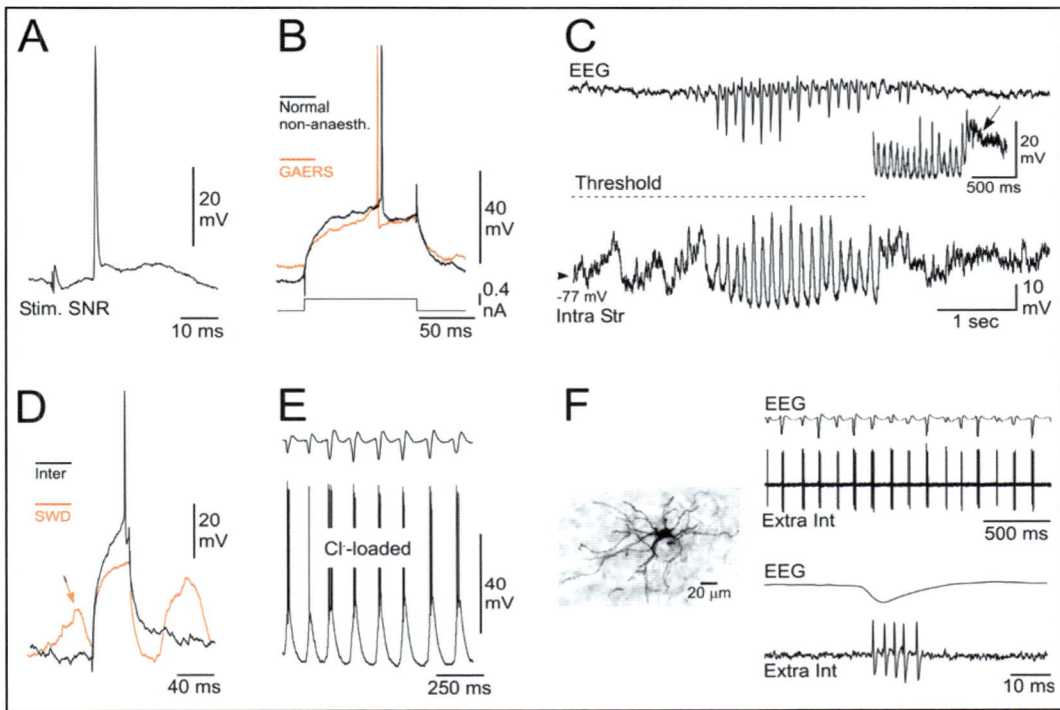

Figure 5. Striatal output neurons are silenced during absence seizure. (A) Antidromic activation of a striatal output neuron by electrical stimulation of the SNR (Stim. SNR), identifying the recorded cell as a striatonigral neuron. (B) Superimposition of current-induced responses in GAERS (red trace) and normal, anaesthetic-free, rat (black trace) striatal output neurons. Note that the cellular excitability, including the characteristic slow ramp depolarization preceding action potential firing, is not modified in the epileptic animal. (C) The occurrence of a SWD in the EEG (top trace) is accompanied, in the recorded striatal output neuron (bottom trace), by rhythmic membrane depolarizations that remain subthreshold for action potential firing (dashed line). The mean membrane potential during interictal periods is indicated. As depicted in the inset, the end of ictal activity can be succeeded by a rebound of membrane depolarization (oblique arrow). (D) The injection of a depolarizing current pulse elicits in the striatal cell an action potential during the interictal epoch (Inter) whereas it remains subthreshold when coincident with a large membrane depolarization (arrow) occurring during the SWD. (E) In contrast with the recordings obtained with KAc electrodes (C), striatal output neurons recorded with KCl electrodes (bottom trace) exhibit rhythmic depolarizing potentials that generate bursts of action potentials, indicating the presence during the seizure activity of a powerful chloride-dependent conductance. (F) Microphotograph of a GABAergic striatal interneuron labeled by juxtacellular injection of neurobiotin. (Top) This cell displays during the cortical seizure recurrent bursts of action potentials. (Bottom) The expanded record clearly shows that the burst of action potential is concomitant with the spike-component in the EEG. (D), (E) and (F) are modified from Slaght *et al.*, 2004.

■ Subthalamonigral neurons as the victorious pathway

Corticosubthalamic neurons display during cortical seizures rhythmic bursts of action potentials (see above). These cortical paroxysms are reflected in the STN by synchronized, rhythmic, high-frequency bursts of action potentials (Paz *et al.*, 2005; Paz *et al.*, in press). Intra-burst pattern in STN neurons is composed by an early, cortically-generated, depolarizing synaptic potential, followed by a short hyperpolarization, originating from rhythmic bursting in pallidosubthalamic neurons, and a rebound of depolarization due to a mixture of intrinsic and synaptic mechanisms.

Intracelluar recordings in GAERS show that STN neurons projecting to SNR *(Figure 6A)* exhibit passive and active membrane properties similar to those described *in vitro* from non-epileptic rats (Beurrier *et al.*, 1999; Bevan and Wilson, 1999; Bevan *et al.*, 2002), indicating a "normal" intrinsic excitability of STN neurons in the epileptic animal (Paz *et al.*, 2005). Unlike the striatal output neurons, the firing rate of STN neurons doubles during SWDs (Paz *et al.*, 2005), with a firing profile switching from an irregular interictal pattern to high-frequency bursts of action potentials during cortical paroxysms *(Figure 6B)*. The initial discharge of STN neurons during bursting activity *(Figure 6C)* is generated by a short depolarizing potential likely due to the early discharge of CSth neurons (see *Figure 4E, G*). The brief inhibition within the STN burst reflects a transient (~17 ms) synaptic hyperpolarization that reversed in polarity at a membrane potential (~-73 mV; *Figure 6D*) consistent with the chloride equilibrium potential of $GABA_A$ current in STN neurons (Bevan *et al.*, 2000). Given the temporal coherence between the STN inhibition and the bursting firing of GABAergic pallidal neurons *(Figure 6E)*, it is very likely that the chloride-dependent hyperpolarizing potentials in STN during seizures result from propagated activities in the subthalamo-pallido-subthalamic loop (Paz *et al.*, 2005). The post-inhibitory rebound of firing in STN neurons may result from synergistic interactions between active membrane properties and excitatory synaptic inputs. Indeed, STN neurons possess low-threshold calcium channels responsible, at least in part, for the generation of burst activity following membrane hyperpolarization (Bevan *et al.*, 2000). In addition, the sustained firing of CSth neurons during SWD *(Figure 4E, G)* would provide an additional excitatory synaptic mechanism amplifying the post-inhibitory rebound of excitation in STN neurons.

These findings showing that absence seizures are accompanied by repetitive discharges in STN neurons, which reflect complex interactions between intrinsic properties and mixed synaptic inputs, suggest that the propagation of cortical paroxysms in the basal ganglia might convey powerful excitation to SNR *via* the STN.

■ Conclusions and future challenges

Our recent findings obtained from *in vivo* electrophysiological recordings in GAERS, a well-established genetic model of absence epilepsy, demonstrate a severe functional imbalance between the cortico-striato-nigral and cortico-subthalamo-nigral pathways during SWDs *(Figure 7)*. The propagation of powerful epileptic discharges in the corticosubthalamic pathway leads to a sustained bursting activity in glutamatergic subthalamonigral neurons whereas the seizure activity in corticostriatal neurons produces a feed-forward inhibition of GABAergic striatonigral neurons. This might result in a change in the balance between the ongoing synaptic excitation and inhibition to the SNR. The sudden reinforcement of the synaptic excitation originating from the STN would promote repetitive firing in SNR cells. Such a hypothesis, combining

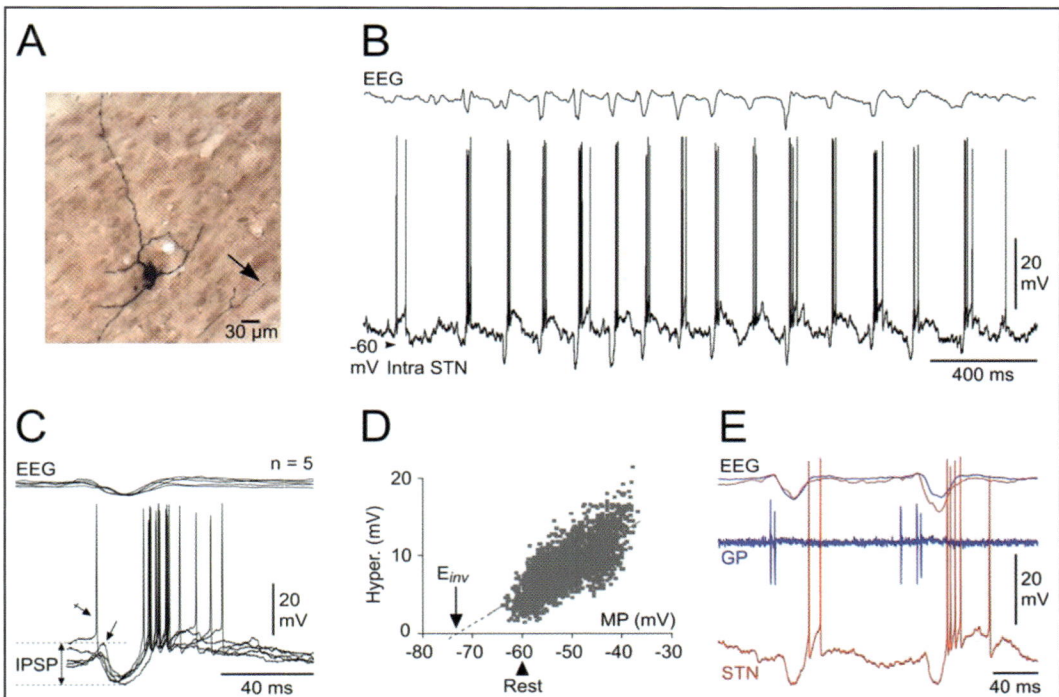

Figure 6. **Rhythmic bursting in the subthalamo-pallidal network during absence seizure.** (A) Microphotograph of a GAERS STN neuron intracellularly injected with neurobiotin. The arrow indicates the posterior axonal collateral projecting to the SNR. (B) Intracellular recording of a STN neuron (bottom trace) during a cortical SWD (top trace) showing rhythmic burst firing concomitant with the EEG spike. (C) DC superimposition (n = 5) of the STN intracellular activities (bottom traces) and the corresponding spike-wave complexes (top traces). The peak of the EEG spike was used to align the intracellular and the EEG records. An early depolarization (arrow), which could generate an action potential (crossed arrow), was followed rapidly by a transient IPSP and then a rebound excitation. (D) Amplitude of IPSPs (measured as indicated in (C) by the double arrow) as a function of the membrane potential (MP). The extrapolated reversal potential (E_{inv} = –73 mV) is consistent with a chloride-dependent mechanism. (E) Examples of two successive EEG spike-wave complexes (top traces) and the corresponding intracellular activity of a STN neuron (red trace) and extracellular firing of a GABAergic pallidal neuron (blue trace), indicating the coherent timing between the STN IPSPs and the bursting activity in pallidal neurons. Results depicted in panels (A-D) are modified from Paz *et al.*, 2005.

permissive (interruption of inhibitory inputs) and active processes (exacerbation of excitatory inputs), is supported by recent experiments performed in freely moving GAERS demonstrating a synchronized bursting in SNR neurons concomitant with SWDs (Deransart et al., 2003).

The possibility that a modulation in the activity of the SNR could control absence seizures has emerged from pharmacological studies in GAERS showing that intranigral injections of $GABA_A$ agonists or NMDA antagonists in the SNR have antiepileptic effects (Depaulis et al., 1988; Depaulis et al., 1989; Deransart et al., 1996; Deransart et al., 1998; Deransart et al., 2001) whereas aggravation of absence seizures is induced by application of GABA$_A$ antagonist in the SNR (Deransart et al., 1998). Thus, the repetitive discharge of SNR neurons, resulting from synchronized bursting in subthalamonigral neurons during SWDs, could prolong seizures *via* recurrent inhibition of thalamocortical neurons. Such a positive control process, responsible for an aggravation of the abnormal thalamocortical oscillations, could occur through a resonance phenomenon when the nigral-induced thalamic rhythmicity is in-phase with SWDs. In contrast, the recovery of the desynchronized firing in STN neurons at the end of the SWD, together with the rebound of excitation in striatal projection neurons (Slaght et al., 2004), could initiate the post-ictal decrease in the activity of nigrothalamic neurons (Deransart et al., 2003) and, so participate in the termination of the seizure.

These attractive, but putative, mechanisms of remote control of absence seizures by the BG have to be validated by further experiments. In particular, it will be crucial to determine the functional impact of the SNR activity in the thalamocortical loops and its causal implication in the propensity of cerebral cortex, at the level of cortical focus as well as in other cortical regions, to generate and propagate electrical paroxysms *(Figure 7)*.

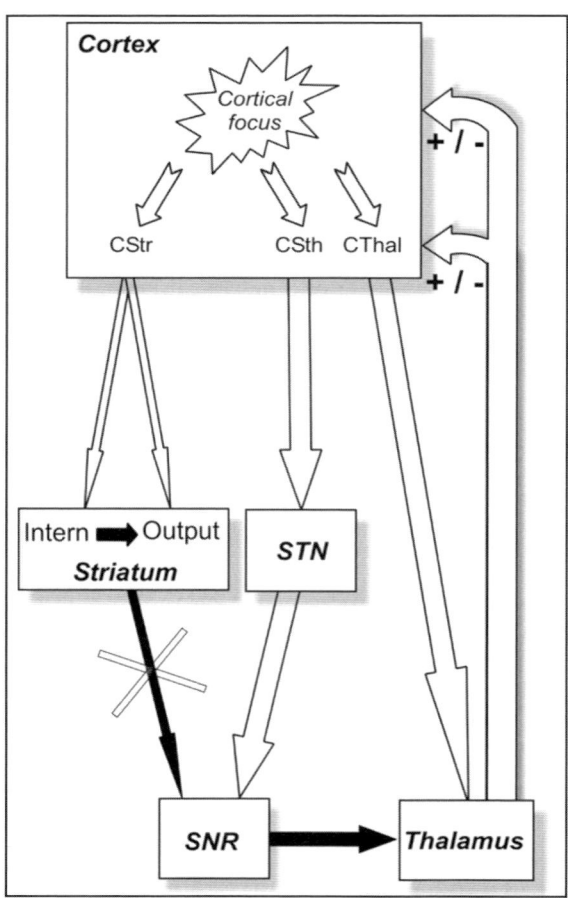

Figure 7. Propagation of epileptic discharges in basal ganglia networks and possible scenario for the control of absence seizures. Following our current hypothesis, seizure activity is initiated in a cortical focus then rapidly propagates to corticostriatal (CStr), corticosubthalamic (CSth) and corticothalamic (CThal) neurons. Cortical paroxysms spread to the striatum and excite the GABAergic interneurons (Intern) which, in turn, preclude the generation of action potential (white cross) in striatal output neurons (Output). In parallel, the propagation of bursting discharges in CSth neurons induces repetitive firing in the substantia nigra pars reticulata (SNR). The modulation of the thalamic activity by nigrothalamic neurons could, as a function of the imposed phase relationships between cortical and thalamic oscillations (see text for details), attenuate (-) or aggravate (+) the electrical paroxysms in the cortical focus and/or in other cortical regions.

Acknowledgements: This work was supported by the Ministère Français de la Recherche and l'Institut National de la Santé et de la Recherche Médicale. We thank A. Menetrey for assistance with the histological processing.

References

Albin RL, Young AB, Penney JB. The functional anatomy of basal ganglia disorders. *Trends Neurosci* 1989; 12 (10): 366-75.

Bar-Gad I, Bergman H. Stepping out of the box: information processing in the neural networks of the basal ganglia. *Curr Opin Neurobiol* 2001; 11 (6): 689-95.

Beurrier C, Congar P, Bioulac B, Hammond C. Subthalamic nucleus neurons switch from single-spike activity to burst-firing mode. *J Neurosci* 1999; 19 (2): 599-609.

Bevan MD, Magill PJ, Terman D, Bolam JP, Wilson CJ. Move to the rhythm: oscillations in the subthalamic nucleus-external globus pallidus network. *Trends Neurosci* 2002; 25 (10): 525-31.

Bevan MD, Wilson CJ. Mechanisms underlying spontaneous oscillation and rhythmic firing in rat subthalamic neurons. *J Neurosci* 1999; 19 (17): 7617-28.

Bevan MD, Wilson CJ, Bolam JP, Magill PJ. Equilibrium potential of GABA(A) current and implications for rebound burst firing in rat subthalamic neurons *in vitro*. *J Neurophysiol* 2000; 83 (5): 3169-72.

Charpier S, Leresche N, Deniau JM, Mahon S, Hughes SW, Crunelli V. On the putative contribution of GABA(B) receptors to the electrical events occurring during spontaneous spike and wave discharges. *Neuropharmacology* 1999; 38 (11): 1699-706.

Chevalier G, Deniau JM. Spatio-temporal organization of a branched tecto-spinal/tecto-diencephalic neuronal system. *Neuroscience* 1984; 12 (2): 427-39.

Coenen AM, van Luijtelaar EL. Genetic animal models for absence epilepsy: a review of the WAG/Rij strain of rats. *Behav Genet* 2003; 33 (6): 635-55.

Connors BW, Gutnick MJ. Intrinsic firing patterns of diverse neocortical neurons. *Trends Neurosci* 1990; 13 (3): 99-104.

Crunelli V, Leresche N. Childhood absence epilepsy: genes, channels, neurons and networks. *Nat Rev Neurosci* 2002; 3 (5): 371-82.

Danober L, Deransart C, Depaulis A, Vergnes M, Marescaux C. Pathophysiological mechanisms of genetic absence epilepsy in the rat. *Prog Neurobiol* 1998; 55 (1): 27-57.

Deniau JM, Chevalier G. The lamellar organization of the rat substantia nigra pars reticulata: distribution of projection neurons. *Neuroscience* 1992; 46 (2): 361-77.

Deniau JM, Thierry AM. Anatomical segregation of information processing in the rat substantia nigra pars reticulata. *Adv Neurol* 1997; 74: 83-96.

Depaulis A, Snead OC, 3rd, Marescaux C, Vergnes M. Suppressive effects of intranigral injection of muscimol in three models of generalized non-convulsive epilepsy induced by chemical agents. *Brain Res* 1989; 498 (1): 64-72.

Depaulis A, Vergnes M, Marescaux C, Lannes B, Warter JM. Evidence that activation of GABA receptors in the substantia nigra suppresses spontaneous spike-and-wave discharges in the rat. *Brain Res* 1988; 448 (1): 20-9.

Deransart C, Depaulis A. The control of seizures by the basal ganglia? A review of experimental data. *Epileptic Disord* 2002; 4 (Suppl 3): S61-72.

Deransart C, Hellwig B, Heupel-Reuter M, Leger JF, Heck D, Lucking, CH. Single-unit analysis of substantia nigra pars reticulata neurons in freely behaving rats with genetic absence epilepsy. *Epilepsia* 2003; 44 (12): 1513-20.

Deransart C, Le-Pham BT, Hirsch E, Marescaux C, Depaulis A. Inhibition of the substantia nigra suppresses absences and clonic seizures in audiogenic rats, but not tonic seizures: evidence for seizure specificity of the nigral control. *Neuroscience* 2001; 105 (1): 203-11.

Deransart C, Riban V, Le B, Marescaux C, Depaulis A. Dopamine in the striatum modulates seizures in a genetic model of absence epilepsy in the rat. *Neuroscience* 2000; 100 (2): 335-44.

Deransart C, Vercueil L, Marescaux C, Depaulis A. The role of basal ganglia in the control of generalized absence seizures. *Epilepsy Res* 1998; 32 (1-2): 213-23.

Gerfen CR, Staines WA, Arbuthnott GW, Fibiger HC. Crossed connections of the substantia nigra in the rat. *J Comp Neurol* 1982; 207 (3): 283-303.

Groenewegen HJ, Berendse HW. Anatomical relationships between the prefrontal cortex and the basal ganglia in the rat. In: Thierry AM, Glowinski J, Goldman-Rakic PS, Christen Y, eds. *Motor and cognitive functions of the prefrontal cortex*. Berlin: Springer, 1994; 51-77.

Grofova I, Zhou M. Nigral innervation of cholinergic and glutamatergic cells in the rat mesopontine tegmentum: light and electron microscopic anterograde tracing and immunohistochemical studies. *J Comp Neurol* 1998; 395 (3): 359-79.

Gulledge AT, Stuart GJ. Excitatory actions of GABA in the cortex. *Neuron* 2003; 37 (2): 299-309.

Gutnick MJ, Crill WE. The cortical neuron as an electrophysiological unit. In: Gutnick MJ, Mody I, eds, *The cortical neuron*. Oxford: Oxford University Press; 1995; 33-52.

Kincaid AE, Zheng T, Wilson CJ. Connectivity and convergence of single corticostriatal axons. *J Neurosci* 1998; 18 (12): 4722-31.

Kita H. Physiology of two disynaptic pathways from the sensorimotor cortex to the basal ganglia output nuclei. In: Percheron G, McKenzie JS, Feger J, eds. *The basal ganglia IV*. New York: Plenum, 1994; 263-76.

Kitai ST, Deniau JM. Cortical inputs to the subthalamus: intracellular analysis. *Brain Res* 1981; 214: 411-5.

Kolomiets BP, Deniau JM, Glowinski J, Thierry AM. Basal ganglia and processing of cortical information: functional interactions between trans-striatal and trans-subthalamic circuits in the substantia nigra pars reticulata. *Neuroscience* 2003; 117 (4): 931-8.

Koos T, Tepper JM. Inhibitory control of neostriatal projection neurons by GABAergic interneurons. *Nat Neurosci* 1999; 2 (5): 467-72.

Krout KE, Loewy AD, Westby GW, Redgrave P. Superior colliculus projections to midline and intralaminar thalamic nuclei of the rat. *J Comp Neurol* 2001; 431 (2): 198-216.

Mahon S, Deniau JM, Charpier S. Relationship between EEG potentials and intracellular activity of striatal and cortico-striatal neurons: an *in vivo* study under different anesthetics. *Cereb Cortex* 2001; 11 (4): 360-73.

Mahon S, Deniau JM, Charpier S. Corticostriatal plasticity: life after the depression. *Trends Neurosci* 2004; 27 (8): 460-7.

Mahon S, Casassus G, Mulle C, Charpier S. Spike-dependent intrinsic plasticity increases firing probability in rat striatal neurons *in vivo*. *J Physiol* 2003; 550 (Pt 3): 947-59.

Manning JP, Richards DA, Leresche N, Crunelli V, Bowery NG. Cortical-area specific block of genetically determined absence seizures by ethosuximide. *Neuroscience* 2004; 123 (1): 5-9.

Maurice N, Deniau JM, Glowinski J, Thierry AM. Relationships between the prefrontal cortex and the basal ganglia in the rat: physiology of the cortico-nigral circuits. *J Neurosci* 1999; 19 (11): 4674-81.

Maurice N, Deniau JM, Menetrey A, Glowinski J, Thierry AM. Prefrontal cortex-basal ganglia circuits in the rat: involvement of ventral pallidum and subthalamic nucleus. *Synapse* 1998; 29 (4): 363-70.

Meeren H, van Luijtelaar G, Lopes da Silva F, Coenen A. Evolving concepts on the pathophysiology of absence seizures: the cortical focus theory. *Arch Neurol* 2005; 62 (3): 371-6.

Meeren HK, Pijn JP, van Luijtelaar EL, Coenen AM, Lopes da Silva FH. Cortical focus drives widespread corticothalamic networks during spontaneous absence seizures in rats. *J Neurosci* 2002; 22 (4): 1480-95.

Panayiotopoulos CP. Absence epilepsies. In: Engel J, Pedley TA, eds, *Epilepsy: a comprehensive textbook*. Philadelphia: Lippincot-Raven, 1997: 2327-46.

Paz JT, Deniau JM, Charpier S. Rhythmic bursting in the cortico-subthalamo-pallidal network during spontaneous genetically determined spike and wave discharges. *J Neurosci* 2005; 25 (8): 2092-101.

Paz JT, Polack PO, Slaght SJ, Deniau JM, Charpier S. Propagation of cortical paroxysms in basal ganglia circuits during absence seizure. In: Bolam P, Magill P, eds. *IBAGS VIII*, 2005: 55-63.

Pinault D, Leresche N, Charpier S, Deniau JM, Marescaux C, Vergnes M, et al. Intracellular recordings in thalamic neurones during spontaneous spike and wave discharges in rats with absence epilepsy. *J Physiol* 1998; 509 (Pt 2): 449-56.

Plenz D, Kitai ST. Up and down states in striatal medium spiny neurons simultaneously recorded with spontaneous activity in fast-spiking interneurons studied in cortex-striatum-substantia nigra organotypic cultures. *J Neurosci* 1998; 18 (1): 266-83.

Ramanathan S, Hanley JJ, Deniau JM, Bolam JP. Synaptic convergence of motor and somatosensory cortical afferents onto GABAergic interneurons in the rat striatum. *J Neurosci* 2002; 22 (18): 8158-69.

Sakai ST, Grofova I, Bruce K. Nigrothalamic projections and nigrothalamocortical pathway to the medial agranular cortex in the rat: single- and double-labeling light and electron microscopic studies. *J Comp Neurol* 1998; 391 (4): 506-25.

Slaght SJ, Leresche N, Deniau JM, Crunelli V, Charpier S. Activity of thalamic reticular neurons during spontaneous genetically determined spike and wave discharges. *J Neurosci* 2002; 22 (6): 2323-34.

Slaght SJ, Paz T, Chavez M, Deniau JM, Mahon S, Charpier S. On the activity of the corticostriatal networks during spike-and-wave discharges in a genetic model of absence epilepsy. *J Neurosci* 2004; 24 (30): 6816-25.

Smith Y, Bevan MD, Shink E, Bolam JP. Microcircuitry of the direct and indirect pathways of the basal ganglia. *Neuroscience* 1998; 86 (2): 353-87.

Steriade M. Neocortical cell classes are flexible entities. *Nat Rev Neurosci* 2004; 5 (2): 121-34.

Sugimoto T, Hattori T. Organization and efferent projections of nucleus tegmenti pedunculopontinus pars compacta with special reference to its cholinergic aspects. *Neuroscience* 1984; 11 (4): 931-46.

Timofeev I, Steriade M. Neocortical seizures: initiation, development and cessation. *Neuroscience* 2004; 123 (2): 299-336.

Williams D. A study of thalamic and cortical rhythms in petit mal. *Brain* 1953; 76 (1): 50-69.

Wilson CJ. The contribution of cortical neurons to the firing pattern of striatal spiny neurons. In: Houk JC, Davies JL, Beiser DG, eds. *Models of Information Processing in the Basal Ganglia*. Cambridge: MIT Press, 1995: 29-50.

Zheng T, Wilson CJ. Corticostriatal combinatorics: the implications of corticostriatal axonal arborizations. *J Neurophysiol* 2002; 87 (2): 1007-17.

Cortical control of absence seizures: focal initiation, spreading and modulation

Gilles van Luijtelaar[1], Evgenia Y. Sitnikova[1,2], Inna S. Midzyanovskaya[2]

[1] NICI-Biological Psychology, Radboud University Nijmegen, Nijmegen
[2] Institute of Higher Nervous Activity and Neurophysiology (RAS), Moscow

The abrupt and brief impairment of consciousness (absence), the concomitant electroencephalographic seizure activity in the form of 2.5-5 Hz spike-wave pattern and the minimal myoclonic jerks of the eyes and peri-oral automatisms in an otherwise quiet person form the essential characteristics of a patient having a typical absence seizure (Panayiotopoulos, 2001). The decrease in the level of consciousness in patients and in rodent models of absence epilepsy is demonstrated experimentally in reaction time studies and in visual and auditory evoked potential studies made during the seizures: increased or even no reaction and the morphology of evoked potentials is reminiscent to those made during deep slow wave sleep but with more afterdischarges (Mirsky and Tecce, 1968, Inoue et al., 1992, Meeren et al., 1998; 2001). Patients and genetic epileptic rats share also the disrupted perception of passage of time in a time estimation task as a consequence of the presence of an absence seizure (van Luijtelaar et al., 1991a;b). However, the impairment of consciousness seems to be incomplete to moderate since humans are sometimes able to recall information that was presented to them during the seizure such as that their name was called and rats are able to discriminate between relevant and less relevant stimuli presented during the seizure (Gloor, 1986; Drinkenburg et al., 2003). Finally, the execution of repetitive, motor automatisms seem to be possible during the presence of an absence seizure. The origin of the decrease of consciousness is currently the topic of brain imaging studies, possible candidates structures or brain regions are specific parts of the cingulate and the cortico-thalamo-cortical circuitry (Blumenfeld, 2005a;b).

The second hallmark of absence seizures, the electroencephalographic signs, *i.e.* characteristic paroxysmal electrical activity, bilateral symmetrical and generalized 2.5-5 Hz spike and wave discharges (SWDs) invading the "whole" brain, has gained much more attention. The SWDs are accompanied by autonomic changes such as a deep inhale, followed by accelerated breathing (van Luijtelaar and Coenen, 1986; Shuykin et al., 2004). These SWDs, 1-30 sec, do not appear randomly in time, they tend to appear in clusters, in humans as well in rats (Kellaway, 1985; Midzyanovskaya et al., 2006). The term pyknolepsy, a term not often used anymore and equivalent for absence epilepsy, refers to the fact that SWDs tend to cluster, in rats in a repetitive series of SWDs that can be seen often during the transition phase from wake to non-REM sleep, more specifically, after a period of wakefulness, the rat lies down, preparing for sleep to come, next some slow activity invade the EEG and than clusters of SWDs may become prominent.

The "centrencephalic" theory describing a subcortical origin of the generalized SWDs associated with absence seizures (Penfield and Jasper, 1947) and its successor, the cortico-reticular theory (Gloor, 1969), have dominated the literature in the last five decades of the previous century. Most of the experiments towards understanding the origin of the brain oscillation have worked within this theoretical framework, for review see Meeren et al. (2005; van Luijtelaar and Sitnikova, 2006). An assumed diffuse increase in excitability of the cortex subserves transformation of normal oscillations (sleep spindles), initiated by the reticular thalamic nucleus (RTN) into SWDs. Most of these studies were done in cats.

In the last decade, genetic rodent models were more often used to study SWDs (Marescaux et al., 1992; Coenen et al., 1991; Danober et al., 1998; van Luijtelaar et al., 2002; Crunelli and Leresche, 2002; Coenen and van Luijtelaar, 2003; Depaulis and van Luijtelaar, 2006). Outcomes of studies in GAERS (Genetic Absence Epilepsy Rats from Strasbourg) (Liu et al., 1991; Marescaux et al., 1992; Avanzini et al., 2000; Aker et al., 2002) and WAG/Rij rats (Inoue et al., 1993), supported the idea that SWDs are triggered in the lateral parts of thalamus, suggesting that cortically recorded SWDs originate from the thalamus. SWDs in GAERS were suppressed after large electrolytic lesions of the lateral thalamus (Vergnes and Marescaux, 1992) and also after more restricted chemical lesions of the RTN (Avanzini et al., 1992; Avanzini et al. 1993). The same was true in WAG/Rij rats: SWDs were completely abolished after ibotenic lesions of large parts of the thalamus including the RTN (Meeren, 2002). Also other parts of the thalamus, such as the intralaminair thalamic neurons, might play a role. It has been proposed that these parts of the thalamus plays a role during synchronization and maintenance of SWDs (Seidenbecher and Pape, 2001). The outcomes of the above mentioned studies fit into the cortico-reticular theory which proposed that a pacemaker of SWDs is located in the (lateral) thalamus. Surprisingly, the synaptic organization of the rostral pole of RTN of the non-epileptic ACI rat appears to be very similar to that of the epileptic WAG/Rij rat (van de Bovenkamp-Janssen et al., 2004a), while also GAERS failed to show any essential structural alterations in neurons of the RTN compared to their non-epileptic control rats, no neuronal loss occurred in RTN of epileptic animals (Sabers et al., 1996). Recently alterations in the AMPA-Glu4 receptor were described in the RTN of 6 months old WAG/Rij rats in comparison with age matched control and much younger WAG/Rij with much less seizures (van de Bovenkamp-Janssen et al., 2006). The outcomes of the latter study may suggest that the cortical excitatory afferents induce more burst firing in the RTN than in control rats.

It needs to be remarked that some physiological and anatomical properties in rodents' brains are crucially different from the felines' ones (the vast majority of the neurophysiological studies were traditionally done in the sixties and seventies in cats) and this might provide some particularities of rodent models of epilepsy such as the intraspike frequency in a train of SWDs from 3 to 4.5 Hz in cats and 7-11 Hz in rats and the presence and absence of GABA-ergic inhibitory interneurons throughout the thalamus in cats and rats respectively (Jones, 1985; Ohara et al., 1983). Therefore intrinsic inhibition is absent in the largest part of rat thalamus and the vast majority of thalamic nuclei receive only external inhibitory inputs from the RTN. These factors may significantly influence proneness of oscillatory activity of thalamic neurons and general properties of thalamo-cortical networks in initiation, synchronizing and spreading of SWDs.

■ A global role of the cortex in absence seizures

A diffuse and global role of the cortex in the transformation of sleep spindles to SWDs was proposed by those who adhered to the reticulo-cortical theory, but also by others (Gloor, 1969; Gloor et al., 1990; Bancaud, 1969, 1972; Niedermeyer, 1996). The whole neocortex was considered to play a role in the origin of or in the transformation of normal to pathological oscillations, and there was no reason to assume that one cortical region could be more favorable for epileptogenesis than another. Studies in GAERS and WAG/Rij rats suggested initially also a global role of the cortex in absence epilepsy: cortical deactivation by the spreading depression technique (unilateral diffusion of KCl) resulted in immediate abolishment of SWDs not only in the injected cortex but also in the ipsilateral thalamus (Vergnes and Marescaux, 1992; Meeren, 2002), in agreement with outcomes of spreading depression studies in the penicillin model (Avoli and Gloor, 1981; Gloor, 1990). This had led to the development of the hypothesis that an intact thalamo-cortical network is a prerequisite for the occurrence of SWDs and that any interference in this network may be detrimental for the initiation of SWDs. This hypothesis is also supported by the fact that surgical removal of the cortex abolishes SWDs, that cortical slices do not show spontaneous widely synchronized bursting activity, and that only in a thalamo-cortical slice preparation with preserved thalamocortical connectivity some stimuli can elicit oscillatory activity (Avoli and Gloor, 1982; Kostopoulos, 2000; Tancredi et al., 2000).

Surprisingly few studies have directly tested the increased cortical excitability theory, a second assumption of the reticulo-cortical theory of absence epilepsy, *in vitro* or *in vivo*. In one study in the penicillin feline model it was shown that subthreshold EPSP underlying SWDs produce more effectively action potentials than those underlying sleep spindles (Kostopoulos and Avoli, 1983). We investigated the excitability of the sensory-motor cortex interictally in WAG/Rij rats by establishing thresholds and afterdischarges for various types of electrical stimulation, for methods see Mares et al. (2002). Only the threshold for electriically induced limbic seizures was reduced in WAG/Rij rats, but no differences were found in the thresholds and afterdischarges for other seizure types in comparison with ACI rats (Tolmacheva et al., 2004). *In vitro*, some basic electrophysiological properties of cortical excitability in GAERS, WAG/Rij and in non-epileptic control rats were investigated but turned out not to be principally different. This mainly concerns passive cortical properties such as the complex waveform of the evoked local field potentials, the percentage of pyramidal neuron populations (intrinsically bursting and regular spiking cells) and intrinsic membrane properties. (Luhmann et al., 1995; Avanzini et al., 1996; D'Antuono et al., 2006).

■ A cortical focus

A comprehensive study of network mechanisms, responsible for the immediate onset, widespread generalization and high synchrony of SWDs has challenged this view that the cortex plays only a global role (Meeren et al., 2002). Field potentials were simultaneous recorded from multiple cortical and thalamic sites in free moving WAG/Rij rats. The cortico-cortical, intrathalamic, and cortico-thalamic interrelationships between these field potentials were quantified using non-linear association analysis (Pijn et al., 1989) by measurements of the association strength (as the degree of correlation) and the time delay between signals recorded at different cortical and thalamic sites. These parameters together characterized functional coupling between populations of interacting neuronal populations.

Figure 1 illustrates a generalized spike-wave discharge in a WAG/Rij rat and the results of the non-linear analyses, the existence of a cortical focus originating from

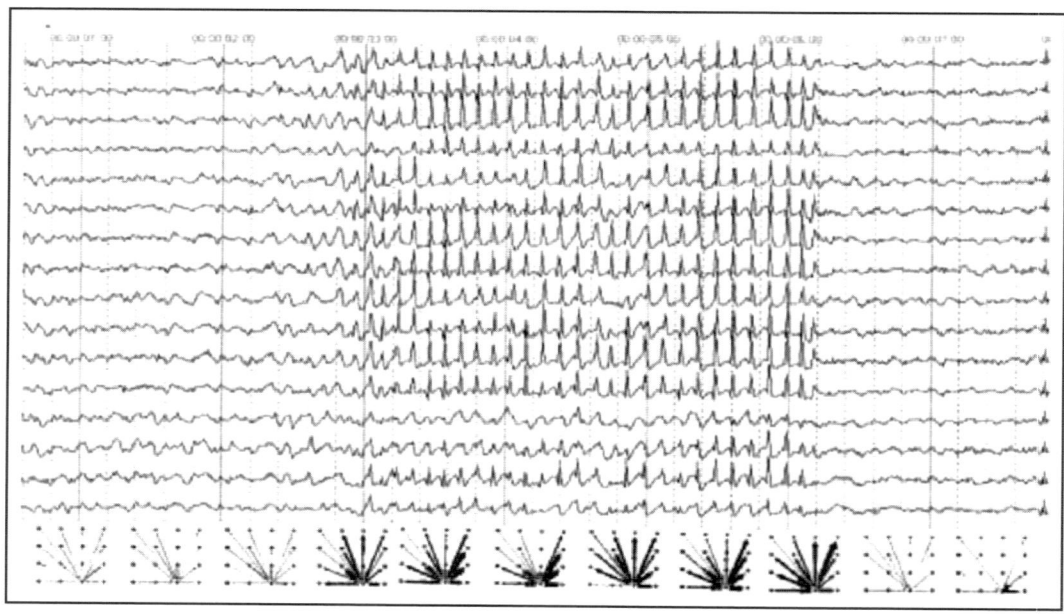

Figure 1. A generalized SWD recorded from the lateral convexity of the neocortex of a WAG/Rij rat. Results of the non-linear association analysis are presented underneath; calculations are done on EEG epochs of 500 msec. The thickness of the arrows represents the strength of the association, while the arrowheads point into the direction of the lagging site. The results of the analysis consistently suggest a cortical focus located at the projection area of upper lip. SWDs recorded at other cortical sites lag the focal site with time delays that increase with electrode distance (Adapted from Meeren et al., 2002).

one of the 16 electrodes in the SmI (somatosensory cortex) (it is shown in graphs at the bottom, the start point of arrows reflects the beginning of activity at the SmI in all eleven time frames). SWDs recorded at other cortical sites consistently lagged behind this focal site. Intra-thalamic relationships were more complex and could not account for the observed cortical propagation pattern. Functionally interconnected cortical and thalamic sites appeared to influence each other, while the direction of this bi-directional coupling could vary throughout one seizure. However, during the first five hundred milliseconds the cortical focus was consistently leading its thalamic counterpart. Thereafter, cortex and thalamus were found to alternately lead and lag unpredictably. These results are incompatible with the common assumption that the thalamus acts as the primary driving source for SWDs. Instead, a cortical focus leads the generation of generalized SWDs. The cortical origin was stationary throughout the seizure and among different seizures in the same animal, however the exact site of origin of different subject varied slightly, as was determined with functional topography. Despite the individual variation, all sites of origin were located in the peri-oral region of the somatosensory cortex (Meeren *et al.*, 2002) (Figure 2).

Other evidence for the cortical focus theory, coming from studies in GAERS and WAG/Rij's, was collected by other, independent laboratories, as well as by ourselves. Many different experimental techniques were used such as immunocytochemistry, morphometry, fMRI, neurophysiology and pharmacology.

Cytoarchitectural abnormalities in the neocortex

It is common belief that typical absence epilepsy is a purely "functional" disease since no structural lesion of any kind has been identified (Berkovic *et al.*, 1987; Niedermeyer, 1996). Morphological studies are extremely scare; however, microdysgenesis was demonstrated in childhood absence epilepsy with an increased number of dystrophic neurons in neocortex and sub-cortical white matter of the frontal lobe (Meencke, 1989). The cellular structure of cortical tissue appears to have not been considered in animal models of absence epilepsy. In the framework of our cortical focal theory of absence seizures, Karpova *et al.* (2005) examined the cytoarchitecture of the Golgi stained anterior part of neocortex in WAG/Rij rats, paying attention to the frontal (motor) region and to the somatosensory cortex, including the perioral region of the SmI.

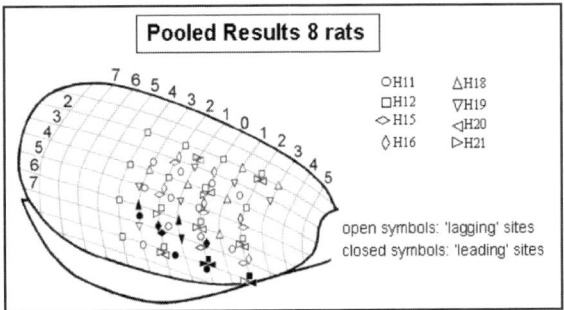

Figure 2. Pooled data from eight rats, in all animals leading sites of SWDs, filled symbols, locate in the somatosensory cortex. Open symbols represent lagging sites. The numbers represent the coordinates of the cortical surface in mm with zero point at the Bregma. Leading sites of SWDs occupy an area with the anterior-posterior coordinates from 2 (anterior to the bregma) to 3 (posterior to the bregma) mm, extending laterally from 6 to 8 mm (Adapted from Meeren *et al.*, 2002).

Typical for both the SmI and motor cortex of WAG/Rij rats was a disorder in distribution of pyramidal cells in the superficial cortical layers (I-III) (only the neurons in layer I-III were investigated). Apical dendrites of superficial pyramidal cells were often split in two branches, declined and went in non-perpendicular direction *(Figure 3)*. Quantitative morphometric measurements of dendrites such as total length of dendrites, mean length of dendritic segment and size of dendritic arbor were increased in the SmI, indicating an abnormal pattern of dendritic arborization in the epileptic zone in WAG/Rij rats. Disturbances in dendritic trees, a receptive part of pyramidal neurons, may cause an impairment of communications between individual neurons. As mentioned, the differences were found in the superficial pyramidal cells, which, owing to long-range projections to the remote cortical regions, may synchronize intrinsic cortical oscillations (Gray and McCormick, 1996). Therefore, the perioral area of the SmI may express corrupted associations with other cortical areas and facilitate synchronization and propagation of SWDs.

Pharmacological studies in the neocortex

The role of the SmI in the incidence of SWDs was studied using unilateral microinjections of lidocaine into the vibrissal area of the SmI. Lidocaine temporary deactivates neuronal activity. A temporal decrease in the number of SWDs followed the injection of lidocaine, indicating that pharmacological deactivation of the driving cortical source caused a temporal reduction of SWDs (Sitnikova and van Luijtelaar, 2004). Bilateral local injections of the sodium channel blocker phenytoin in the peri-oral region of the SmI in WAG/Rij and in GAERS rats showed an clear abolishment of SWDs, while systemic administration of the drug increased SWDs (*Figure 4*, van Luijtelaar *et al.*, 2005; Gurbanova *et al.*, 2006). The increase in SWDs after systemic administration of PHT is classical in absence epileptic patients and in rats (Peeters *et al.*, 1988), which might be putatively referred to its action in the ventral basal part of the thalamus (O'Brien *et al.*, 2005).

After bilateral injection of the anti-absence drug ethosuximide at multiple cortical and thalamic loci in GAERS, the incidence of SWDs was diminished only in case of administration to the SmI but not or much less at other cortical or thalamic (RTN or basal complex) areas. Therefore, treatment in the targeted thalamic nuclei is insufficient for ethosuximide to have a large anti-absence effect comparable to systemic administration; instead, the action of this agent may reside primarily in the focal cortical zone (Manning *et al.*, 2003; 2004). The outcome of these studies demonstrated that the WAG/Rij rats are not unique in the existence and location of the focal cortical origin of SWDs but that a comparable locus exists in GAERS as well. Therefore it seems that the two most commonly used and well described genetic rodent models of absence epilepsy share the existence of a cortical area at which local injections of PHT and ethosuximide abolish SWDs, suggesting a crucial role in initiating SWDs (*Figure 4*).

In a combined EEG, in situ hybridization and immunocytochemical studies in WAG/Rij rats, it was found that two types of sodium channels (Nav1.1 and Nav1.6) were up-regulated and overexpressed selectively at ML +6 mm in the transverse plane at bregma (Klein *et al.*, 2004). This region of the cortex closely matches the

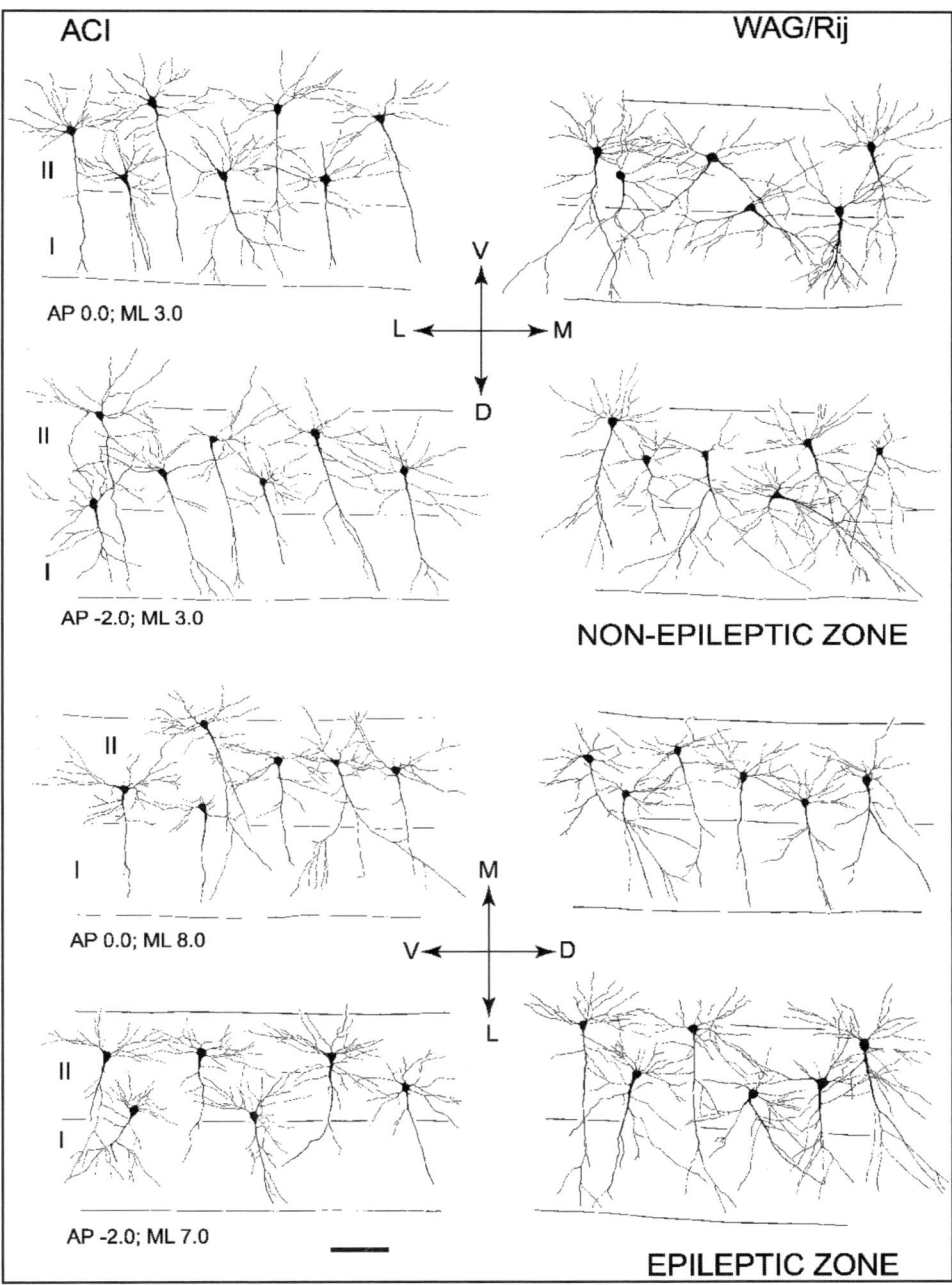

Figure 3. Composite extended drawings of Golgi-impregnated neurons in ACI (non-epileptic) and WAG/Rij rats of two cortical areas: frontal (presumably less-epileptic) and somatosensory (epileptic) areas. Coordinates of each zone are given below pictures according to the atlas of rat brain (Paxinos and Watson, 1998). Dendritic spines are not drawn; cortical layers are shown in roman numerals. Scale = 100 μm (From Karpova et al., 2005, reprinted with permission).

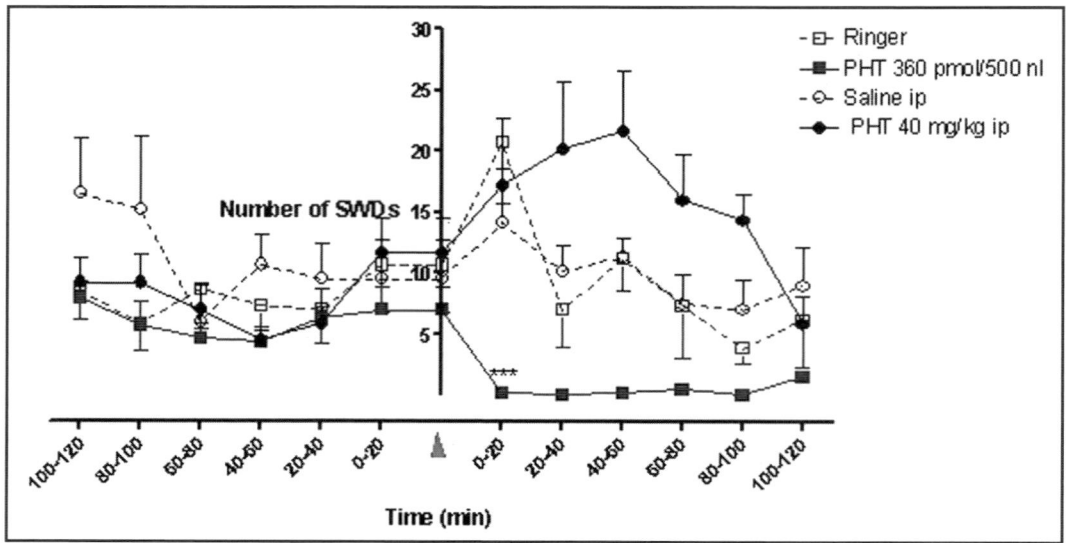

Figure 4. Local injections in WAG/Rij rats (n=6) with Phenytoin (PHT) in the focal cortical area suppress SWDs, systemic injections show the typical aggravating effects in the number of SWDs (Gurbanova, et al., 2006).

electrophysiological determined region of seizure onset (Meeren et al., 2002). The up-regulation was age dependent and this corresponds with the well documented age-dependent increase of SWDs (Coenen and van Luijtelaar, 1987; Schridde and van Luijtelaar, 2004; Klein et al., 2004). The Klein et al. study demonstrates that the age dependent increase in SWDs is closely related to the age dependent upregulation of certain types of sodium channels in the superficial layers of the perioral part of the somatosensory cortex. Moreover, it suggest that an upregulation of certain types of sodium channels can be held responsible for an assumed increased excitability in WAG/Rij rats and perhaps also in GAERS. As was described above, local blocking of sodium channels with PHT abolished SWDs, completely in line with the outcomes of Klein et al. (2004) (Figure 5).

Functional differences in excitability were very recently found in the somatosensory cortex of WAG/Rij's. An increase in NMDA mediated excitability in pyramidal shaped cells in deep layers of the neocortex was found in slices (D'Antuono et al., 2006). Inherent properties of hyperpolarisation-activated currents of pyramidal neurons (layer II-III) in the somatosensory cortex of WAG/Rij rats differed from those of two other strains (Wistar and ACI), and this modification of physiological properties of neurons was accompanied by a reduced protein expression (Strauss et al., 2004). It was proposed by the diverse authors that the above-mentioned changes increase the excitability of the SmI, and facilitate the initiation of SWDs.

A functional change in the BOLD signal during SWDs was found in fully conscious WAG/Rij rats. Significant increase in signal was found in widespread thalamic areas and the neocortex, including the SmI (Tenney et al., 2004). Other fMRI

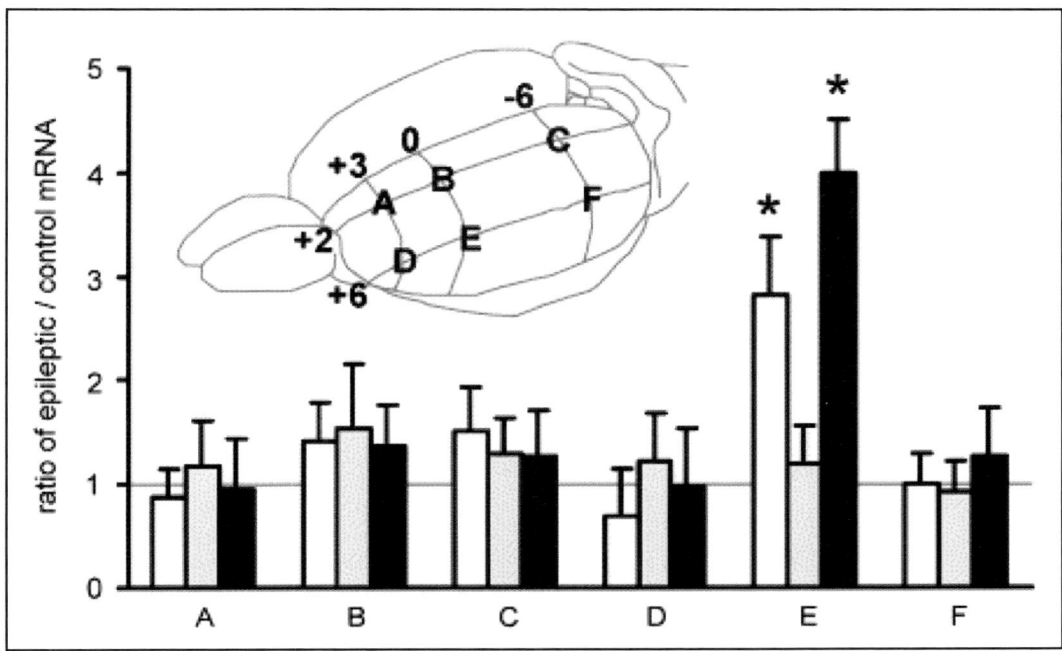

Figure 5. Sodium channel mRNA in WAG/Rij and Wistar cortex. Anatomical locations of tissue plugs used for quantitative PCR analysis are indicated on inset drawing of rat brain. The histogram shows the ratio of sodium channel mRNA levels in the neocortex of 6-month-old WAG/Rij (epileptic) rats compared to age-matched Wistar (control) rats. At anatomical location "E", there is a statistically significant increase in Nav1.1 (white bars) and Nav1.6 mRNA (black bars), but not Nav1.2 mRNA (gray bars), in the epileptic animals compared to control animals. Data is plotted as mean ± S.E.; $n=8$ animals, $*=p<0.05$. (reprinted with permission from Klein et al., 2004).

measurements were performed in WAG/Rij under fentanyl-haloperidol anesthesia in combination with simultaneous local field potentials recordings (Nersesyan et al., 2004a; 2004b). It was shown that spontaneous SWDs intensively involve the thalamus and left and right somatosensory areas. Appearance of SWDs in these regions was accompanied by an intense neuronal activity and an increased blood flow, as measured in a 7 Tesla scanner *(Figure 6)*.

■ Cortical propagation and synchronization

The outcomes of the Meeren et al. study (2002) showed that the electroencephalographic seizure activity is initiated at the perioral region of the somatosensory cortex and is quickly propagated over the cortex. The propagation of seizure activity from a focal origin over the cortex occurs through cortico-cortical connections since it may be disrupted by deep transcortical cuts, as has been shown in cats (Neckelmann et al., 1998). Visual inspection of the EEG often fails to identify any remarkable EEG activity that may precede fully developed bilateral synchronized and generalized appearing spike-wave activity, yielding to the conventional belief that SWDs are unpredictable. However, there is a *transitional* period during which absence seizure

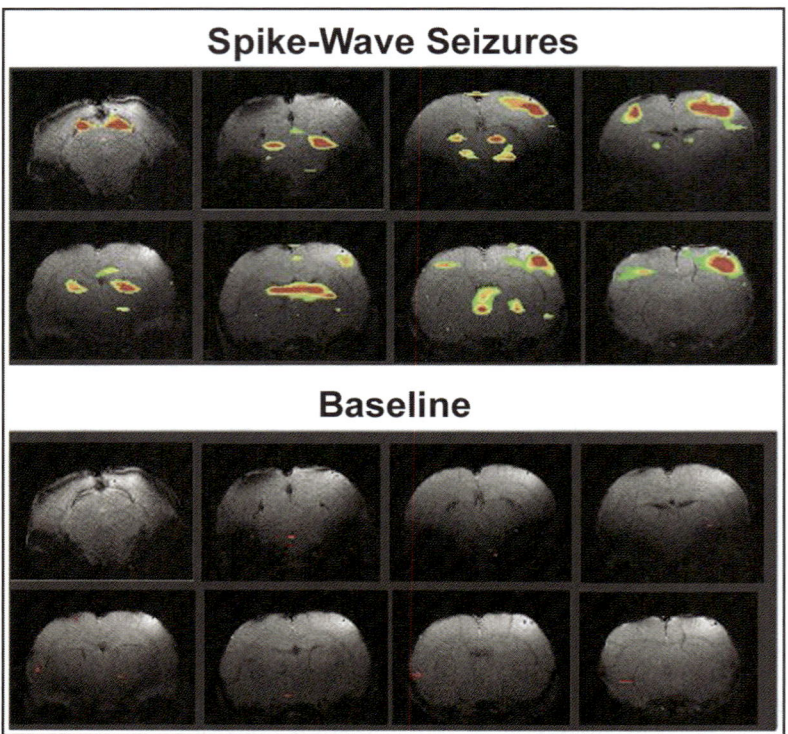

Figure 6. Increased BOLD response in the thalamus and somatosensory cortex in fentanyl/haloperidol anesthetized WAG/Rij rats accompanying EEG recorded spike-wave discharges (upper) and in control periods (Nersesyan et al., 2004, reprinted with permission).

become fully generalized (Rodin and Ancheta, 1987; Rodin, 1999). During this *transitional* period, more and more neuronal populations get involved in paroxysmal activity and the synchrony of neuronal networks is gradually increased (Steriade and Amzica, 1994; Steriade, 2003). The amount of synchrony can be assessed quantitatively by computational EEG analysis, such as coherence analysis.

We measured cortico-cortical coherence in two epochs, 1 sec before the onset of SWDs (defined by the presence of the first undisputable spike) and 1 sec after its onset (Sitnikova and van Luijtelaar, 2006). The difference in coherence (intra-hemispheric coherence) in the two epochs was calculated between electrodes in the frontal cortex, two locations within the somatosensory cortex (the projection area of the vibrissae and the paws), and the occipital cortex. Next, the inter-hemispheric coherence difference between symmetrical electrode pairs was calculated. It was hypothesized here that SWDs emerge due to an interplay between the focal epileptic zone in the SmI(vib) and its closest neighboring zone, due to either abnormal and excessive synchronization and excitation or reduced inhibition. It has been established that the degree of synchrony progressively increases from an early stage of the seizure to a later state (Steriade and Amzica, 1994). Here we focused on unilateral intra-hemispheric and bilateral inter-hemispheric cortico-cortical coherence during the *transitional* period in epochs – 1 sec before the onset of SWDs and during SWDs (immediately after the onset of a spike-wave discharge). The onset was defined at the first undisputable spike in a train of spike and waves.

Changes of coherence which accompanied the onset of SWDs were statistically analyzed. First, unilateral cortico-cortical coherence was calculated between electrodes at the frontal cortex, two locations within the somatosensory cortex (the projection area of the vibrissae and the paws), and the occipital cortex. Second, the bilateral coherence between symmetrical electrodes was analyzed. We assumed that if SWDs might emerge in the perioral region of SmI (Meeren *et al.*, 2002) they will show a more increased coherence between this zone and its closest neighboring electrode than between two other equally distant electrodes. Based on the analysis of coherence we specified changes of short-distant and long-distant intracortical synchronization in the cortex that accompanied the onset of SWDs.

Intra-hemispheric cortico-cortical coherence

The occurrence of SWDs was accompanied by a frequency-specific increase of intra-hemispheric coherence (range 0.11-0.28) between all electrode pairs. The increase of coherence was found generally between 6 and 40 Hz *(Figure 7)*. The largest increase was found in *SmI(paws) – frontal* EEG pair. Noteworthy, this pair showed also more synchrony in frequencies from 40-60 Hz. The increase in coherence was largest in all electrode pairs for the frequency of the SWDs (8-11.5 Hz) and its first harmonic (16-21.5 Hz). Coherence in 12-16 and 22-40 Hz also increased, although only in the anterior EEG derivations. There was also a small but significant decrease of coherence in the low frequencies (< 6 Hz) in *SmI(vib)-frontal* and *SmI(vib)-SmI(paws)* pairs *(Figure 7)*. It seems that the whole somatosensory cortex including the focal epileptic zone (Meeren *et al.*, 2002) and functionally related areas such as the adjacent parietal and frontal areas are engaged in specific local interactions that might be critical for the initiation of SWDs. The more remote electrode pairs, *i.e. fronto-occipital* and *SmI(vib)-occipital*, revealed a smaller, albeit significant, increase of coherence associated with SWDs onset *(Figures 7 and 8)*.

Trans-hemispheric cortico-cortical coherence

As compared to intra-hemispheric pairs, trans-hemispheric pairs showed a larger (0.17-0.40) increase on coherence pre vs after the onset of SWDs and also this effect was frequency-specific. The increase was largest in SWDs-specific frequencies (8-11.5 and first harmonic) in all trans-hemispheric pairs, but not at the *occipital* site. The coherence change in SWDs-nonspecific frequencies (12-16 and 22-40 Hz) was lower than the SWDs-specific frequencies, again with an exception of the occipital pairs, in which the magnitude of the coherence change in SWDs-specific and SWDs-nonspecific frequencies was about the same. A small but significant decrease in the change of coherence in the lower (< 6 Hz) frequencies was found between the two homologous pairs in the SmI (paws and vibrissal regions). The outcomes suggests that bilateral interaction between frontal and somatosensory cortex intensively involve physiological frequencies of SWDs, in contrast to the occipital trans-hemispheric associations, which were lower and not specific for certain frequencies *(Figure 8)*.

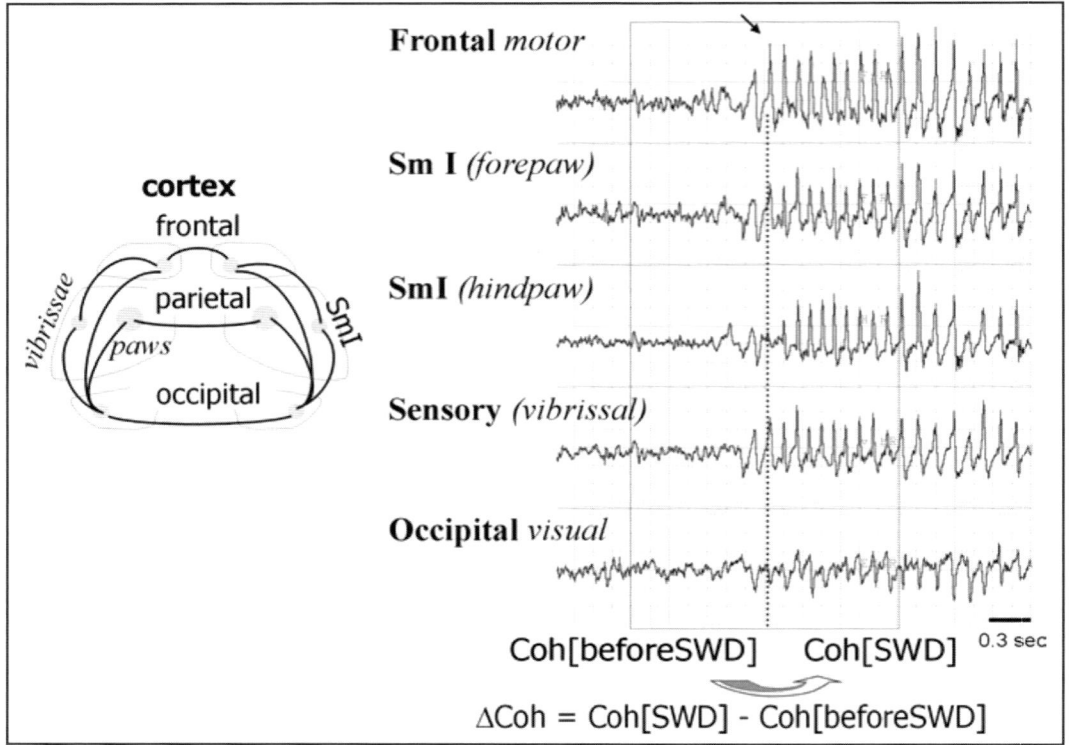

Figure 7. The left schema shows positioning of cortical electrodes and outlines electrode pairs (thick black lines) in which coupling has been measured. The right plate shows a typical spike-wave discharge (SWD). Small black arrow at the frontal EEG track points to the first spike (the assumable marker of the onset of a SWD). This time marker has been applied to all recording channels (dotted vertical line shows). Coherence was computed in two subsequent epochs, one sec before and 1 sec after SWD-onset. The coefficients of differential coherence was statistically analyzed.

The bilateral coherence change did not decay with electrode distance. Distances between symmetrical bilateral electrodes decreasing in the sequence SmI(vib) > occipital > SmI(paws) > frontal, that did not correspond to the differences in coherence. Therefore it seems that the occurrence of SWDs relates to the stronger bilateral communications between symmetrical (and functionally homogenous) frontal cortical sites as compared to unilateral associations between functionally heterogeneous and even more proximate areas. The large-scale increase of bilateral coherence runs in parallel with the bilateral propagation of SWDs and this could account for the fact that SWDs are bilateral symmetrical and generalized. Another conclusion based on the cortical pattern of the changes in coherence, larger changes in coherence between more remote left and right frontal and somatosensory electrode pairs than between more nearby occipital pairs, is that the outcomes are incompatible with a massive and simultaneous induction of SWDs by a thalamic oscillator. This implies that also the coherence pattern is more in favor of a role of the somatosensory cortex as an initiator for SWDs than the lateral thalamus including the RTN.

It seems that, on the level of EEG, SWDs constitute complex resonant phenomena, in which network synchronization involves not only frequencies 8-11.5 Hz and its first harmonic, but also less for SWDs specific frequencies. These changes of network associations signify hyper-synchronization of ~10 Hz rhythm and transformation of normal background rhythmic activity to spike-wave paroxysms. A small series of frequencies showed a decrease in coherence change. It is possible that attenuation of low-frequency coherence facilitates the increase of higher-frequency synchrony. It might be important that bidirectional changes of coherence (decrease in low and increase in 8-11.5 Hz band and first harmonic) are characteristic for the somatosensory area, suggesting that the somatosensory cortex builds up a specific pattern of network associations primarily involved in paroxysmal rhythmogenesis giving rise to SWDs.

The trans-hemispheric cortical coherence increase was larger than the intra-hemispheric cortical but also larger than the cortico-thalamic and thalamo-thalamic coherence (Sitnikova, personal observation). This may imply that the *corpus callosum* is crucially involved in the pathophysiology of absence seizures. The thalamus is a less good candidate for intrahemisperic transfer considering few left-right projections. It is thought that the *corpus callosum* is the major anatomical substrate involved in bilateral transfer of SWDs. Transcallosal cuts prevents bilaterally symmetrical SWDs: after callosomectomy SWDs occurred independently in the two hemispheres (Vergnes *et al.*, 1989).

We believe that SWDs are initiated due to the functional integration of global and local network processes. First, a global increase of coherence in SWDs-specific frequencies (~ 10 Hz and the first harmonic) found in widespread uni- and bilateral pairs. Second, a relatively local (in the SmI and the frontal regions) reduction of coherence in the low frequencies. Normally, the SmI in rodents may initiate 10 Hz rhythm itself and independently from other cortical regions (Nicolelis *et al.*, 1995). In case of SWDs, nearby and remote cortical areas need synchrony in order for local oscillations to develop into SWDs, for this process the synchrony in the SWDs-specific frequencies are imperative. Moreover, a reduction of low-frequency coherence between SmI (paws and vibrissal) and frontal cortical areas may further encourage SWDs. Since 8-11.5 Hz (sigma) activity is not compatible with 1-4.5 Hz (delta), high delta synchronization may prevent genesis of sigma activity (*i.e.* it precludes sigma synchronization) and vice versa (Terman *et al.*, 1996; Destexhe and Sejnowski, 2002). We assume that reduction of delta coherence in the local fronto-parietal cortical circuit may further promote sigma synchronization in this particular area and facilitate the occurrence of SWDs. It is possible that the decrease of delta coherence (delta desynchronization) may imply a down-regulation of slow inhibitory GABAb-ergic mechanisms. As known, GABA-b-mediated IPSPs with kinetics around 300 ms (~3 Hz) are incompatible with fast GABAa-ergic (10 Hz) mediated IPSPs (Contreras *et al.*, 1997). Therefore a shift from delta to sigma synchrony during the transitional period of SWDs may be caused by a reduction of GABAb-ergic inhibition at the expense of GABA-a-ergic inhibition, and this may contribute to triggering SWDs. How this is compatible with the fact that local injections at the somatosensory cortex with GABAb antagonists in the cortex of GAERS reduce SWDs (Manning *et al.*, 2004), needs to be established.

Neocortical GABA-ergic interneurons: targets for modulation

The $GABA_A$ receptor is of primary importance in absence epilepsy due to the role of the GABA-ergic RTN in synchronization and desynchronization cortico-thalamo-cortical pathways. For over ten years it is already known that synaptic network properties in the neocortex of WAG/Rij rats are impaired in comparison to non-epileptic Wistar control. More precisely, both the excitability of cortical cells and the efficiency of GABAergic inhibition, as measured with extra- and intracellular recordings in slices is considerably reduced in the fronto-parietal cortex (Luhmann et al., 1995). The fact that SWDs can be elicited in cats by cortical application of $GABA_A$-receptor antagonists (e.g. Steriade en Contreras, 1998; Kostopoulos, 2000) is in line with the reduction of inhibition in cortical tissue of WAG/Rij rats. As known, inhibitory GABA-ergic interneurons form 20-30% of the neocortical population (Peters and Jones, 1984; Markram et al., 2004). Inhibitory interneurons are subdivided into several classes and about 50% of all inhibitory interneurons are basket cells (for review see Markram et al., 2004). Basket cells are "local circuit neurons", they effectively control firing activity of pyramidal cells and other interneurons by synchronizing the activity in neuronal networks. Basket cells typically express the two calcium-binding proteins, parvalbumin (PV) and calbindin (CB). PV is co-expressed with GABA in 90% of GABA-ergic neurons (Miettinen et al., 1996; Celio, 1986) and PV-immunostaining is an appropriate way to mark basket cells (Kawaguchi and Kubota, 1997). The network of GABA-ergic interneurons in general and PV-containing cells in particular are engaged in cortical oscillations and play a role in determining cortical (hyper)excitability (Bacci et al., 2003; 2005).

PV immunostaining has been used in WAG/Rij rats to study the distribution of GABA-ergic neurons over various brain regions (van de Bovenkamp-Janssen et al., 2004b). It was suggested that an increase of cortical excitability and/or low efficacy of GABAergic inhibitory system could be due to a smaller amount of inhibitory neurons or from the impairment of metabolism of GABA in GABA-ergic neurons. All WAG/Rij and (non-epileptic control) ACI rats showed large cortical regions that hardly show any PV-immunoreactive cells. These cortical regions were not devoid of neurons but they simply could not be stained with the anti-PV serum presumably these cells do not contain enough PV to become immunopositive. No specific cortical area was consistently unstained in each rat examined, demonstrating that there are individual differences in the affected regions. Quantification of PV-positive cells showed that WAG/Rij rats have 2 times less PV-positive cells in the parietal (Par1) and in the forelimb area of the somatosensory cortex (FL) as age-matched ACI rats. Par1 and FL are parts of the somatosensory cortex, Par1 contains the peri-oral projections. The lack of PV in these regions may destabilize intraneuronal Ca^{2+} homeostatic processes such as excitability and inhibition, intracellular signaling and neurotransmitter release. Considering the co-localization of PV with GAD and GABA, we assume that the cortex contains areas with a lesser amount or even a lack of GABA-ergic cells in both strains while at some cortical regions, e.g. Par1 and FL WAG/Rij, show less PV-stained cells. This might cause local cortical alterations of inhibition. This suggestion is in agreement with the neurophysiological data demonstrating an impairment of GABA-ergic inhibition in frontal cortex

(Luhmann et al., 1995) or in the perioral region of the somatosensory cortex of WAG/Rij rats in comparison to control Wistar rats (D'Antuono et al., 2006). An impairment of inhibitory processes in the frontal cortex of WAG/Rij rats in a strain comparative study, as measured with auditory evoked potentials was also found in a double click paradigm (De Bruin et al., 2001).

Interestingly, PV containing cells, in the cortex, e.g. in layer 5 of the somatosensory cortex, are specifically or preferentially targeted by several ascending neurotransmitter systems including those containing Acetylcholine, serotonin, dopamine and noradrenaline. They modulate interneurons either by classical synapses, or neuromodulatory or by diffuse non-synaptic transmission. The latter way is quite efficient since multiple cells can be reached. The PV containing cells are Fast Spiking (FS) cells, sensitive for loreclezole and zolpidem, suggesting the presence of the Beta2-3 and alpha1 subunit in their $GABA_A$ receptor (Bacci et al., 2003). Interestingly, zolpidem and loreclezole are both effective against SWDs (Depoortere et al., 1996; Ates et al., 1992). These FS cells target the soma and axonal hillcock of pyramidal neurons, ideal locations for controlling the output and oscillatory synchronization of groups of principal cells (Bacci et al., 2005). Autoradiographic and immunocytochemical studies of the somatosensory cortex showed a decreased enhancement of 3H-flunitrazepam binding and of beta2 – beta3 subunits of the $GABA_A$ receptor in GAERS at the somatosensory cortex compared to controls (Spreafico et al., 1993). All this may suggest that FS spiking PV containing cells in the somatosensory cortex of genetic epileptic rats are less efficient in fulfilling their inhibitory role.

Cortical target of neuromodulatory control of SWDs: dopaminergic and serotonergic systems

The brain aminergic systems have been recognized as important modulators of spike-wave activity for almost twenty years (Warter et al., 1988). Chlonidine, an alpha-2 adrenoreceptor agonist that inhibits the release of noradrenaline, induces drowsiness and aggravates absence seizures, is a good example of a SWDs modulating drug (Buzsaki et al., 1991; Sitnikova and van Luijtelaar, 2005). In a series of experiments, basal levels of monoamines were investigated in WAG/Rij rats and Wistar control rats in the neocortex before and after exposure to an intense sound. These series of experiments were performed in close collaboration of Dr. Tuomisto's lab in Kuopio. A first incidental observation was that tissue content (noradrenaline) of the frontal cortex was higher in WAG/Rij compared to control rats (Midzyanovskaya et al., in prep). More attention was paid to the brain dopaminergic system as neuromodulator by others and us (Warter et al., 1988; Depaulis et al., 1992; Deransart et al., 1998; de Bruin et al., 2000; Midzianovskaia et al., 2001; Deransart et al., 2001; Riban et al., 2004; Birioukova et al., 2005). Experimental manipulations, leading to decrease of brain dopaminergic tone such as the systemic administration of various types of DA antagonists, easily facilitate absence seizures in GAERS and WAG/Rij rats (Warter et al., 1988; de Bruin et al., 2000; Midzianovskaya et al., 2001). The frontal cortex receives DA-ergic terminals of a particular subpopulation of Ventral Tegmental Area neurons, which comprise the so called mesocortical dopaminergic system. Since absence paroxysms in rats were shown to start from the frontal somatosensory cortex

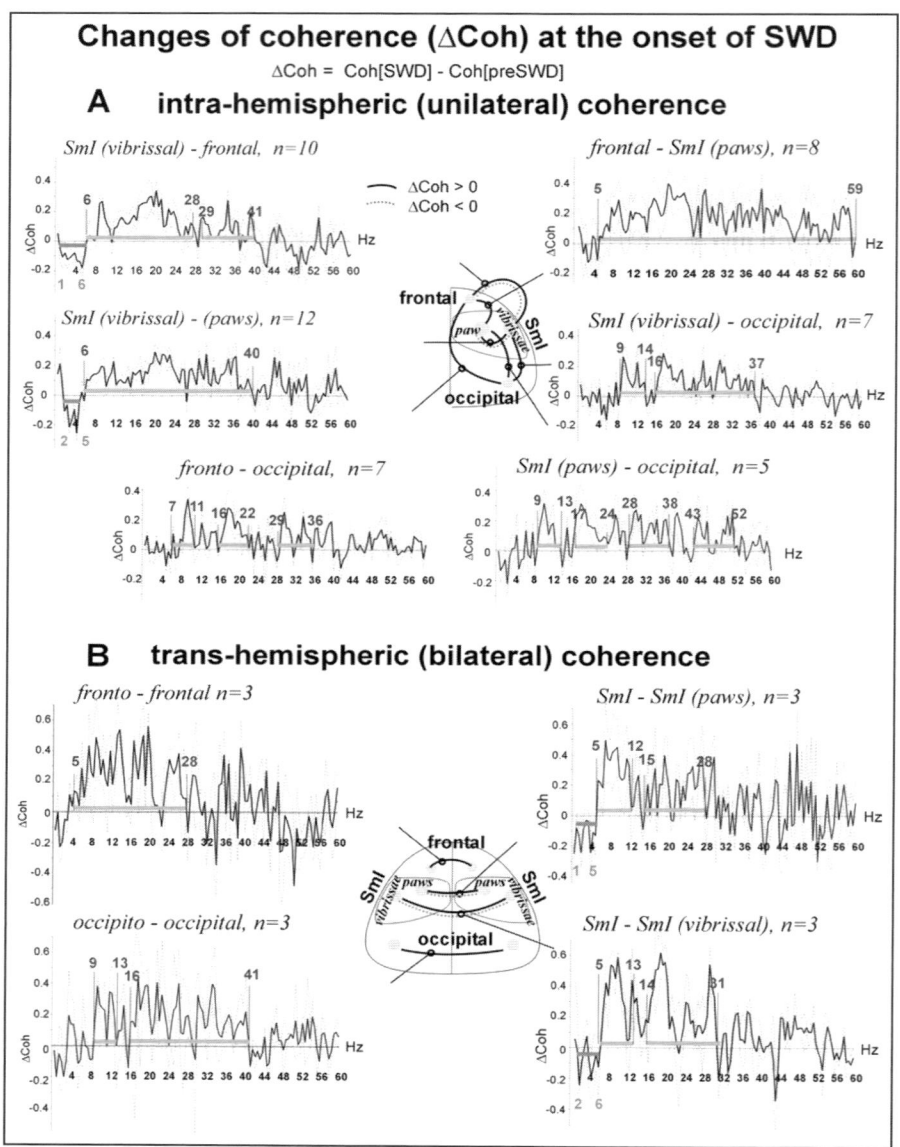

Figure 8. Occurrence of SWDs corresponds to strengthening of intra- and interhemispheric synchronization between various cortical loci. Coherence between 6 Hz and 40-60 increased with SWDs onset, as estimated by statistical analysis of coherence spectra. During fully developed SWDs, synchronization in low frequency band decreased but only between EEG pairs that include SmI. Probably, low frequency synchronization is higher at the time before the onset of SWDs, when SmI triggers SWDs. At the time when fully developed mature SWDs are present in the cortex, high frequency synchronization between all EEG pairs was strengthened; this likely reflects the generalized pattern of a seizure. Interestingly, the interhemispheric coherence difference is higher than the intra coherence difference, emphasizing a large role of the corpus callosum in bilateral synchronization of SWDs.

area (Meeren et al., 2002), one can expect that the cortical aminergic tone has a significant impact on susceptibility to absence epilepsy. Indeed, our data show that the density of D2-like dopamine receptors in the frontal and parietal cortex were higher in absence-epileptic WAG/Rij rats as compared to non-epileptic ACI rats (Birioukova et al., 2005) and moreover, this parameter significantly correlated with individual scores of spike-wave paroxysms (SWI) in WAG/Rij rats (Figure 9).

The increased density of D2-like receptors points to a putative dopaminergic deficiency of frontal cortex in rats with a genetic predisposition to develop and show SWDs. Subsequent neurochemical experiments (Midzyanovskaya et al., 2006; subm.) provided us with arguments partly supporting this hypothesis. As mentioned, we measured tissue concentrations of noradrenaline, dopamine and serotonin as well as some of their metabolites such as 5-HIAA, HVA, DOPAC and tryptophan (TRT), a precursor of serotonin in frontal and parieto-occipital regions of necortex of WAG/Rij and Wistar rats, in control or immediately after exposure to an emotional stressor (aversive sound). Although no strain differences were observed, we found that the metabolic rate of dopamine (assessed by ratios of dopamine metabolites' tissue concentrations to the tissue concentration of dopamine itself (HVA/DA and DOPAC/DA), as measured in the frontal or parieto-occipital cortex respectively) showed significant negative correlations with the number of SWDs (Spike-Wave Index (SWI), Figure 10A, B). These complementary lines of evidence show that a high number of SWDs is accompanied by an insufficient dopaminergic tone in the neocortex. Presumably, a poor dopaminergic activity can facilitate the origin of pathological oscillations in either the somatosensory cortex or in the circuitry between the somatosensory cortex and the frontal cortical areas.

A third aminergic system also shows signs of insufficient cortical control. TRT, as measured in the frontal cortex, displayed also a highly significant negative correlation with SWI (Figure 10C). In addition, the metabolic rate of serotonin in the parieto-occipital cortex, as assessed by means of the ratio of 5HIAA/5HT, correlated negatively with SWI (Figure 10D) (Midzyanovskaya et al., 2006). Serotonin in the cortex blocks synchronized ECoG activity and facilitates processing of external information from the environment by a local mechanism that is not mediated by secondary systems (Dringenberg and

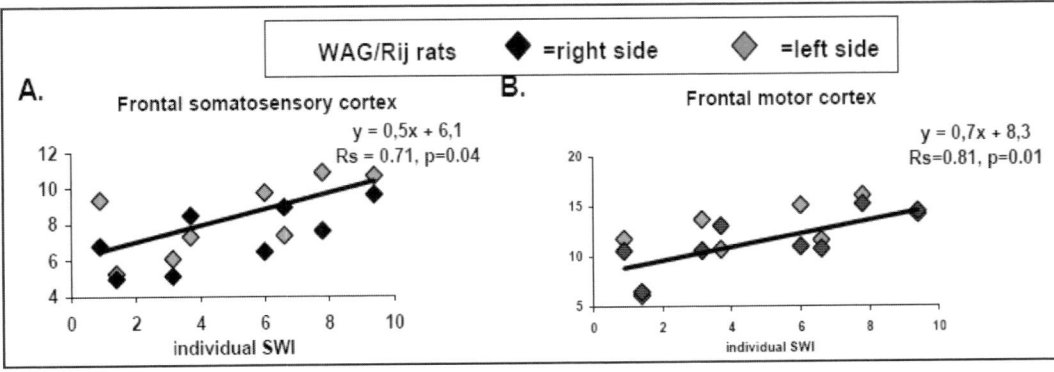

Figure 9. Optical density of D2-like dopamine receptors as measured in the frontal part of the somatosensory (A) and frontal motor (B) cortical regions correlates positively with the index of spike-wave activity (SWI).

Vanderwolf, 1998). This let us expect that a poor serotonergic activity in the neocortex facilitates oscillations that will lead to SWDs, and causes a decrease in the ability of cortical neurons to process information. Indeed, our experiments with emotional stress let us suggest that a deficient cortical filtering of stressful information takes place in absence epileptic rats (Midzyanovskaya et al., 2006). Pharmacological data does show that the brain serotonin is able to modulate SWDs but does not let a definite conclusion on its role. Experiments with i.p or i.c.v. administration of serotonergic compounds demonstrated that activation of $5\text{-}HT_{1A}$, $5\text{-}HT_7$ and $5\text{-}HT_{2C}$ suppress this type of epileptic activity, whereas stimulation of $5\text{-}HT_{1A}$ receptors activates the generation of SWDs in WAG/Rij rats (Jakus et al., 2003, Graf et al., 2004). Experiments with local application of serotoninergic compounds on neocortex are still lacking *(Figure 10)*.

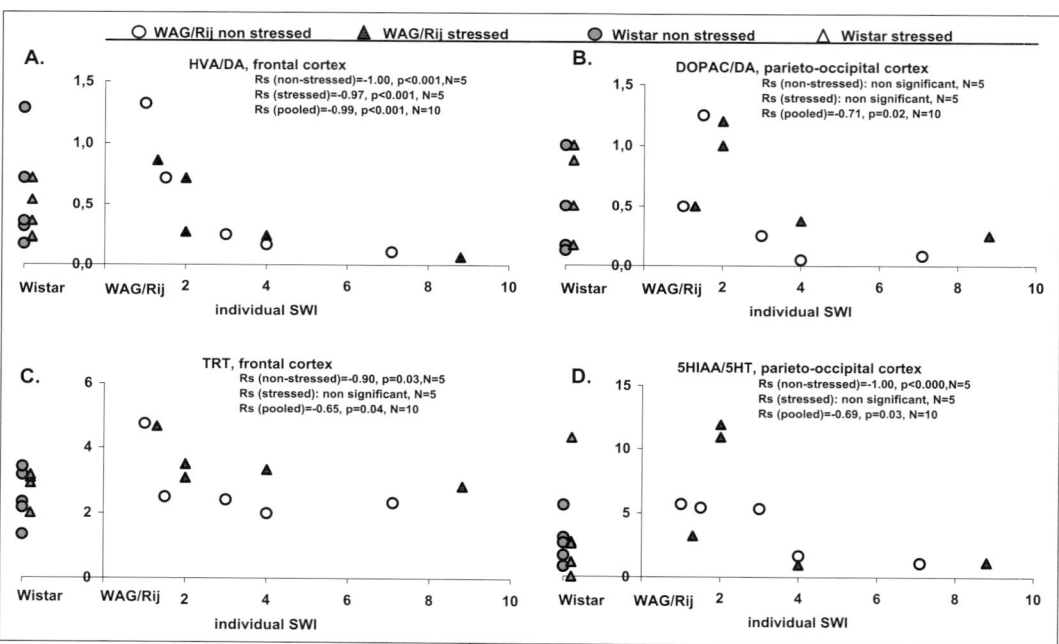

Figure 10. Individual concentrations of (A) HVA/DA ratio in frontal cortex in control and stressed WAG/Rij and Wistar rats and a scatter plot of this parameter and individual score for spike-wave discharges (SWI); (B) DOPAC/DA in parieto-occipital cortex in control and stressed WAG/Rij and Wistar rats and a scatter plot of this parameter and individual SWI; (C) TRT in frontal cortex in control and stressed WAG/Rij and Wistar rats and a scatter plot of this parameter and individual SWI; (D) 5HIAA/5HT ratio in parieto-occipital cortex in control and stressed WAG/Rij and Wistar rats. Correlation coefficients for the stressed and control rats are given above each scatter plot. Stress was induced by exposure to an oversive noise.

Conclusions

The concepts on the origin of absence epilepsy are evolving since the middle of the last century. The SWDs accompanying absence seizures are not likely to appear due to a general increase in cortical excitability, while also a thalamic origin of SWDs is less likely, as predicted by the cortico-reticular theory. Instead, a focal cortical area is assumed to be the origin for SWDs: the paroxysmal activity in rats (WAG/Rij and GAERS) might arise from the somatosensory cortex. The RTN and the relay nuclei are getting quickly involved in generating SWDs through descending cortico-thalamic pathways.

Outcomes of recent fMRI studies, local application of drugs, neurophysiological, immunocytochemical, in situ hybridization and morphometric data show a global and a focal role of the cortex. A global role and diffuse role since enhanced excitation and reduced inhibition are found in unspecified frontal locations, a local-focal role because some molecular changes were unique for the perioral region of the somatosensory area. Neurophysiological studies of the various types of cortical cells are necessary to characterize in which way cells in this focal zone differ from other cortical areas and from the same functional areas in non-epileptic rats.

Mechanisms of synchrony in cortical networks were analysed with coherence analyses. It seems that during the onset of SWDs, the homologous zone in the other hemisphere is synchronized through frequency specific activity. The intrahemispheric coherence at the onset remains smaller.

The GABA-ergic PV containing cells, most likely basket cells, are putative candidates as targets for modulation by ascending monoaminergic and cholinergic neurotransmitter systems. Dopaminergic, adrenergic and serotonergic stimulation on, to few, PV containing neurons might facilitate the oscillatory drive of the cortex, perhaps more in the peri-oral region than anywhere else. It is greatly acknowledged that besides cortical cells in the forebrain, also subcortical structures regions and brainstem and regions modulate the propensity of cortico-thalamo-cortical circuits to oscillate (Buzsaki et al., 1990; Deransart et al., 2001; Charpier, this volume).

Whether the same mechanisms, among others a cortical zone from which SWDs are initiated and quickly spread over the cortex, may underlie the pathophysiology of seizures in human primary idiopathic generalized epilepsies needs to be established. There is more and more evidence that also in patients absence seizures are not "generalized" in the sense of homogeneous cortical activation but involve highly localized discharges from frontal and parietal sources.

The discovery of a focal cortical zone in GAERS and WAG/Rij rats opens new reasons to reinvestigate those specific parts of the neocortex. Whether surgical bilateral removal of these area would prove of falsify the cortical focus theory, seems doubtful considering that parallel cortico-thalamo-cortical networks exist. The interruption of a single pathway does not prevent the (further) activation of the next one.

References

Aker RG, Özkara C, Dervent A, Onat FY. Enhancement of spike and wave discharges by microinjection of bicuculline into the reticular nucleus of rats with absence epilepsy. *Neurosci Lett* 2002; 322: 71-4.

Ates N, van Luijtelaar EL, Drinkenburg WH, Vossen JM, Coenen AM. Effects of loreclezole on epileptic activity and on EEG and behaviour in rats with absence seizures. *Epilepsy Res* 1992; 13: 43-8.

Avanzini G, de Curtis M, Marescaux C, Panzica F, Spreafico R, Vergnes M. Role of the thalamic reticular nucleus in the generation of rhythmic thalamo-cortical activities subserving spike and waves. *J Neural Transm Suppl* 1992; 35: 85-95.

Avanzini G, Vergnes, M, Spreafico, R, Marescaux, C. Calcium-dependent regulation of genetically determined spike and waves by the RTN of rats. *Epilepsia* 1993; 34: 1-7.

Avanzini G, de Curtis M, Franceschetti, S, Sancini, G, Spreafico, R. Cortical *versus* thalamic mechanisms underlying spike and wave discharges in GAERS. *Epilepsy Res* 1996; 26: 37-44.

Avanzini G, Panzica F, de Curtis M. The role of the thalamus in vigilance and epileptogenic mechanisms. *Clin Neurophysiol* 2000; 111: S19-26.

Avoli M, Gloor P. The effects of transient functional depression of the thalamus and on spindles and on bilateral synchronous epileptic discharges of feline generalized penicillin epilepsy. *Epilepsia* 1981; 22: 443-52.

Avoli M, Gloor P. Role of the thalamus in generalized penicillin epilepsy: observations on decorticated cats. *Exp Neurol* 1982; 77: 386-402.

Bacci A, Huguenard JR, Prince DA. Modulation of neocortical interneurons: extrinsic influences and exercises in self-control. *Trends Neurosci* 2005; 28: 602-10.

Bacci A, Rudolph U, Huguenard JR, Prince DA. Major differences in inhibitory synaptic transmission onto two neocortical interneuron subclasses. *J Neurosci* 2003; 23: 9664-74.

Bancaud J. Physiopathogenesis of generalized epilepsies of organic nature (Stereoencephalographic study). In: Gastaut H, Jasper HH, Bancaud J, Waltregny, A eds. *The Physiopathogenesis of the Epilepsies*. Springfield, IL: Charles C. Thomas, 1969: 158-85.

Bancaud J. Mechanisms of cortical discharges in "generalized" epilepsies in man. In: Petsche H, Brazier MAB, eds. *Synchronization of EEG activity in epilepsies*. New York: Springer, New York, 1972: 368-81.

Berkovic SF, Andermann F, Andermann E, Gloor P. Concepts of absence epilepsies: discrete syndromes or biological continuum? *Neurology* 1987; 37: 993-1000.

Birioukova LM, Midzyanovskaya IS, Lensu S, Tuomisto L, van Luijtelaar G. Distribution of D1-like and D2-like dopamine receptors in the brain of genetic epileptic WAG/Rij rats. *Epilepsy Res* 2005; 63: 89-96.

Blumenfeld H. Consciousness and epilepsy: why are patients with absence seizures absent? *Prog Brain Res* 2005a; 150: 271-86.

Blumenfeld H. Cellular and network mechanisms of spike-wave seizures. *Epilepsia* 2005b; 46 S9: 21-33.

Buzsaki G, Kennedy B, Solt VB, Ziegler M. Noradrenergic control of thalamic oscillation: the role of alpha-2 receptors. *Eur J Neurosci* 1991; 3: 222-9.

Buzsaki G, Smith A, Berger S, Fisher LJ, Gage FH. Petit mal epilepsy and parkinsonian tremor: hypothesis of a common pacemaker. *Neuroscience* 1990; 36: 1-14.

Celio MR. Parvalbumin in most gamma-aminobutyric acid-containing neurons of the rat cerebral cortex. *Science* 1986; 231: 995-7.

Coenen AM, van Luijtelaar EL. The WAG/Rij rat model for absence epilepsy: age and sex factors. *Epilepsy Res* 1987; 1: 297-301.

Coenen AM, Drinkenburg WH, Peeters BW, Vossen JM, van Luijtelaar EL. Absence epilepsy and the level of vigilance in rats of the WAG/Rij strain. *Neurosci Biobehav Rev* 1991; 15: 259-63.

Coenen AML, van Luijtelaar ELJM. Genetic Animal models for absence epilepsy: a review of the WAG/Rij strain of Rats. *Behavioral Genetics* 2003; 33: 635-55.

Contreras D, Destexhe A, Steriade M. Intracellular and computational characterization of the intracortical inhibitory control of synchronized thalamic inputs *in vivo*. *Neurophysiol* 1997; 78: 335-50.

Crunelli V, Leresche N. Childhood absence epilepsy: genes, channels, neurons and networks. *Nat Rev Neurosci* 2002; 3: 371-82.

Danober L, Deransart C, Depaulis A, Vergnes M, Marescaux C. Pathophysiological mechanisms of genetic absence epilepsy in the rat. *Prog Neurobiol* 1998; 55: 27-57.

D'Antuono M, Inaba Y, Biagini G, D'Argancelo V, Avoli M. Synaptic hyperexcitability of deep layer neocortical cells in a genetic model of absence seizures. *Genes, Brain and Behavior* 2006; 5: 73-84.

de Bruin NM, van Luijtelaar EL, Jansen SJ, Cools AR, Ellenbroek BA. Dopamine characteristics in different rat genotypes: the relation to absence epilepsy. *Neurosci Res* 2000; 38: 165-73.

Depaulis A. The inhibitory control of the substantia nigra over generalized non-convulsive seizures in the rat. *J Neural Transm Suppl* 1992; 35: 125-39.

Depaulis A, van Luijtelaar, G. Genetic models of absence epilepsy in the rat. In: Pitkanen A, Schwartzkroin P, Moshe S, eds. *Models of seizures and Epilepsy*. San Diego CA: Elsevier, CA, 2006: 223-48.

Depoortere H, Francon D, van Luijtelaar EL, Drinkenburg WH, Coenen AM. Differential effects of midazolam and zolpidem on sleep-wake states and epileptic activity in WAG/Rij rats. *Pharmacol Biochem Behav* 1995; 51: 571-6.

Deransart C, Landwehrmeyer GB, Feuerstein TJ, Lucking CH. Up-regulation of D3 dopaminergic receptor mRNA in the core of the nucleus accumbens accompanies the development of seizures in a genetic model of absence-epilepsy in the rat. *Brain Res Mol Brain Res* 2001; 94: 166-77.

Deransart C, Vercueil L, Marescaux C, Depaulis A. The role of basal ganglia in the control of generalized absence seizures. *Epilepsy Res* 1998; 32: 213-23.

Destexhe A, Sejnowski TJ. The initiation of burst in thalamic neurons and the cortical control of thalamic sensitivity, *Phil Tranl R Soc Lond B* 2002 ; 357: 1649-57.

Dringenberg HC, Wanderwolf CH. Involvement of direct and indirect pathways in electrocorticographic activation. *Neurosci Biobehav Rev* 1998; 22: 249-57.

Drinkenburg WH, Schuurmans ML, Coenen AM, Vossen JM, van Luijtelaar EL. Ictal stimulus processing during spike-wave discharges in genetic epileptic rats. *Behav Brain Res* 2003; 143: 141-6.

Gurbanova AA, Aker R, Berkman K, Onat FY, van Rijn CM, van Luijtelaar G. Effects of systemic and intracortical administration of phenytoin in two genetic models of absence epilepsy. Submitted.

Gloor P, Avoli M, Kostopoulos G. Thalamo-cortical relationships in generalized epilepsy with bilaterally synchronous spike-and-wave discharge. In: Avoli M, Gloor P, Naquet R, Kostopoulos G, eds. *Generalized Epilepsy: Neurobiological Approaches*. Boston: Birkhäuser Boston Inc, 1990: 190-212.

Gloor P. Neurophysiological bases of generalized seizures termed centrencephalic. In: Gastaud H, Jasper HH, Bancaud J, Waltregny A, eds. *The physiopathogenesis of the epilepsies*. Springfield, IL: Charles C. Thomas, 1969: 209-36.

Gloor P. Consciousness as a neurological concept in epileptology: a critical review. *Epilepsia* 1986; 27 S2: 14-26.

Golshani P, Liu XB, Jones EG. Differences in quantal amplitude reflect GluR4- subunit number at corticothalamic synapses on two populations of thalamic neurons. *Proc Natl Acad Sci USA* 2001; 98: 4172-7.

Graf M, Jakus R, Kantor S, Levay G, Bagdy G. Selective 5-HT1A and 5-HT7 antagonists decrease epileptic activity in the WAG/Rij rat model of absence epilepsy. *Neurosci Lett* 2004; 359: 45-8.

Gray CM, McCormick DA. Chattering cells: superficial pyramidal neurons contributing to the generation of synchronous oscillations in the visual cortex. *Science* 1996; 274: 109-13.

Inoue M, van Luijtelaar EL, Vossen JM, Coenen AM. Visual evoked potentials during spontaneously occurring spike-wave discharges in rats. *Electroencephalogr Clin Neurophysiol* 1992; 84: 172-9.

Inoue M, Duysens J, Vossen JM, Coenen AM. Thalamic multiple-unit activity underlying spike-wave discharges in anesthetized rats. *Brain Res* 1993; 612: 35-40.

Jakus R, Graf M, Juhasz G, Gerber K, Levay G, Halasz P, Bagdy G. 5-HT2C receptors inhibit and 5-HT1A receptors activate the generation of spike-wave discharges in a genetic rat model of absence epilepsy. *Exp Neurol* 2003; 184: 964-72.

Jasper HH, Kershman J. Electroencephalographic classification of the epilepsies. *Arch Neurol Psychiat* 1941; 45: 903-43.

Jones EG. *The thalamus*. New York: Plenium Press, 1985, 955 p.

Karpova AV, Bikbaev AF, Coenen AM, van Luijtelaar G. Morphometric Golgi study of cortical locations in WAG/Rij rats: the cortical focus theory. *Neurosci Res* 2005; 51: 119-28.

Kellaway P. Sleep and epilepsy. *Epilepsia* 1985; 26 S1: 15-30.

Kawaguchi Y, Kubota Y. GABAergic cell subtypes and their synaptic connections in rat frontal cortex. *Cereb Cortex* 1997; 7: 476-86.

Klein JP, Khera DS, Nersesyan H, Kimchi EY, Waxman SG, Blumenfeld H. Dysregulation of sodium channel expression in cortical neurons in a rodent model of absence epilepsy. *Brain Res* 2004; 1000: 102-9.

Kostopoulos G, Avoli M. Enhanced response of cortical neurons to thalamic stimuli precedes the appearance of spike and wave discharges in feline generalized penicillin epilepsy. *Brain Res* 1983; 278: 207-17.

Kostopoulos GK. Spike-and-wave discharges of absence seizures as a transformation of sleep spindles: the continuing development of a hypothesis. *Clin Neurophysiol* 2000; 111 S2: 27-38.

Liu Z, Vergnes M, Depaulis A, Marescaux C. Evidence for a critical role of GABAergic transmission within the thalamus in the genesis and control of absence seizures in the rat. *Brain Res* 1991; 545: 1-7.

Luhmann HJ, Mittmann T, van Luijtelaar G, Heinemann U. Impairment of intracortical GABAergic inhibition in a rat model of absence epilepsy. *Epilepsy Res* 1995; 22: 43-51.

Manning JP, Richards DA, Leresche N, Crunelli V, Bowery NG. Cortical-area specific block of genetically determined absence seizures by ethosuximide. *Neuroscience* 2004; 123: 5-9.

Manning JP, Richards DA, Bowery NG. Pharmacology of absence epilepsy. *Trends Pharmacol Sci* 2003 ; 24: 542-9.

Mares P, Haugvicova H, Kubova H. Unequal development of thresholds for various phenomena induced by cortical stimulation in rats. *Epilepsy Res* 2002 ; 49 : 35-43.

Marescaux C, Vergnes M, Depaulis A. Genetic absence epilepsy in rats from Strasbourg – a review. *J Neural Transm Suppl* 1992; 35: 37-69.

Markram H, Toledo-Rodriguez M, Wang Y, Gupta A, Silberberg G, Wu C. Interneurons of the neocortical inhibitory system. *Nat Rev Neurosci* 2004 ; 5 : 793-807.

Meeren HK, van Luijtelaar EL, Coenen AM. Cortical and thalamic visual evoked potentials during sleep-wake states and spike-wave discharges in the rat. *Electroencephalogr Clin Neurophysiol* 1998; 108: 306-19.

Meeren HK, van Cappellen van Walsum AM, van Luijtelaar EL, Coenen AM. Auditory evoked potentials from auditory cortex, medial geniculate nucleus, and inferior colliculus during sleep-wake states and spike-wave discharges in the WAG/Rij rat. *Brain Res* 2001; 898: 321-31.

Meeren HKM. *Cortico-thalamic mechanisms underlying generalized spike-wave discharges of absence epilepsy. A lesional and signal analytical approach in the WAG/Rij rat*. Nijmegen University, PhD thesis, 2002.

Meeren HK, Pijn JP, van Luijtelaar EL, Coenen AM, Lopes da Silva FH. Cortical focus drives widespread corticothalamic networks during spontaneous absence seizures in rats. *J Neurosci* 2002; 22: 1480-95.

Meeren H, van Luijtelaar G, Lopes da Silva F, Coenen A. Evolving concepts on the pathophysiology of absence seizures: the cortical focus theory. *Arch Neurol* 2005; 62: 371-6.

Meencke HJ. Pathology of childhood epilepsies. *Cleveland Clin J Med* 1989; 56: S111-120.

Midzianovskaia IS, Kuznetsova GD, Coenen AM, Spiridonov AM, van Luijtelaar EL. Electrophysiological and pharmacological characteristics of two types of spike-wave discharges in WAG/Rij rats. *Brain Res* 2001; 911: 62-70.

Midzyanovskaya I, Strelkov V, van Rijn CM, Budziszewska B, van Luijtelaar ELJM, Kuznetsova G. Measuring clusters of spontaneous spike-wave discharges in absence epileptic rats. *J Neurosci Methods* 2006, feb 8, Epub ahead of print.

Midzyanovskaya IS, Kuznetsova GD, van Luijtelaar ELJM, van Rijn CM, Tuomisto L, MacDonald E. The brain 5HTergic response to an acute sound stress in rats with generalized (absence and audiogenic) epilepsy. *Brain Res Bull* 2006; 69: 631-8.

Midzyanovskaya IS, Birioukova LM, Kuznetsova GD, van Luijtelaar ELJM, Tuomisto L, MacDonald E. The brain catecholaminergic response to an acute sound stress in rats with generalized (absence and audiogenic) epilepsy. subm.

Miettinen M, Koivisto E, Riekkinen P, Miettinen R. Coexistence of parvalbumin and GABA in nonpyramidal neurons of the rat entorhinal cortex. *Brain Res* 1996; 706: 113-22.

Mirsky AF Tecce, JJ. The analysis of visual evoked potentials during spike-wave EEG activity. *Epilepsia* 1968; 9: 211-20.

Neckelmann D, Amzica F, Steriade M. Spike-wave complexes and fast components of cortically generated seizures. III. Synchronizing mechanisms. *J Neurophysiol* 1998; 80: 1480-94.

Nersesyan H, Hyder F, Rothman DL, Blumenfeld H. Dynamic fMRI and EEG recordings during spike-wave seizures and generalized tonic-clonic seizures in WAG/Rij rats. *J Cereb Blood Flow Metab* 2004; 24: 589-99.

Nersesyan H, Herman P, Erdogan E, Hyder F, Blumenfeld H. Relative changes in cerebral blood flow and neuronal activity in local microdomains during generalized seizures. *J Cereb Blood Flow Metab* 2004; 24: 1057-68.

Nicolelis MA, Baccala LA, Lin RC, Chapin JK. Sensorimotor encoding by synchronous neural ensemble activity at multiple levels of the somatosensory system. *Science* 1995; 268: 353-1358.

Niedermeyer E. Primary (idiopathic) generalized epilepsy and underlying mechanisms. *Clin Electroencephalogr* 1996; 27: 1-21.

O'Brien TJ, Lige L, Wallengren C, Lohman RJ, Morris MJ. Carbamazepine aggravates absence seizures in GAERS by acting on the ventrobasal thalamus *via* GABA-A mediated mechanism, Epilepsy congress Washington, dec 2005.

Ohara PT, Lieberman AR, Hunt SP, Wu JL. Neuronal elements containing GAD in the dorsal LGN of the rat: immunocytochemical studies by light and electron microscopy. *Neurosci* 1983; 8: 189-211.

Panayiotopoulos CP. Treatment of typical absence seizures and related epileptic syndromes. *Paediatr Drugs* 2001; 3: 379-403.

Peeters BWMM, Spooren WPJM, van Luijtelaar, ELJM, Coenen, AML. The WAG/Rij model for absence epilepsy : anticonvulsant drug evaluation. *Neurosci Res Commun* 1988 ; 2 : 93-7.

Peinado MA, Quesada A, Pedrosa JA, Martinez M, Esteban FJ, Del Moral ML, Peinado JM. Light microscopic quantification of morphological changes during aging in neurons and glia of the rat parietal cortex. *Anat Rec* 1997; 247: 420-5.

Penfield WG, Jasper HH. Highest level seizures. *Assoc Res Nerv Ment Dis Proc* 1947; 26: 252-71.

Peters A, Jones EG. (eds) *Cerebral Cortex, vol. 1, Cellular Components of the Cerebral Cortex*, New York, Plenum, 1984.

Polack PO, Charpier S. Intracellular activity of cortical and thalamic neurons during High Voltage Rhythmic spike discharges in Long Evans rats *in vivo*. *J of Physiology* 2006; jan 12, Epub ahead of publication.

Pijn JP, Vijn PCM, Lopes da Silva FH, Van Ende Boas W, Blanes W. The use of signal analysis for the location of an epileptogenic focus: a new approach. *Adv Epileptology* 1989; 17: 272-6.

Riban V, Pereira de Vasconcelos A, Pham-Le BT, Ferrandon A, Marescaux C, Nehlig A, Depaulis A. Modifications of local cerebral glucose utilization in thalamic structures following injection of a dopaminergic agonist in the nucleus accumbens – involvement in antiepileptic effects? *Exp Neurol* 2004; 188: 452-60.

Rodin E. Decomposition and mapping of generalized spike-wave complexes. *Clin Neurophysiol* 1999; 110: 1868-75.

Rodin E, Ancheta O. Cerebral electrical fields during petit mal absences. *Electroencephalogr Clin Neurophysiol* 1987 ; 66: 457-66.

Sabers A, Moller A, Scheel-Kruger J, Mouritzen Dam A. No loss in total neuron number in the thalamic reticular nucleus and neocortex in the genetic absence epilepsy rats from Strasbourg. *Epilepsy Res* 1996; 26: 45-8.

Schridde U, van Luijtelaar G. The influence of strain and housing on two types of spike-wave discharges in rats. *Genes Brain Behav* 2004; 3: 1-7.

Seidenbecher T, Pape HC. Contribution of intralaminar thalamic nuclei to spike-and-wave-discharges during spontaneous seizures in a genetic rat model of absence epilepsy. *Eur J Neurosci* 2001; 13: 1537-46.

Shyukin NN, Nikolay AA, Kuznetsova GD. Spike-wave discharges and breathing pattern. In: van Luijtelaar G, Kuznetsova GD, Coenen A, Chepurnov SA, eds. *The WAG/Rij model of absence epilepsy : The Nijmegen – Russian Federation papers*. Nijmegen, Netherlands: NICI, 2004: 263-5.

Sitnikova E, van Luijtelaar G. Cortical control of generalized absence seizures: effect of lidocaine applied to the somatosensory cortex in WAG/Rij rats. *Brain Res* 2004; 1012: 127-37.

Sitnikova E, van Luijtelaar G. Reduction of adrenergic neurotransmission with clonidine aggravates spike-wave discharges and alters activity in cortex and thalamus in WAG/Rij rats. *Brain Res Bull* 2005; 64: 533-40.

Sitnikova E, van Luijtelaar G. Cortical and thalamic coherence during spike-wave seizures in WAG/Rij rats. *Epilepsy Res* 2006; in press.

Spreafico R, Mennini T, Danober L, Cagnotto A, Regondi MC, Miari A, De Blas A, Vergnes M, Avanzini G. GABA-a receptor impairment in the genetic absence epilepsy rats from Strasbourg (GAERS): an immunocytochemical and receptor binding autoradiographic study. *Epilepsy Res* 1993; 15: 229-38.

Steriade M, Amzica F. Dynamic coupling among neocortical neurons during evoked and spontaneous spike-wave seizure activity. *J Neurophysiol* 1994; 72: 2051-69.

Steriade M, Contreras D. Spike-wave complexes and fast components of cortically generated seizures. I. Role of neocortex and thalamus, *J Neurophysiol* 1998; 80: 1439-55.

Steriade M. *Neuronal substrates of sleep and epilepsy*. Cambridge, Cambridge University Press, 2003.

Strauss U, Kole MH, Brauer AU, Pahnke J, Bajorat R, Rolfs A, Nitsch R, Deisz RA. An impaired neocortical Ih is associated with enhanced excitability and absence epilepsy. *Eur J Neurosci* 2004; 19: 3048-58.

Tancredi V, Biagini G, D'Antuono M, Louvel J, Pumain R, Avoli M. Spindle-like thalamocortical synchronization in a rat brain slice preparation. *J Neurophysiol* 2000; 84: 1093-7.

Tenney JR, Duong TQ, King JA, Ferris CF. FMRI of brain activation in a genetic rat model of absence seizures. *Epilepsia* 2004; 45: 576-82.

Terman D, Bose A, Kopell N. Functional reorganization in thalamocortical networks: transition between spindling and delta sleep rhythms. *Proc Natl Acad Sci USA* 1996; 93: 15417-22.

Tolmacheva EA, van Luijtelaar G, Chepurnov SA, Kaminskij Y, Mares P. Cortical and limbic excitability in rats with absence epilepsy. *Epilepsy Res* 2004; 62: 189-98.

van de Bovenkamp-Janssen MC, Akhmadeev A, Kalimullina L, Nagaeva DV, van Luijtelaar EL, Roubos EW. Synaptology of the rostral reticular thalamic nucleus of absence epileptic WAG/Rij rats. *Neurosci Res* 2004a; 48: 21-31.

van de Bovenkamp-Janssen MC, Korosi A, Veening JG, Scheenen WJJM, van Luijtelaar ELJM, Roubos, EW. Neuronal parvalbumin and absence epilepsy in WAG/Rij rats. In: Luijtelaar G, Kuznetsova GD, Coenen AM, Chepurnov SA, eds. *The WAG/Rij model of absence epilepsy: the Nijmegen-Russian federation papers*. Van Nijmegen, the Netherlands: Nijmegen University Press, 2004b, 29-36.

van de Bovenkamp-Janssen MC, van der Kloet YC, van Luijtelaar G, Roubos EW. NMDA-R1 and-NMDA-NR1 and AMPA-GluR4 receptor subunit immunoreactivities in the absence epileptic WAG/Rij rat. *Epilepsy Research* 2006; 69: 119-28.

van Luijtelaar, ELJM, Coenen AML. Two types of electrocortical paroxysms in an inbred strain of rats. *Neurosci Lett* 1986; 70: 393-7.

van Luijtelaar EL, van der Werf SJ, Vossen JM, Coenen AM. Arousal, performance and absence seizures in rats. *Electroencephalogr Clin Neurophysiol* 1991a; 79: 430-4.

van Luijtelaar EL, de Bruijn SF, Declerck AC, Renier WO, Vossen JM, Coenen AM. Disturbances in time estimation during absence seizures in children. *Epilepsy Res* 1991b; 9: 148-53.

van Luijtelaar EL, Ates N, Coenen AM. Role of L-type calcium channel modulation in nonconvulsive epilepsy in rats. *Epilepsia* 1995; 36: 86-92.

van Luijtelaar EL, Drinkenburg WH, van Rijn CM, Coenen AM. Rat models of genetic absence epilepsy: what do EEG spike-wave discharges tell us about drug effects? *Methods Find Exp Clin Pharmacol* 2002; 24(Sl D): 65-70.

van Luijtelaar G, Azizova A, Onat F. The role of the cortex in absence epilepsy: focal and systemic effects of phenytoin. *Epilepsia* 2005; 46(S8): 304-5.

van Luijtelaar G, Sitnikova EY. Focal and global aspects of cortical control of absence seizures, the contribution of rodent models. *Neurosci Biobehav Rev* 2006; 29: Epub ahead of print].

Vergnes M, Marescaux C, Lannes B, Depaulis A, Micheletti G, Warter JM. Interhemispheric desynchronization of spontaneous spike-wave discharges by corpus callosum transection in rats with petit mal-like epilepsy. *Epilepsy Res* 1989; 4: 8-13.

Vergnes M, Marescaux C. Cortical and thalamic lesions in rats with genetic absence epilepsy. *J Neural Transm Suppl* 1992; 35: 71-83.

Warter JM, Vergnes M, Depaulis A, Tranchant C, Rumbach L, Micheletti G,Marescaux C. Effects of drugs affecting dopaminergic neurotransmission in rats with spontaneous petit mal-like seizures. *Neuropharmacol* 1988; 27: 269-74.

Willoughby JO, Mackenzie L. Nonconvulsive electrocorticographic paroxysms (absence epilepsy) in rat strains. *Lab Anim Sci* 1992; 42: 551-4.

Zhang L, Jones EG. Corticothalamic inhibition in the thalamic reticular nucleus. *J Neurophysiol* 2004; 91: 759-66.

Systems and networks in absence seizures and epilepsies in humans

Edouard Hirsch, Maria-Paola Valenti

Department of Neurology, University of Strasbourg Hospital, Strasbourg, France

---

A network is a functionally and anatomically connected set of cortical and subcortical brain regions in which activity in any one part affects activity in all others. A System is a group of independent but interrelated elements (networks) comprising a unified whole. A considerable amount of evidence supports the existence of specific cortical and subcortical networks in the genesis, expression, control of typical absences seizures (TA). Generalized seizures correspond to a manifestation whose initial semiology indicates, or is consistent with, more than minimal involvement of both cerebral hemispheres (Commission of ILAE, 1989). Spike-Waves Discharges (SWDs) in TA are characterized by a short period of increased cortical excitation corresponding to the spike on the EEG which is followed by a longer-lasting period of cortical inhibition corresponding to the wave component. Electro-clinical signs occurring during TA could result from the activation of two interdependent networks: cortico-thalamic (generation), basal ganglia (control) constituting a system *(Figure 1)*.

■ Typical absences: the symptom

Typical absences (TA), by definition, are epileptic seizures manifested with impairment of consciousness and 2.5- to 4-Hz generalized spike and slow wave discharges (Hirsch et al., 2005). Impairment of consciousness may be mild (requiring special testing) (Aarts et al., 1984; Jus et al., 1962) or severe and may be associated with other clinical manifestations, such as automatisms (Penry et al., 1969), regional or widespread myoclonia (rhythmic or random), and autonomic disturbances (Hirsch et al., 2005). Furthermore, the electroencephalographic (EEG) discharge may be brief or long, continuous or fragmented, with multiple or single spikes that are consistently associated or not associated with the slow wave. The intra discharge frequency may be relatively constant or vary (Panayiotopoulos, 2005).

Thus, the term "typical absences" does not refer to a stereotyped symptom but to a cluster of clinico-EEG manifestations that may be syndrome-related.

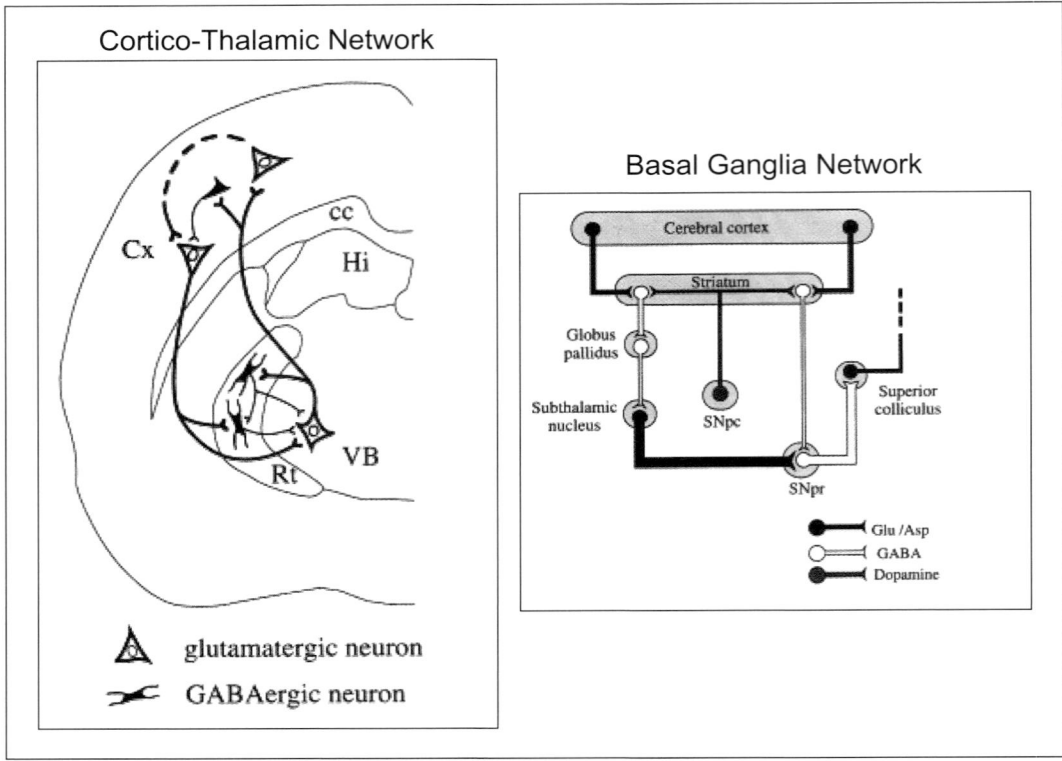

Figure 1. Left (cortico-thalamic), Right (basal ganglia) networks.

■ Epileptic syndromes with typical absences

An epileptic syndrome, by definition, requires the nonfortuitous clustering of many symptoms and signs (Commission of ILAE, 1989).

Four epileptic syndromes with TA have been recognized by the International League Against Epilepsy (Commission of ILAE, 1989): childhood absence epilepsy (CAE), juvenile absence epilepsy (JAE), juvenile myoclonic epilepsy (JME), and myoclonic absence epilepsy (MAE). The first three (CAE, JAE, JME) are considered as part of idiopathic generalized epilepsies, whereas the fourth (MAE) is categorized among the symptomatic or probably symptomatic generalized epilepsies. There may be more epileptic syndromes with TA, such as eyelid myoclonia with absences (EMA), perioral myoclonia with absences, and others awaiting further studies and confirmation (Panayiotopoulos et al., 1994). Many of these syndromes are different in presentation, severity, and prognosis.

Childhood Absence Epilepsy

Childhood Absence Epilepsy (CAE) represents an idiopathic generalized epilepsy defined as follows: "pyknolepsy" occurs in children of school age (peak manifestation age 6-7 years), with a strong genetic predisposition in otherwise normal children. It appears more frequently in girls than in boys. It is characterized by very frequent (several to many per day) absences. The EEG reveals bilateral, synchronous symmetrical spike-waves, usually 3 Hz, on a normal background activity. During adolescence, generalized tonic-clonic seizures often develop. Otherwise, absences may remit or, more rarely, persist as the only seizure type (Commission of ILAE, 1989).

This brief definition of the Commission mainly based on retrospective studies can be a source of confusion. Many authors make the arbitrary interpretation that any type of epilepsy with onset of absences in childhood corresponds to CAE. A more precise definition of childhood absence epilepsy has been recently proposed by the ILAE Task Force on Classification defining inclusion and exclusion criteria. It takes into account several important diagnostic points, such as the degree of impairment of consciousness, the morphology of spike-wave discharges and the presentation of generalized tonic-clonic seizures. Clear exclusion criteria are also proposed (Loiseau and Panayiotopoulos 2005): the presence of eyelid myoclonia (which is predominantly myoclonic with minimal consciousness impairment) and typical absence seizures consistently provoked by specific stimuli. The same applies for multiple spikes (more than three spikes per wave) that also indicate a bad prognosis and co-existent myoclonic jerks or generalized toic-clonic seizures (Panayiotopoulos *et al.*, 1989).

Juvenile Absence Epilepsy

According to the Revised International Classification of Epilepsies and Epileptic Syndromes (Commission of ILAE, 1989), Juvenile Absence Epilepsy (JAE) is one of the age-related idiopathic generalized epilepsies. The following description is given: absences in JAE have the same electroclinical characteristics as in pyknolepsy, but absences with retropulsive movements are less common. Manifestations occur around puberty. TA frequency is lower than in pyknolepsy, occurring less frequently than every day, mostly sporadically. Association with GTCS is frequent, and precedes the absence manifestations more often than in childhood absence epilepsy, often occurring on awakening. Not infrequently, the patients also have myoclonic seizures. So there is an overlap between JAE and JME.

■ Systems and networks in typical absences

Typical absence seizures are characterized by the spontaneous occurrence of Spike-Waves Discharges (SWDs) that usually occur in quiet wakefulness or drowsiness. Numerous findings (Spiegel *et al.*, 1951) support the proposal by Jasper and Kershman (1941) that the cortico-thalamic system is involved in the generation of SWDs that appears on a normal background of cortical activity. Thalamic neurons have the unique ability to shift between the oscillatory and tonic firing mode. Alertness state is characterized by a desynchronized EEG caused by the tonic firing of cortico-thalamic neurons. During the transition from wakefulness to drowsiness or sleep, firing pattern of cortico-thalamic network shifts to an oscillatory, rhythmic, synchronized mode of electrical activity which underlies the shift from a desynchronized to a synchronized state of the EEG (McCormick, 1992; Steriade *et al.*, 1993; Sherman *et al.*, 1996). Whether SWDs originate in the thalamus or the cortex is still a matter of debate. A recent study in a rat model of absence epilepsy, the WAG/Rij rat argues for a focal cortical dysfunction that drives widespread cortico-thalamic networks during spontaneous absences (Meeren et al., 2002). However, as shown in various animal models, SWDs occur only in the cortex and thalamus and cannot be recorded from limbic areas (Danober et al., 1998). Apart the cortico-thalamic network, it is demonstrated in several animal models that basal ganglia network play a role in control of TA (Danober et al., 1998; see also chapter by Paz et al. in this volume).

Systems and networks involved in the expression of symptoms during typical absence seizures in human

Signs observed during TA vary and may depend of the area of the cortex involved during cortico-thalamic network oscillations. Severe impairment of consciousness with complete loss of awareness, responsiveness and cessation of on-going activities could be explained by the involvement of the cortico-thalamic network. Clinically, the patient stops talking, eating, walking. The child may remain motionless, with vacant eyes (Loiseau & Panayiotopoulos, 2005). In some patients, SWDs are of maximal amplitude in regard of orbito-frontal or fronto-polar region (Holmes et al., 2004). Consequently, it can be speculated, that the projection of a cortico-thalamic network on orbito-frontal or fronto-polar cortices could participate to impairment of consciousness. An argument supporting this hypothesis is that "frontal pseudo absences seizures" are reported during focal seizures initiating in the fronto-polar cortex (Chauvel et al., 1995).

Mild clonic symptoms often occur during TA. These motor phenomena could be related, as in animal models (Danober et al., 1998), to an involvement of the motor cortex during cortico-thalamic network oscillation *(Figure 2)*.

Other associated ictal clinical features such as automatisms are common in TA. In *perseverative automatisms*, the patient persists in what he is doing, i.e. eating, walking, handling objects. These activities can be correctly done but are often distorted (walking more slowly, pouring water in a full glass). *De novo* automatisms are in the great majority of cases very simple: lip licking, swallowing, face rubbing, scratching, and fumbling with clothes. Sometimes, they can be more complex: catching objects, grunting, mumbling, humming or singing but are less elaborate than in focal seizures. Automatisms occur in more than 60 per cent of attacks and are related to the long duration of seizures (Penry et al., 1975). A speculative hypothesis to explain automatisms during TA is an imbalance of activation between frontal cortex and temporo-limbic cortex *(Figure 2)* as observed during ictal SPECT of TA.

Tonic up gaze is frequently reported during TA *(Figure 3)*. To our knowledge, this clinical sign does not occur in focal seizures. In humans, physiological involuntary vertical gaze movement is related to activation of brainstem structures (superior colliculus...) (Bhidayasiri et al., 2000). So, in TA, this sign could be related in short duration TA to a sustained activation of the remote control basal ganglia (nigro-striato-colliculus-thalamic) network.

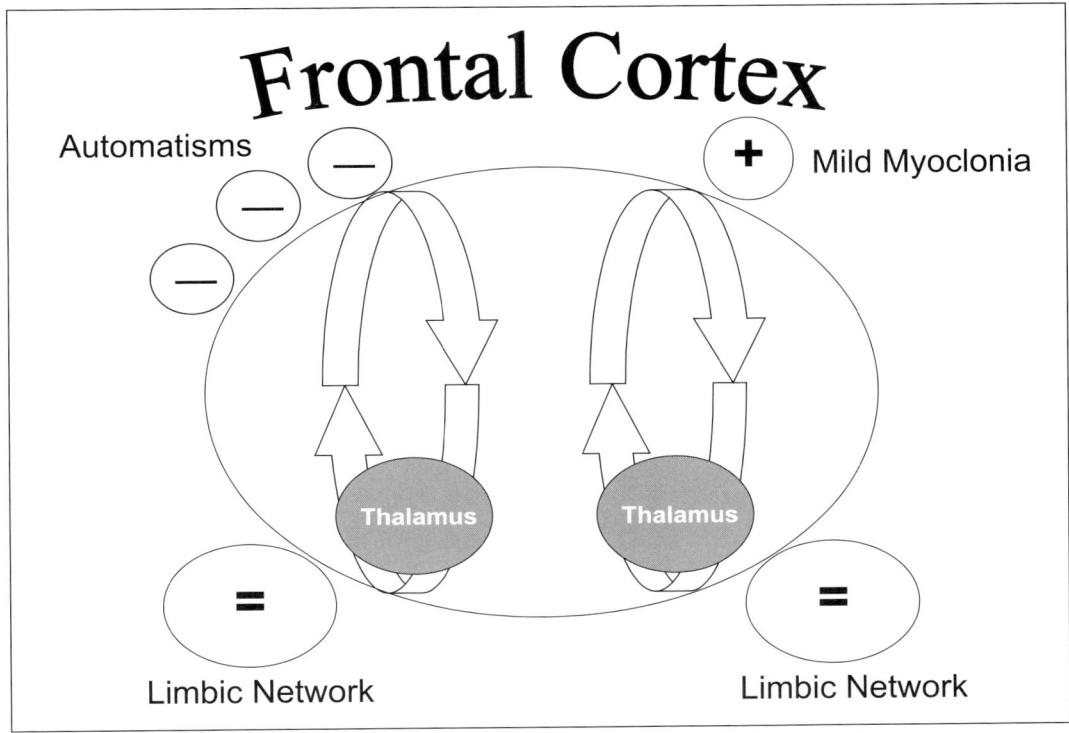

Figure 2. Pathophysiological hypothesis for Left *Automatisms* (imbalance of activation between frontal cortex and limbic cortex), Right *Mild Myoclonia* (involvement of the motor cortex during cortico-thalamic oscillation).

Functional Neuro-Imaging and typical absences in Human

[18F] fluorodeoxyglucose (FDG) tomography (PET) studies were performed during 10 minutes of hyperventilation induced TA. It was reported a 2.5- to 3.5-fold diffuse ictal increase in global glucose uptake evident when ictal studies were compared with hyperventilation control studies in which no seizures occurred (Engel et al., 1985). No specific anatomical substrate of TA was identified. The result of this pioneer work should be discussed in order that the glucose increase uptake reflects ictal and post ictal states. In a $H_2^{15}O$ PET study, Prevett et al. (1995) found a mean global increase in blood flow during TA. In addition, authors reported a focal activation of thalamus during absences which was attributed to the key role played by this structure in the pathogenesis of absence seizures. On the perfusion point of view, several studies report a decrease during absence seizures in blood flow velocities measured by transcranial Doppler ultrasonography in the middle cerebral artery of children with TA (Bode, 1992; Nehlig et al., 1996; De Simone et al., 1998; Diehl et al., 1998; Sanada et al., 1988), SPECT (Yeni et al., 2000; Nehlig et al., 2004) or by ^{133}xenon clearance technique (Sperling et al., 1995). Likewise, a decrease in cortical blood flow was measured by Laser flow Doppler technique in GAERS during each episode of SWD (Nehlig et al., 1996).

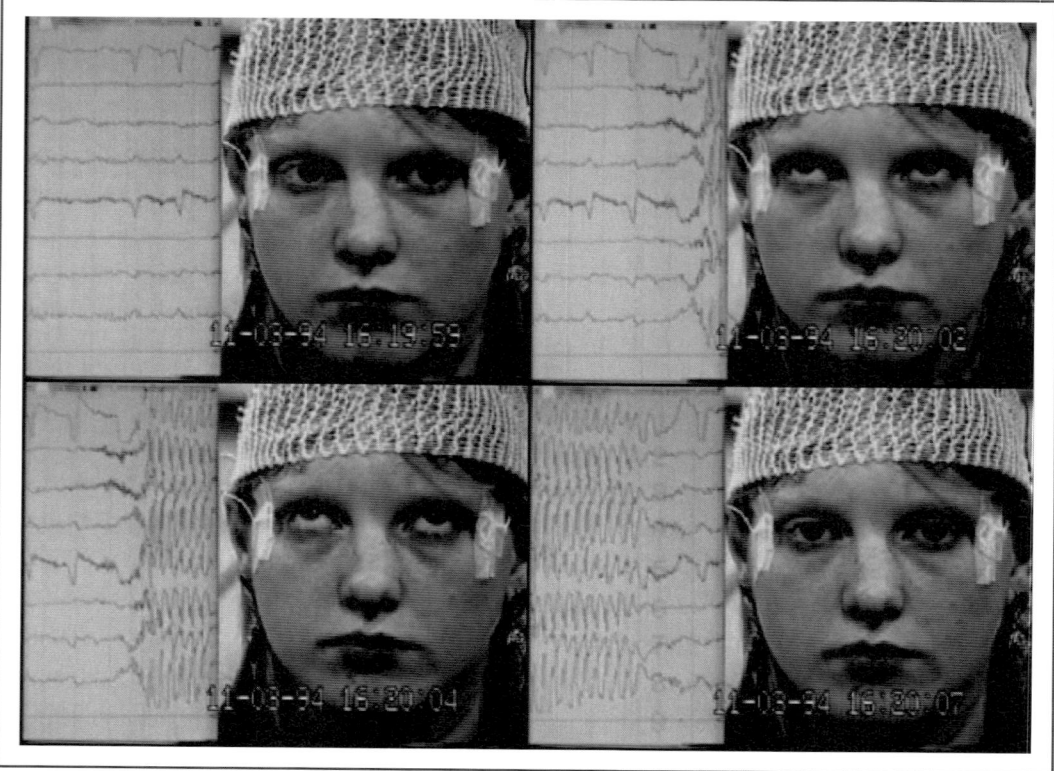

Figure 3. Typical Absence with Tonic Upgaze.

These results are in accordance with recent studies using fMRI, showing that seizure-related BOLD (blood oxygen level dependent) changes, time-locked to the occurrence of SWD induced profound negative changes in all brain areas with the exception of the thalamus (Salek-Haddadi *et al.*, 2003, Labate *et al.*, 2005).

■ Conclusion

Typical Absences represent an abnormal response pattern of cortical neurons to afferent thalamo-cortical volleys that are normally involved in the generation of spindles. SWDs are characterized by a short period of increased cortical excitation corresponding to the spike on the EEG which is followed by a longer-lasting period of cortical inhibition corresponding to the wave component. Electro-clinical signs occurring during TA could result from the activation of two interdependent cortico-thalamic and basal ganglia networks constituting a system. Clinical signs observed during TA varied and may depend of the area of the cortex involved during cortico-thalamic network oscillation. Projections of cortico-thalamic network on orbito-frontal or fronto-polar cortices could participate to impairment of consciousness. Motor phenomena could be related to an involvement of the motor cortex during cortico-thalamic network oscillation. Automatisms during TA could be related to an imbalance of activation between frontal cortex and temporo-limbic cortex. Tonic up gaze could be related to an activation of the remote control basal ganglia (nigro-striato-colliculus-thalamic) network.

References

Aarts HR, Binnie CD, Smit AM, Wilkins AJ. Selective cognitive impairment during focal and generalised epileptiform EEG activity. *Brain* 1984; 107: 293-308.

Bhidayasiri R, Plant GT, Leigh RJ. A hypothetical scheme for the brainstem control of vertical gaze. *Neurology* 2000; 54: 1985-93.

Bode H. Intracranial blood flow velocities during seizures and generalized epileptic discharges. *Eur J Pediatr* 1992; 151: 706-09.

Commission on Classification and Terminology of the International League Against Epilepsy. Proposal for revised classification of epilepsies and epileptic syndromes. *Epilepsia* 1989; 3: 389-99.

Chauvel P, Kliemann F, Vignal JP, Chodkiewicz JP, Talairach J, Bancaud J. The clinical signs and symptoms of frontal lobe seizures. Phenomenology and classification. *Adv Neurol.* 1995; 66: 115-25.

Danober L, Deransart C, Depaulis A, Vergnes M, Marescaux C. Pathophysiological mechanisms of genetic absence epilepsy in the rat. *Progr Neurobiol* 1998; 55: 27-57.

De Simone R, Silvestrini M, Marciani MG, Curatolo P. Changes in cerebral blood flow velocities during childhood absence seizures. *Pediatr Neurol* 1998; 18: 132-35.

Diehl B, Knecht S, Deppe M, Young C, Stodieck, SRG. Cerebral hemodynamic response to generalized spike-wave discharges. *Epilepsia* 1998; 39: 1284-89.

Engel J, Jr, Lubens P, Kuhl DE, Phelps ME. Local cerebral metabolic rate for glucose during petit mal absences. *Ann Neurol* 1985; 17: 121-28.

Hirsch E, Panayiotopoulos.T.Childhood absence epilepsy and related syndromes. In: Roger J, Bureau M, Dravet C, Genton P, Tassinari CA, Wolf P, eds. *Epileptic Syndromes in Infancy, Childhood and Adolescence*. Paris: John Libbey Eurotext; 2005: 315-35.

Holmes MD, Brown M, Tucker DM. Are "generalized" seizures truly generalized? Evidence of localized mesial frontal and frontopolar discharges in absence. *Epilepsia* 2004; 45: 1568-79.

Jasper H, Kershman J. Electroencephalographic classification of the epilepsies. *Arch Neurol Psychiatry* 1941; 45: 903-43.

Jus A, Jus K. Retrograde amnesia in Petit Mal. *Arch Gen Psychiatry* 1962; 6: 163-67.

Labate A, Briellmann RS, Abbott DF, Waites AB, Jackson GD. Typical childhood absence seizures are associated with thalamic activation. *Epileptic Disord.* 2005; 7: 373-77.

Loiseau P, Panayiotopoulos CP. Childhood absence epilepsy. In: Gilman S, ed,. Medlink Neurology. San Diego SA: Arbor Publishing Corp., 2005

McCormick DA. Neurotransmitter actions in the thalamus and cerebral cortex and their role in neuromodulation of thalamocortical activity. *Progr Neurobiol* 1992; 39: 337-88.

Meeren HK, Pijn JP, Van Luijtelaar EL, Coenen AM, Lopes da Silva FH. Cortical focus drives widespread corticothalamic networks during spontaneous absence seizures in rats. *J Neurosci* 2002; 22: 1480-95.

Nehlig A, Vergnes M, Waydelich R, *et al.* Absence seizures induce a decrease in cerebral blood flow: human and animal data. *J Cereb Blood Flow Metab* 1996; 16: 147-55.

Nehlig A, Valenti MP, Thiriaux A, Hirsch E, Marescaux C, Namer IJ. Ictal and interictal perfusion variations measured by SISCOM analysis in typical childhood absence seizures. *Epileptic Disord* 2004; 6: 247-253.

Panayiotopoulos CP, Obeid T, Waheed G. Absences in juvenile myoclonic epilepsy: a clinical and video-electroencephalographic study. *Ann Neurol* 1989; 25: 391-97.

Panayiotopoulos CP, Ferrie CD, Giannakodimos S, Robinson RO. Perioral myoclonia with absences: a new syndrome? In: Wolf P, ed. *Epileptic Seizures and Syndromes*. London: John Libbey; 1994: 143-53.

Panayiotopoulos CP. Idiopathic generalised epilepsies. In: Panayiotopoulos CP, editor. The epilepsies: seizures, syndromes and management.Oxford: Bladon Med 2005: 271-348.

Penry JK, Dreifuss FE. Automatisms associated with the absence of petit mal epilepsy. *Arch Neurol* 1969; 21: 1942-49.

Penry JK, Porter RJ, Dreifuss RE. Simultaneous recording of absence seizures with video tape and electroencephalography. A study of 374 seizures in 48 patients. *Brain.* 1975; 98: 427-40.

Prevett MC, Duncan JS, Jones T, Fish DR, Brooks DJ. Demonstration of thalamic activation during typical absence seizures using $H_2^{15}O$ and PET. *Neurology* 1995; 45: 1396-02.

Salek-Haddadi A, Lemieux L, Merschhemke M, Friston KJ, Duncan JS, Fish DR. Functional magnetic resonance imaging of human absence seizures. *Ann Neurol.* 2003; 53: 663-67.

Sanada S, Murakami N, Ohtahara S. Changes in blood flow of the middle cerebral artery during absence seizures. *Pediatr Neurol* 1988; 4: 158-61.

Sherman SM, Guillery RW. Functional organization of thalamocortical relays. *J Neurophysiol* 1996; 76: 1367-95.

Sperling MR, Skolnick BE. Cerebral blood flow during spike-wave discharges. *Epilepsia* 1995; 36: 156-63.

Spiegel EA, Wycis HT, Reyes V. Diencephalic mechanisms in petit mal epilepsy. *EEG Clin Neurophysiol* 1951; 3: 473-75.

Steriade M, McCormick DA, Sejnowski TJ. Thalamocortical oscillations in the sleeping and aroused brain. *Science* 1993; 262: 679-85.

Yeni SN, Labasakal L, Yalcinkaya C, Nisli C, Dervent A. Ictal and interictal SPECT findings in childhood absence epilepsy. *Seizure* 2000; 9: 265-9.

Spike-wave seizures in corticothalamic systems

Mircea Steriade

Laboratoire de Neurophysiologie, Faculté de Médecine, Université Laval, Québec, Canada

---

Data in this chapter will conclude that electrical seizures with spike-wave (SW) complexes are generated within the neocortex, that they do not occur suddenly but obey the rule of progressive synaptic buildup *via* short- and long-range projection pathways, and that they are associated with inhibition of thalamocortical (TC) neurons, due to cortically evoked excitation of GABAergic thalamic reticular (RE) neurons. This view challenges the classical assumption that SW seizures are suddenly generalized and it also refutes recent *in vitro* results placing emphasis on the thalamus as generator of these paroxysms. SW complexes at 3-4 Hz are the electrographic correlate of absence epilepsy. In the Lennox-Gastaut syndrome pattern (LGS), SW complexes have a lower frequency (1.5-2.5 Hz), often take the form of polyspike-wave (PSW), and are accompanied by fast runs (10-20 Hz). The neuronal substrates of SW/PSW complexes in absence-type seizures and LGS pattern are the same. Although data from our group and other teams were obtained using intracellular and field potential recordings from cortical and thalamic neurons in different animal preparations, the results on the cortical generation of SW seizures in absence epilepsy and LGS are supported by human studies using global methods (see below).

■ Cortical initiation of SW seizures

That SW seizures are generated in the neocortex in the absence of the thalamus was demonstrated in cat by the presence of such electrical paroxysms after thalamectomy (Steriade and Contreras, 1998). In those experiments, bicuculline (an antagonist of $GABA_A$ receptors) was injected in restricted thalamic territories in order to determine the possible co-participation of the thalamus in SW seizures. About 20 minutes after an injection of bicuculline, the number of action potentials per spike-burst during sleep spindles increased, the repetition rate of spike-bursts decreased, the synchrony of spike-bursts between cells increased, and cortical EEG also showed a slowed frequency and increased amplitude of spindles, but no paroxysmal pattern compared to the bona fide SW seizures occurred (Steriade and Contreras, 1998). This result is similar to observations made in rats, in which thalamic injections of bicuculline gave rise to hypersynchronous and slow spindles, but not to SW seizures (Castro-Alamancos, 1999). Importantly, in chronically implanted athalamic monkeys, SW seizures discharges were associated with impairment of awareness during the SW complexes (Marcus et al., 1968). All the above data demonstrate that seizures with SW complexes at about 3 Hz, accompanied by behavioral signs that are similar to those occurring in human *petit mal* epilepsy, may be generated in the absence of the thalamus.

In humans, macaque monkeys and cats, SW seizures mainly occur during drowsiness or light slow-wave sleep (Steriade, 1974; Kellaway, 1985; Steriade et al., 1998a; Shouse, 2001) but not in REM sleep (Frank, 1969). The transition from slow-wave sleep or anesthesia patterns of electrical activity to SW seizures is progressive and the paroxysms often appear without discontinuity from the normal slow sleep oscillations (see *Figure 3*). In keeping with the idea that such seizures may develop without discontinuity from the slow sleep oscillation, wave-triggered averages during hypsarrhythmia show that the relationships between field potential and intracellular activities are very similar during the epoch preceding the seizure and during the seizure, the only difference being the increased amplitude and frequency of SW complexes, compared to the alternating depolarization-hyperpolarization sequences during the slow oscillation (Amzica and Steriade, 1999). The seizure evolves with a progressive neuronal depolarization that reaches a maximum value during the fast runs. In general, SW seizures are dramatically reduced or abolished with transition from slow-wave sleep to spontaneous or sensory-elicited arousal as well as during repetitive brainstem reticular formation stimulation, and they are increased after administration of low doses of a cholinergic receptor antagonist (Danober et al., 1993, 1995).

Multi-site recordings of intracellular activities, extracellular discharges and field potentials showed time-lags as short as 3-10 ms, but up to 50 ms or longer (100-150 ms) intervals between various neocortical areas during SW seizures (Steriade and Amzica, 1994). The degree of synchrony progressively increases from pre-seizure (sleep-like) patterns to the early stage of the paroxysm and, further, to its late stage. A typical SW seizure may start in cortical association area 7, is followed by tonic depolarization and rhythmic spike-bursts in a neuron from area 5 (which is connected monosynaptically with area 7), is further reflected by field EEG potentials recorded from motor area 4, only lastly reaching the thalamus (*Figure 1*). As shown below, however, most TC neurons do not fire during cortically generated seizures. Dual intracellular recordings during spontaneous seizures reinforced the notion of intracortical synchronization of SW seizures (Neckelmann et al., 1998). The synaptic delays between corresponding events in simultaneously recorded cortical neurons were reduced during spontaneously occurring seizures, as compared to the preceding epochs of slow sleep oscillation. The range of values observed during seizures had decreased variability, as well as a central tendency closer to zero. This was most pronounced for the 3-Hz SW complexes. Thus, SW seizures obey the rule of sequential distribution through synaptic pathways, initiated within given cortical fields, spreading to other cortical areas, and eventually to thalamus.

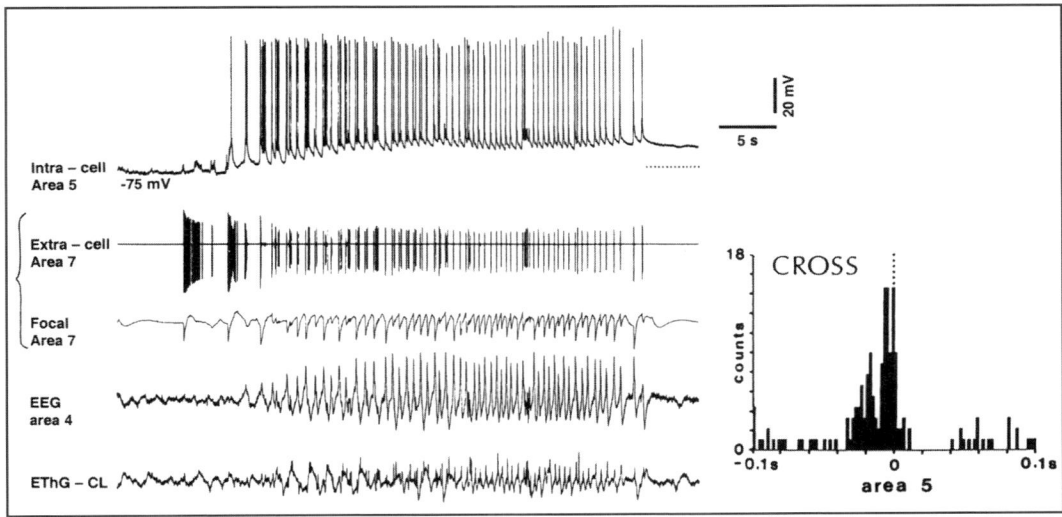

Figure 1. Intracortical and corticothalamic relations during spontaneously occurring electrical seizure with SW complexes at ~2 Hz. Cat under urethane anesthesia. Five simultaneously recorded traces represent intracellular recording from area 5 neuron, unit discharges and field potentials from area 7, EEG from postcruciate area 4, and EThG (electrothalamogram) from ipsilateral thalamic rostral intralaminar centrolateral (CL) nucleus. Dotted line at extreme right of intracellular recording indicates membrane potential before the seizure (-75 mV). At right, cross-correlogram between areas 7 and 5 neurons. Further explanations in text. Modified from Steriade and Amzica (1994).

These data show that cortical SW seizures are *not* generated simultaneously over widespread territories in thalamocortical systems but arise in neocortical areas in which metabolic and network factors render neurons more excitable. With simultaneous intracellular and field potential recordings from different neocortical areas, we observed progressively increased amplitudes of excitatory postsynaptic potentials (EPSPs), leading to action potentials in one area, hundreds of milliseconds or even seconds preceding the first overt paroxysmal depolarization in other areas, which preceded the appearance of full-blown SW seizures (Steriade *et al.*, 2003; Timofeev and Steriade, 2004). EEG recordings in humans with absence epilepsy have also presented evidence for independent sources of these paroxysms (Petsche, 1962; Rodin, 1999).

The development of epileptiform activity may result from either overexcitation due to blockage of inhibition (by focal injection of inhibition blockers, *e.g.* bicuculline) or disfacilitation (produced by deafferentation procedures that mainly interrupt excitatory pathways). The latter factor was much less explored than the former in epilepsy research and we recently focused on it. It is indeed known that reduction in synaptic activity within some cortical foci leads to increase in the sensitivity of cortical neurons in those and surrounding areas (Abbott *et al.*, 1997; Desai *et al.*, 1999). The deafferentation as factor underlying SW seizures is in line with experimental and clinical evidence that such seizures preferentially occur during transition from waking to slow-wave sleep or during slow-wave sleep, states that are characterized by the presence of long-lasting periods of disfacilitation associated with neuronal hyperpolarization (Steriade, 2003). Also, penetrating wounds in humans (Dinner, 1993) or experimental deafferentation through cortical undercut (Topolnik et al., 2003a-b) are factors that promote seizures. In these cases, many axons impinging onto postsynaptic neurons are damaged, which creates a partial deafferentation and enhances the effectiveness of incoming synaptic inputs. The changing patterns of the slow sleep oscillation and its tendency to develop into seizure activity consisting of SW complexes at 2-4 Hz was investigated at different time-intervals after cortical undercut (Nita et al., 2006). Multi-site field potentials and single or dual intracellular recordings from the whole extent of the deafferented cortical gyrus were used. The field and neuronal components of the slow sleep-like oscillation increased in amplitudes and were transformed into paroxysmal patterns, expressed by increased firing rates and tendency to neuronal bursting. The propagation delay of low-frequency activities decreased, with transition from semi-acute (week 1) to chronic (up to week 5) stages following cortical undercut (Figure 2).

Among different cortical neuronal types, characterized intracellularly by their responses to depolarizing current pulses, fast-rhythmic-bursting (FRB) neurons have the highest propensity to develop seizures. Ripples are generated within the neocortex, as shown by their occurrence in isolated neocortical slabs in vivo (Grenier et al., 2001, 2003). These neurons fire high-frequency (300-400 Hz) spike-bursts at fast rates (30-40 Hz), are located in all layers from 2 to 6, and are pyramidal-shaped as well as local-circuit basket-type cells (Steriade et al., 1998b). The evidence that FRB neurons (20-25% of the total cortical neuronal population) have a decisive role in the generation of cortical seizure activity is the following. (a) FRB neurons have a major role in triggering very fast oscillations (80-200 Hz, but also higher frequencies), termed ripples, whose presence at the onset of seizures in epileptic patients has led to the proposal that they could be involved in their initiation (Fisher et al., 1992; Traub et al., 2001). The selective occurrence of FRB neurons over the depolarizing component of the slow sleep oscillation and the progressively increased firing during this phase appears in parallel with increased amplitudes of ripples (Figure 3). The slow oscillation develops without discontinuation into SW/PSW seizures (see Figure 4). There is a close relationship between the fast action potentials of FRB neurons and the wavelets of ripples during paroxysmal PSW complexes (Figure 3). (b) In the case of Lennox-Gastaut seizures, regular-spiking cortical neurons fire single action potentials or spike-doublets during either the EEG "spike" component of SW/PSW complexes or the fast runs, whereas FRB neurons discharge spike-bursts consisting of 6-7 action potentials during SW/PSW complexes and the fast runs (Figure 4).

Cortical neuronal substrates of SW complexes and fast runs

The neuronal mechanisms underlying the generation of the "spike" and "wave" field components of SW complexes, which have been investigated intracellularly in animal experiments, are virtually identical in seizures consisting of only SW complexes, as in absence epilepsy, and in those paroxysms resembling the patterns of the clinical Lennox-Gastaut syndrome.

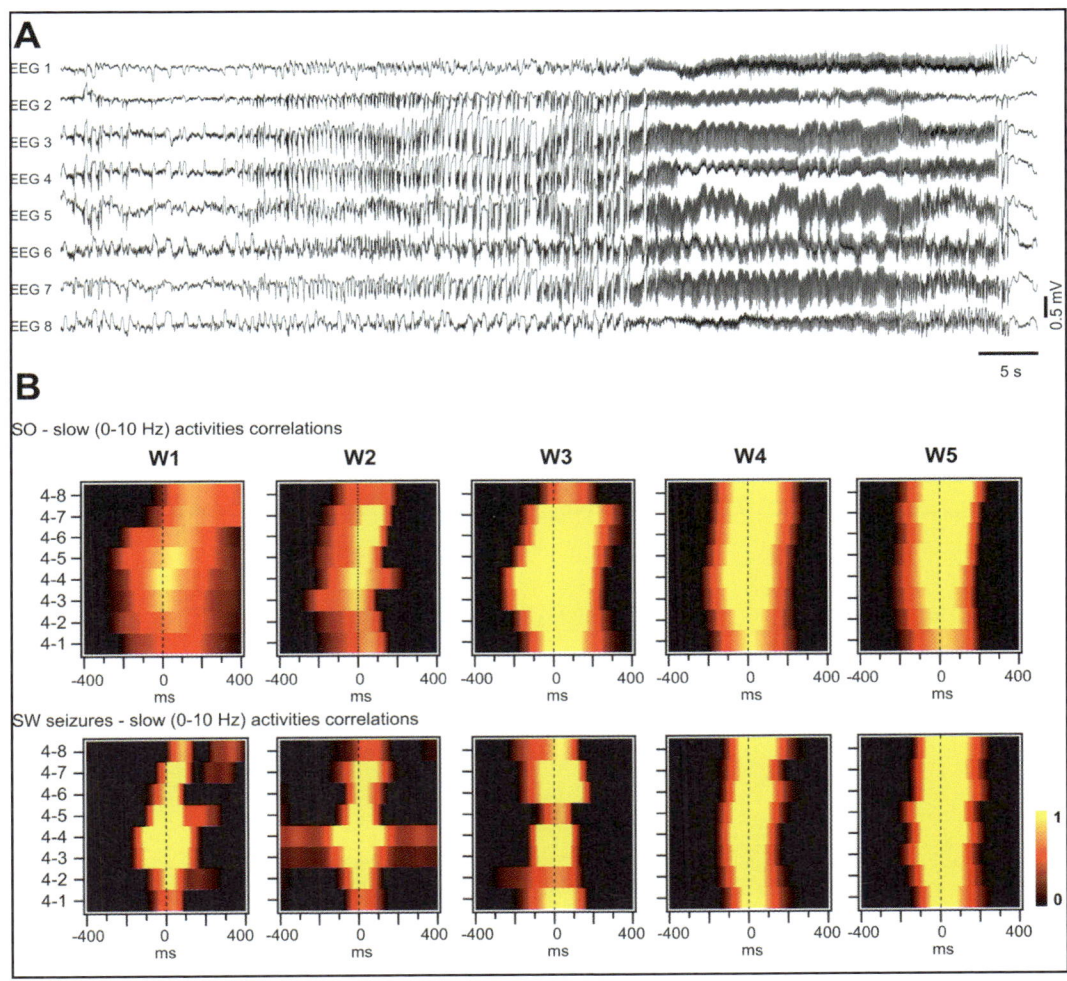

Figure 2. Faster propagation of seizures in deafferented cortex of cat from week 1 (W1) to week 5 (W5). Time correlations across different cortical leads and from W1 to W5 during slow oscillation and seizures. Ketamine-xylazine anesthesia. *A*, development of seizure during W4 consisting of SW/PSW complexes and finishing with fast runs over electrodes EEG1 to EEG8. Note that seizure started in anterior leads (EEG1 to EEG4) and then propagated more posteriorly. *B*, spatio-temporal properties of the slow oscillation (SO) and SW/PSW seizures in the deafferented cortex. One cat is depicted for each week (W1 to W5). Cross-correlations were performed between the most anterior electrode where the seizures occur first (EEG4) and the rest of the electrodes placed over the suprasylvian gyrus. Signal was filtered in the 0-10 Hz range. For both the paroxysmal slow oscillation and the SW/PSW seizures the time-lags diminished from W1 to W5, and the propagation was faster during seizures compared with the paroxysmal slow oscillation (during W1 to W4). Modified from Nita *et al.* (2006).

I shall discuss the contribution of excitatory and inhibitory neurons to the depolarizing ("spike") and hyperpolarizing ("wave") field components of SW/PSW complexes, the neuronal responsiveness during SW/PSW complexes, the cellular mechanisms underlying the fast runs, and the temporal relations between neurons and glial cells.

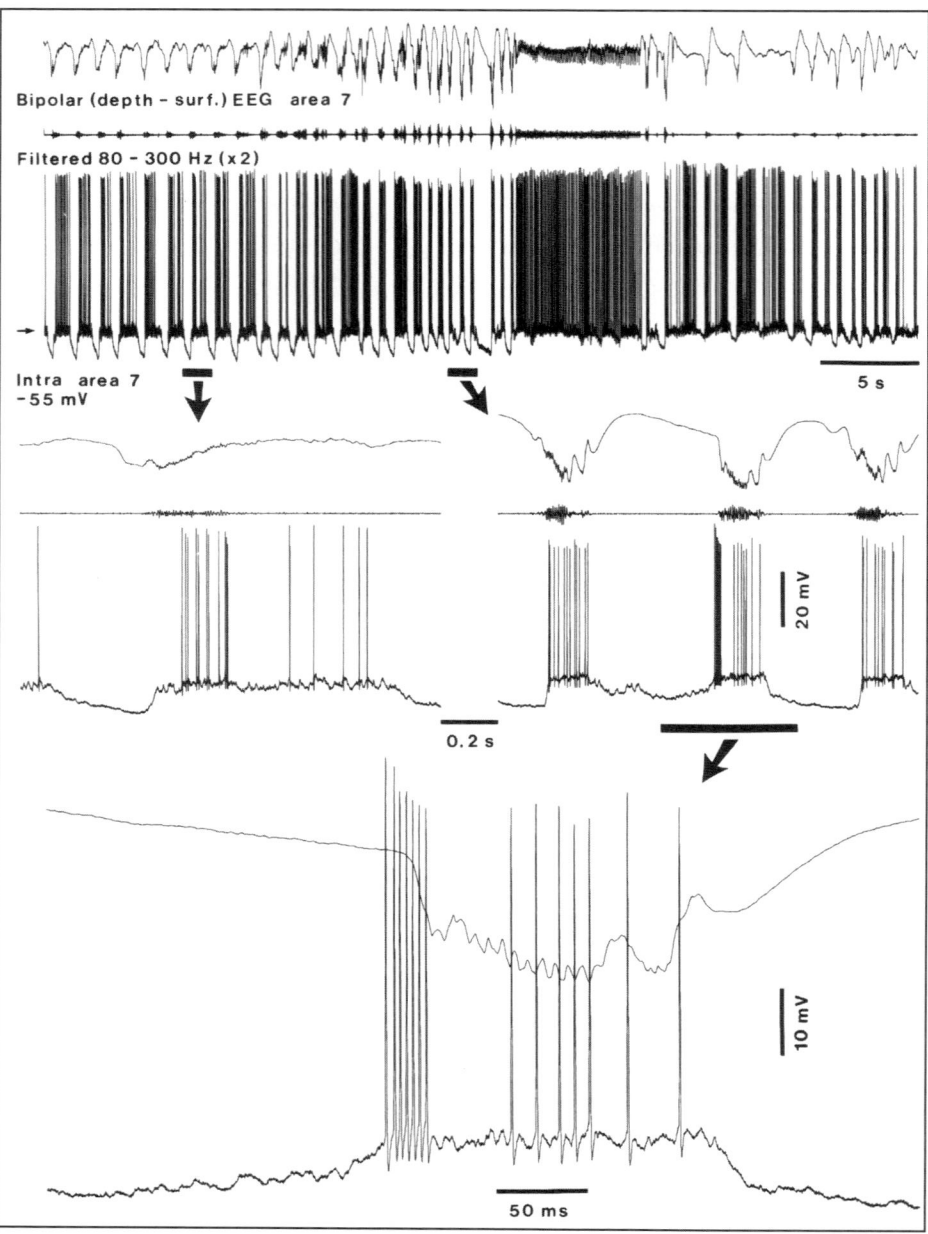

Figure 3. Fast ripples (120 Hz) during spontaneously occurring neocortical seizure. Cat under ketamine-xylazine anesthesia. Intracellular and EEG recording from area 4. Fast-rhythmic-bursting neuron (identified as in *Figure 4*). The 2nd trace in the top panel is depth-EEG filtered for fast events (80-300 Hz) and amplified. Two horizontal bars (below the intracellular trace) indicate the slow sleep-like oscillation (left) and the seizure (right), and are expanded below (arrows). One cycle of the seizure is further expanded below (arrow). Note close time-relation between the action potentials and EEG ripples. Modified from Steriade *et al.* (1998a).

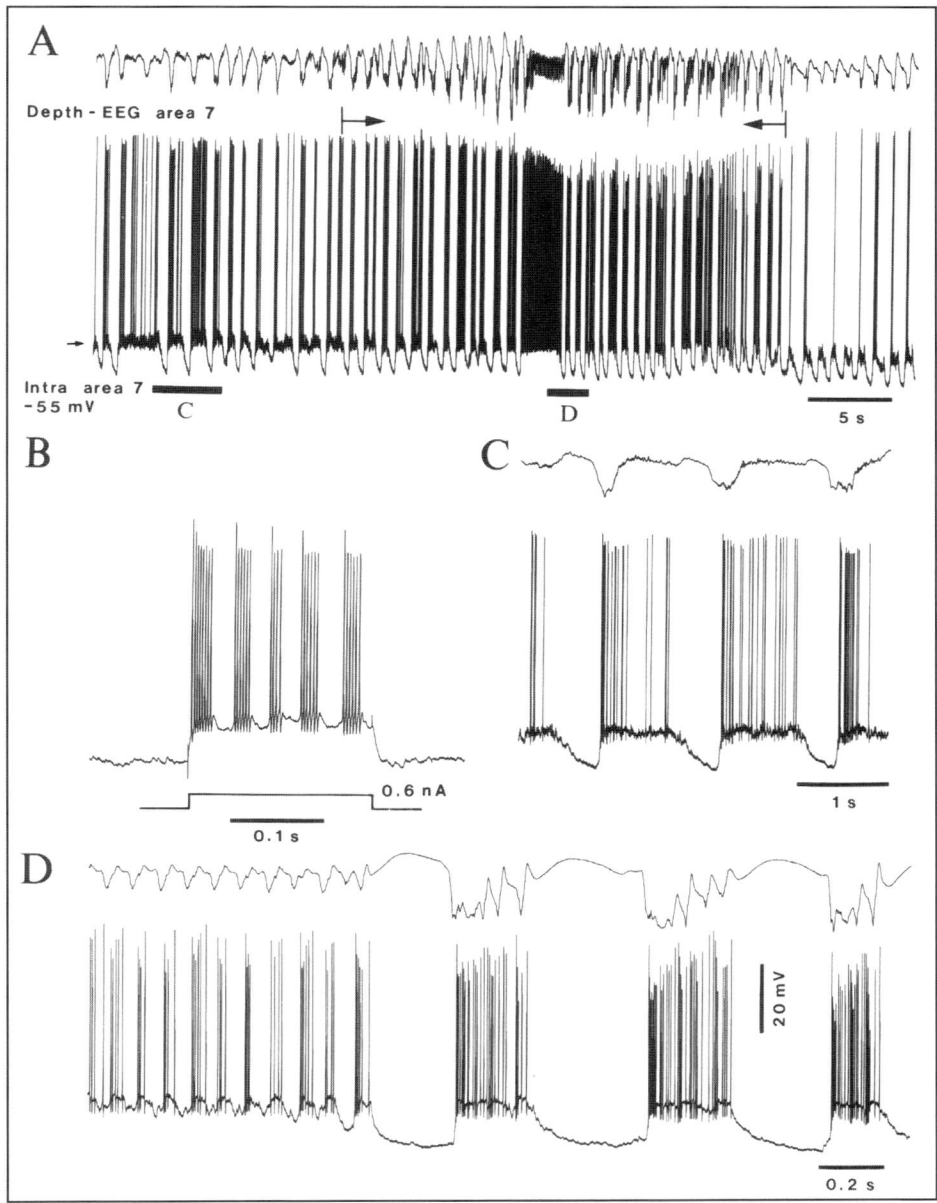

Figure 4. Fast-rhythmic-bursting (FRB) cortical neuron during seizure with polyspike-wave (PSW) complexes and fast runs developing spontaneously from slow sleep-like oscillation. Cat under ketamine-xylazine anesthesia. *A*, top panel illustrates intracellular and depth-EEG recording from cortical area 7. The seizure is indicated by arrows (below the EEG trace) and lasted for ~26 s. *B*, electrophysiological identification of FRB neuron by depolarizing current pulse. *C-D*, expanded periods from parts indicated in the top panel. Panel *C* depicts the slow oscillation before the seizure. Panel *D* shows both fast runs (12 Hz) and PSW complexes (2 Hz). Note high-frequency spike-bursts in neuron during each depth-negativity of fast EEG runs and during components of PSW complexes. Modified from Steriade *et al.* (1998a).

The "spike" component of SW complexes corresponds intracellularly to the paroxysmal depolarizing shift (PDS) (reviewed in McCormick and Contreras, 2001). Firstly isolated, as interictal "spikes", PDSs become rhythmic and progressively evolve into full-blown SW paroxysms (Neckelmann et al., 1998). The PDSs have initially been regarded as giant EPSPs (Johnston and Brown, 1981), enhanced by activation of voltage-dependent currents. The presence of inhibitory processes within the PDS was reported in subsequent experimental studies on animals (Traub et al., 1996; Prince and Jacobs, 1998) as well as in work on human slices maintained in vitro (Cohen et al., 2002). The depolarizing phase of paroxysmal discharges contains a Cl⁻-dependent component that is associated with firing of fast-spiking (FS, presumably local inhibitory) cortical neurons and FS neurons fire at very high frequencies during the PDSs of SW complexes (Timofeev et al., 2002a). Thus, active inhibitory mechanisms participate in the generation of the depolarization component of SW complexes. The inhibitory component in the PDS accounts for the diminished excitability of neocortical neurons to antidromic and synaptic volleys during the "spike" component of SW complexes (Steriade and Amzica, 1999). The decreased responsiveness of neocortical neurons during the PDS is corroborated by a significant decrease in the apparent input resistance during this component of SW complexes (Neckelmann et al., 2000; Timofeev et al., 2002a).

Earlier studies assumed that the "wave" component of SW complexes reflects summated inhibitory postsynaptic potentials (IPSPs) due to GABAergic actions triggered in cortical pyramidal neurons by local-circuit inhibitory cells (Pollen, 1964; Giaretta et al., 1987) and computational models predicted that the "wave" is produced by $GABA_B$-mediated IPSPs (Destexhe, 1998). If so, a decreased input resistance would be detected during the "wave" component. However, the opposite was found during SW seizures in both rat genetic models of absence epilepsy and spontaneous SW seizures in cats (Charpier et al., 1999; Neckelmann et al., 2000; Staak and Pape, 2001; Crunelli and Leresche, 2002). Regarding the hypothesis that $GABA_B$-mediated IPSPs underlie the "wave" component of SW seizures, blocking the G-protein-coupled $GABA_B$-evoked K^+ current did not significantly affect the hyperpolarization in our experiments (see Timofeev and Steriade, 2004). Together, these data suggest that GABA-mediated currents are not important for the hyperpolarization during these cortically generated seizures. The factors generating the "wave" of the SW complexes are some Ca^{2+}-dependent K^+ currents and, especially, disfacilitation (Charpier et al., 1999; Neckelmann et al., 2000) due to the silenced firing of cortical and thalamic neurons.

During the fast runs, which accompany SW/PSW complexes LGS pattern, regular-spiking neurons, which represent the majority of cortical neurons, are steadily depolarized (due to the reduced or silenced firing of local inhibitory cells) that often leads to their spike inactivation *(Figure 5)*.

Considering together the synaptic and intrinsic ionic currents activated by neocortical neurons during SW complexes, the PDS related to the "spike" consists of summated EPSPs and IPSPs as well as an intrinsic current, $I_{Na(p)}$, which was revealed by diminished depolarization in recordings with a blocker of Na^+ current in the recording pipette. The hyperpolarization, related to the "wave", is a combination of K^+ currents,

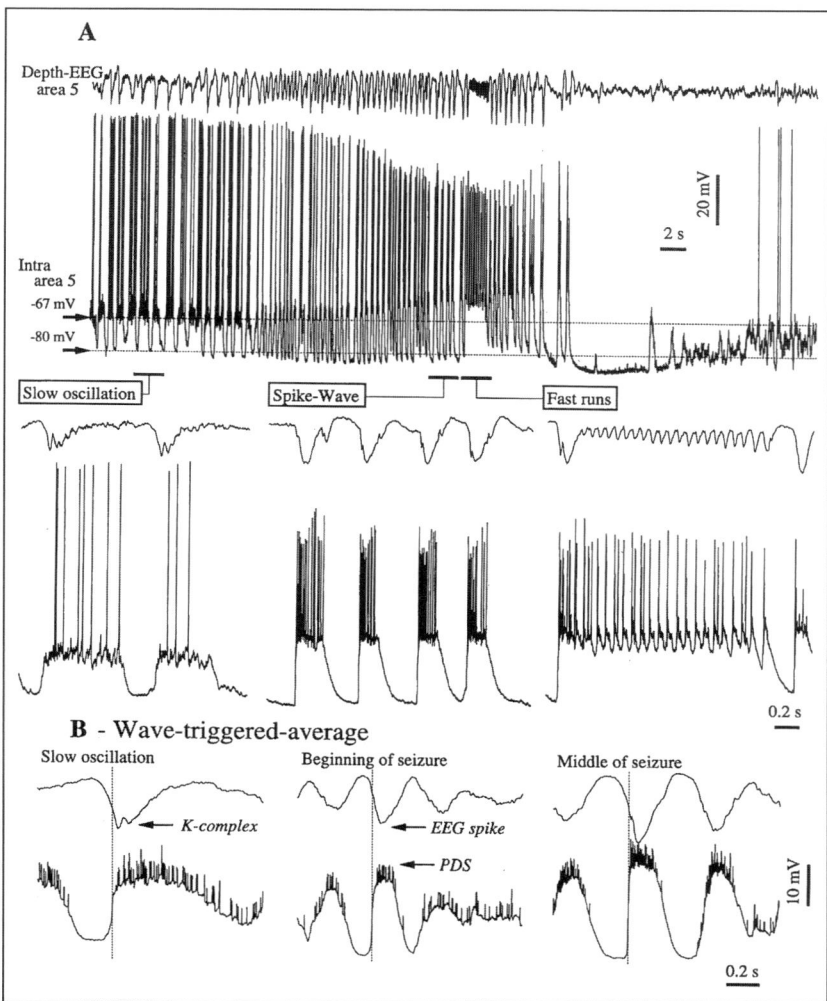

Figure 5. Spontaneously occurring seizure of Lennox-Gastaut pattern type, developing without discontinuity from slow sleep-like oscillation. Similar field-cellular relations during sleep and different components of seizure. Tonic depolarization of cortical neuron during fast runs. Cat under ketamine-xylazine anesthesia. Intracellular recording from regular-spiking area 5 neuron together with depth-EEG from the vicinity in area 5. *A*, smooth transition from slow oscillation to complex seizure consisting of SW complexes at ~2 Hz and fast runs at 15 Hz. The seizure lasted for 25 s. Epochs of slow oscillation preceding the seizure, SW complexes, and fast runs are indicated and expanded below. Note postictal depression (hyperpolarization) in the intracellularly recorded neuron (6 s), associated with suppression of EEG slow oscillation (compare to left part of trace). *B*, wave-triggered-average during the slow oscillation, at the beginning of seizure and during the middle part of seizure. Averaged activity was triggered by the steepest part of the depolarizing component in cortical neuron (dotted lines), during the three epochs. The depth-negative field component of the slow oscillation (associated with cell's depolarization) is termed K-complex. During the seizure, the depolarizing component reaches the level of a paroxysmal depolarizing shift, associated with an EEG "spike". Modified from Steriade *et al.* (1998a).

due to the strong depolarization during the PDS, which supports abundant entry of Na$^+$ and Ca^{2+} into neurons. The hyperpolarization-activated depolarizing sag, due to I$_H$, leads to a new paroxysmal cycle (Timofeev et al., 2002b; Timofeev and Steriade, 2004). Thus, the next paroxysmal cycle originates, at least partically, from the excitation driven by I$_H$ that follows the neuronal silence during the "wave" component in the SW complex.

Finally, glial cells may play a role in cortical seizures through a dialogue with neurons. Most evidence showing that glial cells are endowed with receptors for, and release of, some neurotransmitters stems at this time from experiments in cultures or in slices maintained *in vitro* (Bormann and Kettenmann, 1988; Steinhäuser and Gallo, 1996). Dual intracellular recordings from neurons and glial cells during SW/PSW seizures *in vivo* showed that maximal glial depolarization is reached later than the end of the neuronal depolarization (Amzica and Steriade, 2000). However, the propagation of seizure activity in neocortex through the glial syncytium (Amzica et al., 2002) may contribute to the increased inter-neuronal synchrony during development from the slow sleep oscillation to seizures.

■ Thalamic reticular and thalamocortical cells: opposite behaviors during SW seizures

Absence seizures are defined as a paroxysmal loss of consciousness, with abrupt and sudden onset and offset, without aura or postictal state, accompanied by tonic deviation of gaze. The term absence is only valid for those seizures that occur during wakefulness because during natural sleep, when there is an increased incidence of such paroxysms (see above), or in experimental animals under anesthesia, the subjects prone to these seizures are already quite absent. The definition of these seizures as suddenly generalized and bilaterally synchronous stemmed from the concept of a "centrencephalic" system that would produce bilaterally synchronous SW complexes. However, there are no bilaterally projecting thalamic neurons and brainstem reticular activating neurons rather disrupt SW seizures. Facing the repeated evidence that the "centrencephalic system" cannot account for the generation of generalized seizures and impairment of consciousness, Penfield subsequently excluded the exclusive emphasis on the thalamus and other deeply located structures: "It would be absurd to suppose that this central integration could take place without implication of cortical areas" (cited in a historical note by Jasper, 1990, p. 3-4). A series of experimental studies, discussed above, point to the progressive build-up of SW/PSW seizures at ~3 Hz that obey the rule of synaptic circuits, sequentially distributed through short- and long-range circuits in corticocortical and corticothalamic synaptic networks. Earlier and more recent EEG studies and toposcopic analyses in humans and animals have also indicated that some SW seizures are locally generated and result from multiple, independent cortical foci and topographical analyses of SW complexes in humans showed that the "spike" component of SW complexes propagates from one hemisphere to another with time-lags as short as 15 ms (Lemieux and Blume, 1986; Kobayashi et al., 1994), which cannot be estimated by visual inspection.

The origin of SW seizures within the thalamus or cortex was and continues to be hotly debated. That neocortical excitability represents the leading factor in controlling thalamic events during this type of seizures was documented above.

The two major types of thalamic neurons, which are present in all mammals, are thalamocortical (TC) and thalamic reticular (RE) cells. The former are glutamatergic, thus excitatory, while the latter are GABAergic, thus inhibitory. TC neurons are bushy and their variations are linked mainly to soma size, large neurons projecting to deep and middle cortical layers, whereas small neurons project preferentially to superficial cortical layers. RE neurons have long dendrites, whose secondary and tertiary branches possess vesicle-containing appendages that form synapses on the dendrites of neurons in the same nucleus. It is likely that the long dendrites of RE neurons (up to 1.5-2 mm along the curved axis of the nucleus) are impaired when slices are prepared for studies *in vitro*. Contrary to TC neurons that can communicate only through intermediary of RE or neocortical neurons, RE neurons form an interconnected network (through dendro-dendritic and axo-dendritic connections as well as gap junctions) which is particularly well suited for the generation of some oscillatory types which can occur even in isolated RE nucleus (see Steriade, 2003).

Thalamic reticular and thalamocortical neurons display opposite behaviors during SW seizures. The former are excited and follow faithfully every neocortical PDSs, whereas the latter are inhibited during SW seizures. This is surprising because the corticothalamic axons contact both RE and TC neurons, and the glutamatergic nature of this pathway would implicate excitation at both thalamic targets. The issue is that the numbers of glutamate receptor subunits GluR4 are 3.7 times higher at corticothalamic synapses in RE neurons, compared to TC neurons, and that the mean peak amplitude of corticothalamic excitatory postsynaptic currents (EPSCs) is about 2.5 higher in RE, than in TC, neurons (Golshani *et al.*, 2001). The data mentioned below demonstrate the contrast between RE-cells and TC-cells during SW seizures.

Simultaneous recordings of cortical EEG and RE neurons revealed that spontaneous cortical seizures with SW/PSW complexes at 2-4 Hz, developing without discontinuity from sleep-like patterns, are associated with spike-bursts in RE neurons, which follow each paroxysmal "spike" in cortical EEG *(Figure 6)*. The usual spike-bursts (duration 40 ms) of RE neuron during sleep-like patterns, prior to the paroxysmal episode, developed into longer-duration spike-bursts (200 ms) during the initial part of the seizure with SW complexes at 2 Hz. Thereafter, reduced duration of RE-cell's spike-bursts occurred during the cortical SW complexes at 4 Hz. That RE neurons follow without failure, with prolonged spike-bursts, each cortical paroxysmal discharge during SW seizures was also demonstrated intracellularly (Timofeev *et al.*, 1998). In sum, then, GABAergic RE neurons participate actively during cortically generated SW seizures. This conclusion is drawn from cellular data showing an increased propensity to bursting of RE cells during SW seizures (Steriade and Contreras, 1995; Steriade and Timofeev, 2001), the increase in the ionic current underlying spike-bursts of RE cells in these seizures (Tsakiridou *et al.*, 1995; Avanzini *et al.*, 1999), and the fact that the Cd^{2+}-induced blockage of RE-cells' spike-bursts leads to a decrease in the ipsilateral SW activity (Avanzini *et al.*, 1992).

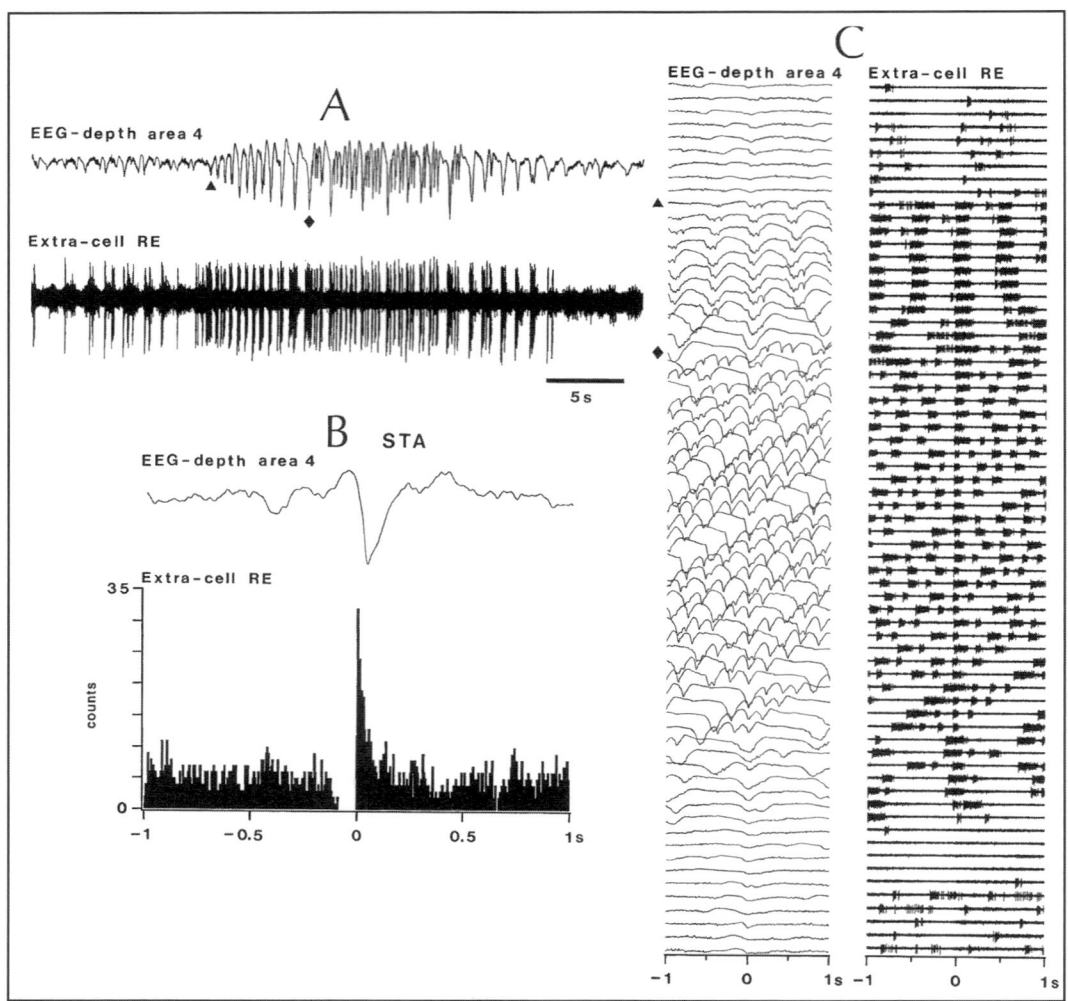

Figure 6. Resonant activities in neocortex and thalamic reticular (RE) neuron. Cat under ketamine-xylazine anesthesia. *A*, spontaneously occurring paroxysmal episode, with SW/PSW complexes at 2-4 Hz, recorded from the depth of cortical area 4 and from rostral RE neuron. *B*, spike-triggered average (STA). RE-cell's spike-bursts aligned at time zero and used to trigger depth-EEG waves. Note correspondence between pre-burst silenced firing and depth-positive (upward) EEG waves of the slow oscillation, and between RE-cell's excitation and depth-negative spiky EEG negative deflection. *C*, sequential analysis of cortical EEG activity and related discharges of RE neuron, triggered by the peak negativity of field potentials in the depth of cortical area 4 (time zero) over a window of 1 s (to be read from top to bottom) ▲ and ◆ in *C* correspond to the same symbols in *A*. Modified from Steriade and Contreras (1995).

The opposite was shown to occur in TC cells. Before presenting more recent intracellular data demonstrating that the majority of TC cells (60% to 90% in various studies) are powerfully inhibited during cortically generated SW seizures, I will mention the results of experiments by Gloor and his team on feline generalized penicillin epilepsy showing that, while SW complexes were induced by systemic administration or cortical application, as it was also obtained with bicuculline (Steriade and Contreras, 1998), penicillin injection in the thalamus did not produce SW seizures (Gloor et al., 1990). Instead, spindles with slowed frequencies were obtained. Another finding, pointing to the requirement of cortex in the generation of SW seizures, was the fact that the thalamus of a decorticated cat exhibited no SW discharge in response to an intramuscular dose of penicillin (Gloor et al., 1990). This explains why the so-called "absence seizures" occurring in thalamic slices after bath applications of a disinhibitory substance (von Krosigk et al., 1993) are not SW paroxysms, but just spindles with increased synchrony and decreased frequencies.

What is the behavior of TC neurons during cortically generated SW seizures? First, a methodological issue should be emphasized: only intracellular recordings can answer this question as, with extracellular recordings, the so-called "spike-bursts" reported in some studies on SW seizures may just represent brisk firing of single action potentials due to prevalent excitation of TC neurons by corticofugal inputs during the depth-negative component of SW complexes. Such activity does not reflect low-threshold bursts de-inactivated by hyperpolarization of TC neurons since these are trains of single spikes at a depolarized level, triggered by depolarizing corticothalamic projections (see Steriade and Contreras, 1995). Then, this firing pattern reflects excitation of TC neurons from cortex, rather than postinhibitory rebound spike-bursts.

Dual simultaneous intracellular recordings from the cortex and thalamus, in vivo, showed that, during cortically generated seizures consisting of SW/PSW complexes at 2-3 Hz, most (60%) TC neurons displayed a steady hyperpolarization as well as phasic IPSPs, closely related to the "spike" component of cortical SW/PSW complexes (Steriade and Contreras, 1995). At the end of the cortical seizure, TC neurons fired at high rates, as if they were released from the inhibition that occurred during the seizure (Figure 7). A similar aspect is illustrated in figure 8, which shows that, following repetitive IPSPs related to cortical paroxysmal discharges, during a short period of quiescence of cortical activity occurring within the SW seizure the TC neuron fired single potentials as they were no longer inhibited by the cortico-RE drive. Thus, the source of inhibition in TC cells should be searched in GABAergic RE neurons that fire spike-bursts during each PDS of cortical neurons (see above). Modeling studies (Lytton et al., 1997) showed that increasing the inhibitory strength from the GABAergic RE neurons onto TC neurons favors the quiescent mode in the latter.

Subsequent research by other teams, using multi-site field potentials and intracellular recordings from TC neurons during spontaneous SW discharges in genetic models of "absence epilepsy", similarly demonstrated that such seizures are initiated in cortex (Meeren et al., 2002) and that the main events which characterize the activity of an overwhelming majority (>90%) of TC neurons are a tonic hyperpolarization and rhythmic IPSPs (Pinault et al., 1998; Crunelli and Leresche, 2002).

140 Generalized Seizures: From clinical phenomenology to underlying systems and networks

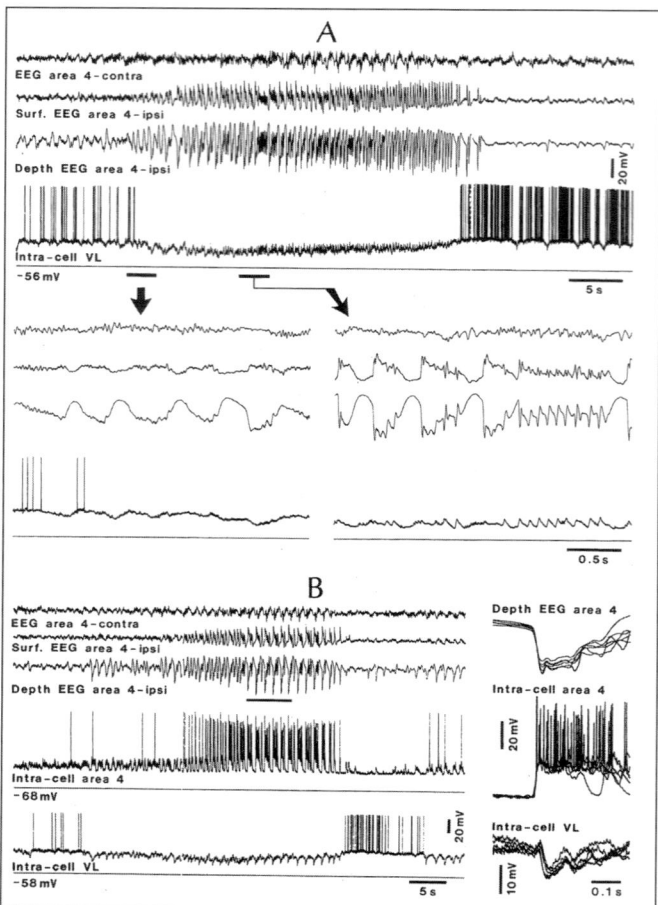

Figure 7. Dual intracellular recordings from neocortical (area 4) and thalamocortical (ventrolateral, VL) neurons demonstrating hyperpolarization of VL neuron during spike-wave (SW) seizure depolarization and spike-bursts in area 4 neuron. Cats under ketamine-xylazine anesthesia. A, four traces depict EEG from the skull over the right area 4, surface and depth EEG from left area 4, and intracellular activity of thalamocortical neuron from left VL nucleus (bottom line shows the current monitor). Two parts are expanded below (arrows). The cortical paroxysm was initiated by progressively increased amplitudes of depth-positive EEG waves in left area 4 (see expanded trace at left) and was characterized by ~2.5 Hz SW/PSW complexes, alternating with activity at 10 Hz. The VL cell was hyperpolarized throughout the seizure and disinhibited at the cessation of cortical paroxysm. B, five traces depict simultaneous recordings of EEG from the skull over the right cortical area 4, surface- and depth-EEGs from the left area 4, as well as intracellular activities of left area 4 cortical neuron and thalamic VL neuron (below each intracellular trace, current monitor). The seizure was initiated by a series of EEG waves at 0.9 Hz in the depth of left area 4, and continued with SW/PSW discharges at ~2 Hz (it also displayed fast runs). These periods were faithfully reflected in the intracellular activity of the cortical neuron, whereas the thalamic VL neuron displayed a tonic hyperpolarization throughout the seizure, with phasic sequences of IPSPs related to the large cortical paroxysmal depolarizations and spike-bursts occurring at the end of the seizure. Note disinhibition of the VL neuron after cessation of cortical seizure. Inset at right shows superimposition of spiky depth-negative EEG deflections associated with depolarization of cortical neuron and rhythmic IPSPs of the thalamic VL neuron. Modified from Steriade and Contreras (1995).

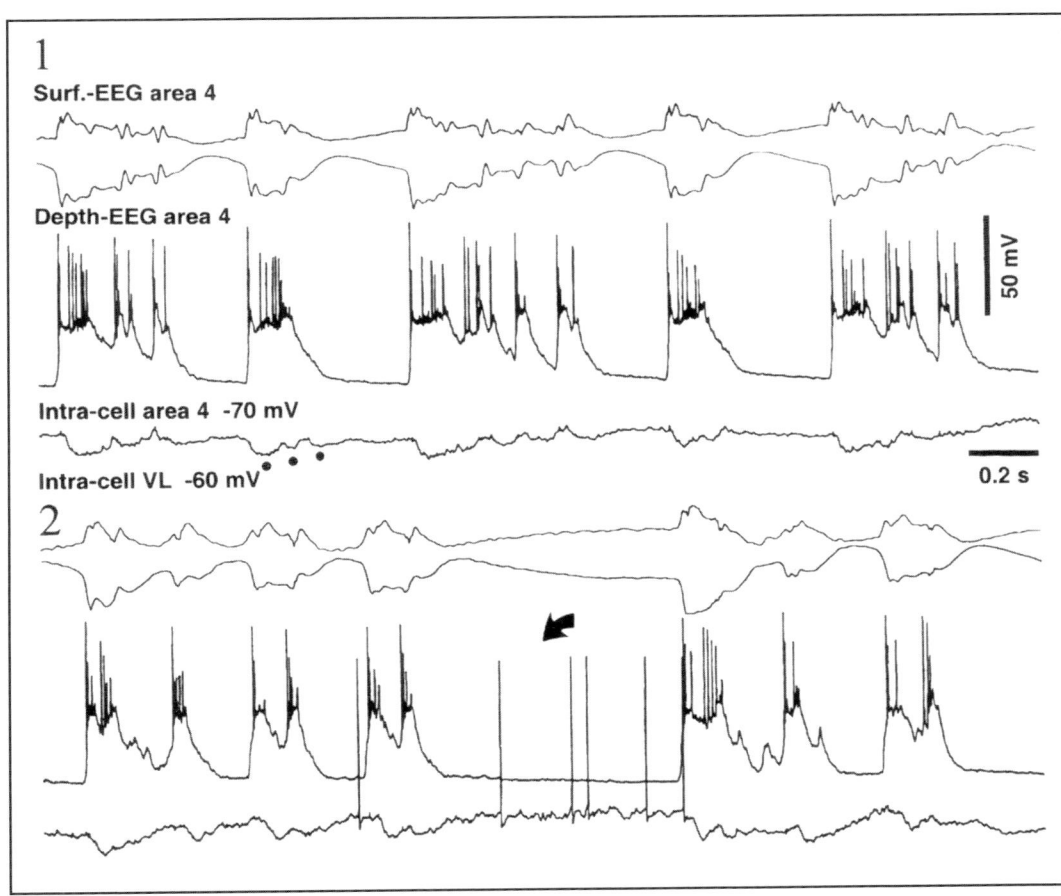

Figure 8. Thalamocortical (TC) neurons are inhibited during cortically generated spike-wave (SW) seizure, display phasic IPSPs but not spike-bursts, and are disinhibited during quiescent period in cortex. Dual intracellular recordings from area 4 cortical neuron and TC neuron from VL nucleus, together with surface- and depth-EEG from cortical area 4. The SW and polyspike-wave (PSW) seizure developed, without discontinuity, from sleep-like EEG patterns. Note paroxysmal depolarizing shifts (PDSs) in cortical neuron, and phasic IPSPs (see dots below the intracellular VL trace) related to cortical PDSs. Also note that, during a brief period of quiescence in cortical SW/PSW seizure (arrow in 2), the hyperpolarization of TC neuron was removed, the TC cell was disinhibited, and the neuron fired single action potentials. Modified from Lytton et al. (1997).

■ Concluding remark

In summary, SW seizures as in absence epilepsy as well as SW/PSW complexes and fast runs as in Lennox-Gastaut syndrome patterns are initiated in the cortex, even in the absence of the thalamus. These cortically generated paroxysms are associated with powerful excitation of thalamic GABAergic RE neurons that, consequently, inhibit TC neurons. The inhibition of TC neurons produces obliteration of external signals at their level and is regarded as the neuronal substrate of unconsciousness during SW seizures.

References

Abbott LF, Varela JA, Sen K, Nelson SB. Synaptic depression and cortical gain control. *Science* 1997; 275: 220-4.

Amzica F, Steriade M. Spontaneous and artificial activation of neocortical seizures. *J Neurophysiol* 1999; 82: 3123-38.

Amzica F, Steriade M. Neuronal and glial membrane potentials during sleep and paroxysmal oscillations in the cortex. *J Neurosci* 2000; 20: 6646-65.

Amzica F, Massimini M, Manfridi A. Spatial buffering during slow and paroxysmal oscillations in cortical networks of glial cells *in vivo*. *J Neurosci* 2002; 22: 1042-53.

Avanzini G, De Curtis M, Marescaux C, Panzica F, Spreafico R, Vergnes M. Role of thalamic reticular nucleus in the generation of rhythmic thalamo-cortical activities subserving spike and waves. *J Neur Trans* 1992; 35 (Suppl): 85-95.

Avanzini G, De Curtis M, Pape HC, Spreafico R. Intrinsic properties of reticular thalamic neurons relevant to genetically determined spike-wave generation. In: Delgado-Escucta AV, Wilson WA, Olsen RW, Porter RJ, eds. *Jasper's Basic Mechanisms of the Epilepsies* (3rd edition). Philadelphia: Lippincott-Williams & Wilkins, 1999: 297-309.

Bormann J, Kettenmann H. Patch clamp study of GABA receptor Cl$^-$ channels in cultured astrocytes. *Proc Natl Acad Sci USA* 1988; 85: 8336-40.

Castro-Alamancos M. Neocortical synchronized oscillations induced by thalamic disinhibition *in vivo*. *J Neurosci* (online) 1999; 19: RC27.

Charpier S, Leresche N, Deniau JM, Mahon S, Hughes SW, Crunelli V. On the putative contribution of GABA$_B$ receptors to the electrical events occurring during spontaneous spike and wave discharges. *Neuropharmacology* 1999; 38: 1699-706.

Cohen I, Navarro V, Clémenceau S, Baulac M, Miles R. On the origin of interictal activity in human temporal lobe epilepsy *in vitro*. *Science* 2002; 298: 1418-21.

Crunelli V, Leresche N. Childhood absence epilepsy: genes, channels, neurons and networks. *Nat Rev Neurosci* 2002; 3: 371-82.

Danober L, Depaulis A, Marescaux C, Vergnes M. Effects of cholinergic drugs on genetic absence seizures in rats. *Eur J Pharmacol* 1993; 234: 263-8.

Danober L, Depaulis A, Vergnes M, Marescaux C. Mesopontine cholinergic control over generalized non-convulsive seizures in a genetic model of absence epilepsy in the rat. *Neuroscience* 1995; 69: 1183-93.

Desai NS, Rutherford LC, Turrigiano GG. Plasticity in the intrinsic excitability of cortical pyramidal neurons. *Nat Neurosci* 1999; 2: 515-20.

Destexhe A. Spike-and-wave oscillations based on the properties of GABA$_B$ receptors. *J Neurosci* 1998; 18: 9099-111.

Dinner D. Posttraumatic epilepsy. In: Wyllie E, ed. *The treatment of epilepsy: Principles*. Philadelphia: Lea & Fibinger, 1993: 654-8.

Fisher RS, Webber WR, Lesser RP, Arroyo S, Uematsu S. High-frequency EEG activity at the start of seizures. *J Clin Neurophysiol* 1992; 9: 441-8.

Frank G. A study of the inter-relations of spike discharge density and sleep stages in epileptic patients. *Electroencephalogr Clin Neurophysiol* 1969; 26: 238.

Giaretta D, Avoli M, Gloor P. Intracellular recordings in precruciate neurons during spike and wabe discharges of feline generalized penicillin epilepsy. *Brain Res* 1987; 405: 68-79.

Gloor P, Avoli M, Kostopoulos G. Thalamocortical relationships in generalized epilepsy with bilaterally synchronous spike-and-wave discharges. In: Avoli M, Gloor P, Kostopoulos G, Naquet R, eds. *Generalized Epilepsies*. Boston: Birkhäuser, 1990: 190-212.

Golshani P, Liu XB, Jones EG. Differences in quantal amplitude reflect GluR4-subunit number at corticothalamic synapses on two populations of thalamic neurons. *Proc Natl Acad Sci USA* 2001; 98: 4172-7.

Grenier F, Timofeev I, Steriade M. Focal synchronization of ripples (80-200 Hz) in neocortex and their neuronal correlates. *J Neurophysiol* 2001; 86: 1884-98.

Grenier F, Timofeev I, Steriade M. Neocortical very fast oscillations (ripples, 80-200 Hz) during seizures: intracellular correlates. *J Neurophysiol* 2003; 89: 841-52.

Jasper HH. Historical introduction. In: Avoli M, Gloor P, Kostopoulos G, Naquet R, eds. *Generalized Epilepsies*. Boston: Birkhäuser, 1990: 1-15.

Johnston D, Brown TH. Giant spike potential hypothesis for epileptiform activity. *Science* 1981; 211: 294-7.

Kellaway P. Sleep and epilepsy. *Epilepsia* 1985; 26 (Suppl 1): 15-30.

Kobayashi K, Nishibayashi N, Ohtsuka Y, Oka E, Ohtahara S. Epilepsy with electrical status epilepticus during slow sleep and secondary bilateral synchrony. *Epilepsia* 1994; 35: 1097-103.

Lemieux JF, Blume WT. Topographical evolution of spike-wave complexes. *Brain Res* 1986; 373: 275-87.

Lytton WW, Contreras D, Destexhe A, Steriade M. Dynamic interactions determine partial thalamic quiescence in a computer network model of spike-and-wave seizures. *J Neurophysiol* 1997; 77: 1679-96.

Marcus EM, Watson CW, Simon SA. Behavioral correlates of acute bilateral symmetrical epileptogenic foci in monkey cerebral cortex. *Brain Res* 1968; 9: 370-3.

McCormick DA, Contreras D. On the cellular and network bases of epileptic seizures. *Ann Rev Physiol* 2001; 63: 815-46.

Meeren HKM, Pijn JPM, van Luijtelaar EJLM, Coenen AML, Lopes da Silva FH. Cortical focus drives widrspread corticothalamic networks during spontaneous absence seizures in rats. *J Neurosci* 2002; 22: 1480-95.

Neckelmann D, Amzica F, Steriade M. Spike-wave complexes and fast components of cortically generated seizures. III. Synchronizing mechanisms. *J Neurophysiol* 1998; 80: 1480-94.

Neckelmann D, Amzica F, Steriade M. Changes in neuronal conductance during different components of cortically generated spike-wave seizures. *Neuroscience* 2000; 96: 475-85.

Nita DA, Timofeev I, Steriade M. Increased propensity to seizures following chronic cortical deafferentation in vivo. *J Neurophysiol* 2006; in press.

Petsche H. Pathophysiologie und Klinik des Petit-Mal. *Wien Zschr Nervenheilkr* 1962; 19: 345-442.

Pinault D, Leresche N, Charpier S, Deniau JM, Marescaux C, Vergnes M, Crunelli V. Intracellular recordings in thalamic neurones during spontaneous spike and wave discharges in rats with absence epilepsy. *J Physiol (Lond)* 1998; 509: 449-56.

Pollen DA. Intracellular studies of cortical neurons during thalamic induced wave and spike. *Electroencephalogr Clin Neurophysiol* 1964; 17: 398-404.

Prince DA, Jacobs K. Inhibitory function in two models of chronic epileptogenesis. *Epilepsy Res* 1998; 32: 83-92.

Rodin E. Decomposition and mapping of generalized spike-wave complexes. *Clin Neurophysiol* 1999; 110: 1868-75.

Shouse MN. Physiology underlying relationship of epilepsy and sleep. In: Dinner DS and Lüders HO, eds. *Epilepsy and Sleep*. San Diego: Academic Press, 2001: 43-62.

Staak R, Pape HC. Contribution of $GABA_A$ and $GABA_B$ receptors to thalamic neuronal activity during spontaneous absence seizures in rats. *J Neurosci* 2001; 21: 1378-84.

Steinhäuser C, Gallo V. News on glutamate receptors on glial cells. *Trends Neurosci* 1996; 19: 339-45.

Steriade M. Interneuronal epileptic discharges related to spike-and-wave cortical seizures in behaving monkeys. *Electroencephalogr Clin Neurophysiol* 1974; 37: 247-63.

Steriade M. *Neuronal substrates of sleep and epilepsy*. Cambridge (UK): Cambridge University Press, 2003, 522 p.

Steriade M, Amzica F. Dynamic coupling among neocortical neurons during evoked and spontaneous spike-wave seizure activity. *J Neurophysiol* 1994; 72: 2051-69.

Steriade M, Amzica F. Intracellular study of excitability in the seizure-prone neocortex in vivo. *J Neurophysiol* 1999; 82: 3108-22.

Steriade M, Contreras D. Relations between cortical and thalamic cellular events during transition from sleep pattern to paroxysmal activity. *J Neurosci* 1995; 15: 623-42.

Steriade M, Contreras D. Spike-wave complexes and fast runs of cortically generated seizures. I. Role of neocortex and thalamus. *J Neurophysiol* 1998; 80: 1439-55.

Steriade M, Timofeev I. Corticothalamic operations through prevalent inhibition of thalamocortical neurons. *Thal & Rel Syst* 2001; 1: 225-36.

Steriade M, Amzica F, Neckelmann D, Timofeev I. Spike-wave complexes and fast runs of cortically generated seizures. II. Extra- and intracellular patterns. *J Neurophysiol* 1998a; 80: 1456-79.

Steriade M, Timofeev I, Dürmüller N, Grenier F. Dynamic properties of corticothalamic neurons and local cortical interneurons generating fast rhythmic (30-40 Hz) spike bursts. *J Neurophysiol* 1998b; 79: 483-90.

Steriade M, Cissé Y, Timofeev I, Crochet S. Synaptic responsiveness during paroxysmal depolarizing shifts of cortical neurons. *Soc Neurosci Abstr* 2003; 29: 10.8.

Timofeev I, Steriade M. Neocortical seizures: initiation, development and cessation. *Neuroscience* 2004; 123: 299-336.

Timofeev I, Grenier F, Steriade M. Spike-wave complexes and fast runs of cortically generated seizures. IV. Paroxysmal fast runs in cortical and thalamic neurons. *J Neurophysiol* 1998; 80: 1495-513.

Timofeev I, Grenier F, Steriade M. The role of chloride-dependent inhibition and the activity of fast-spiking neurons during cortical spike-wave electrographic seizures. *Neuroscience* 2002a; 114: 1115-32.

Timofeev I, Bazhenov M, Sejnowski TJ, Steriade, M. Cortical hyperpolarization-activated depolarizing current takes part in the generation of focal paroxysmal activities. *Proc Natl Acad Sci USA* 2002b; 99: 9533-7.

Topolnik L, Steriade M, Timofeev I. Partial cortical deafferentation promotes development of paroxysmal activity. *Cereb Cortex* 2003a; 13: 883-93.

Topolnik L, Steriade M, Timofeev I. Hyperexcitability of intact neurons underlies acute development of trauma-induced electrographic seizures in cats *in vivo*. *Eur J Neurosci* 2003b; 18: 486-96.

Traub RD, Borck C, Colling SB, Jefferys JG. On the structure of ictal events *in vitro*. *Epilepsia* 1996; 37: 879-91.

Traub RD, Whittington MA, Buhl EH, LeBeau FE, Bibbig A, Boyd S, Cross H, Baldeweg T. A possible role for gap junctions in generation of very fast EEG oscillations preceding the onset of, or perhaps initiating, seizures. *Epilepsia* 2001; 42: 153-70.

Tsakiridou E, Bertollini L, De Curtis M, Avanzini G, Pape HC. T-type calcium conductance in the reticular thalamic nucleus: a contribution to absence epilepsy. *J Neurosci* 1995; 15: 3110-7.

von Krosigk M, Bal T, McCormick DA. Cellular mechanisms of a synchronized oscillation in the thalamus. *Science* 1993; 261: 361-4.

Section IV:
Myoclonic seizures and the frontal lobe

Animal models of myoclonic seizures and epilepsies

Jana Velíšková, Libor Velíšek

Departments of Neurology and Neuroscience, Albert Einstein College of Medicine, Bronx, NY, USA

Myoclonic seizures are an important feature of heterogenous syndromes belonging to myoclonic epilepsies. In humans, the myoclonic seizures are typically brief, involuntary muscle contractions with a sudden onset predominantly in the arms but can involve the entire body. They are often generalized but can have focal origin as well. Based on the classification of the Commission on Pediatric Epilepsy of the International League Against the Epilepsy, there are four types of myoclonus: cortical, thalamocortical, reticular reflex and negative (1997). Cortical myoclonus originates in the sensorimotor cortex and each muscle jerk corresponds to the cortical discharge. Thalamocortical myoclonus involves the thalamocortical loop. The contractions start in muscles innervated by the first cranial nerves and the ones innervated by the last cranial nerves are involved later. In the thalamocortical myoclonus, the myoclonic jerks, which are generalized, occur in the association with EEG generalized spike-wave discharges. This type of myoclonus is identified in nonprogressive generalized epilepsy syndromes such as benign myoclonic epilepsy of infancy, childhood absence epilepsy with myoclonus, or juvenile myoclonic epilepsy, but also in severe progressive myoclonic epilepsy syndromes of infancy (1997). The reflex reticular myoclonus is due to hyperexcitability in the caudal reticular formation. The jerks precede the cortical events and are usually bilateral. They involve first the palatal, superior facial, and jaw muscles with electromyographic (EMG) events correlated with the sequential innervations by the ninth, seventh, and fifth cranial nerves and eventually the whole body (1997). The negative myoclonus is characterized by lapses in muscular activity without losing the posture. Epileptic myoclonus is always accompanied by cortical epileptiform discharches, which distinguishes the epileptic from a non-epileptic myoclonus. The non-epileptic myoclonus includes opsoclonus myoclonus syndrome, sleep myoclonus affecting normal newborns and infants, and startle responses such as hyperekplexia. In addition, non-myoclonic phenomena such as tremor, tics, and chorea also need to be distinguished from the epilepsy syndromes (1997).

Similarly to the criteria for myoclonic seizures in humans, in rats myoclonus has much shorter duration than the tonic-clonic seizures. The other distinction of the myoclonus from the tonic-clonic seizures is preserved righting reflex, which is lost during the tonic-clonic seizures. The origin of myoclonic seizures in the experimental models has been identified in the forebrain. In adult rats, rhythmical movements of forelimbs characterize clonic seizures. The clonic seizures *(Figure 1)* can last seconds to tens of seconds. Head clonus with facial movements may also be observed. During the forelimb clonus, which can be unilateral or bilateral, hindlimbs are widely abducted. Rearing and tail erection (Straub tail) also can be present. During the bilateral clonus the movements are synchronized. A less common behavioral feature of the myoclonic seizures of forebrain origin during the initial phase of the seizure is a short tonus of forelimbs with a twist of the body. It occurs usually during the last myoclonus just prior to progression into the tonic-clonic seizures suggesting an involvement of the brain stem structures. This is characteristic for the flurothyl model of generalized myoclonic seizures. In this model, hindlimbs may be also affected resulting in loss of posture. However, the rat shows an active effort to keep the upright position.

Myolonic seizures in developing animals often progress into tonic-clonic seizures very rapidly, especially during the first two postnatal weeks and thus may be masked by tonic-clonic seizures. Rearing does not occur before the second postnatal week and the synchronization of the movements is poor. The myoclonic seizures rather look like uncoordinated bilateral swimming movements often with hindlimb clonus during the first two postnatal weeks. Unilateral clonus may look like tapping of a forelimb. Also during the development, the righting reflex is always preserved.

■ Models of generalized myoclonus

Electrical stimulation

The myoclonic seizures can be induced by a threshold or just suprathreshold stimulation using corneal electrodes (Mareš and Kubová, 2006). The seizures progress from a facial and mouth movement to rearing with falling and the Racine scale (Racine, 1972), originally developed for kindling, can be used for scoring the seizure stages. The minimal electroshock seizures can be induced also in developing animals (Vernadakis and Woodbury, 1969).

Genetic models

The latest advances in molecular genetics are essential for understanding of underlying mechanisms of seizures and epilepsy. Many spontaneous as well as engineered gene mutations were identified especially in mice and are now an important tool to study epilepsy syndromes. Recently, several excellent reviews on this topic have been written (Noebels, 2003b, a; Burgess, 2006; Noebels, 2006), thus we will not cover this topic in any detail and only some models will be discussed.

Myoclonic seizures are a prominent feature in a small subpopulation of the Senegalese baboon, *Papio papio*, as response to an intermittent light stimulus (Killam *et al.*, 1967; Naquet and Meldrum, 1986; Naquet *et al.*, 1988). The seizures start as bilateral synchronous myoclonus, which may secondary generalize to tonic convulsion (Meldrum *et al.*, 1970). Pharmacological studies in the epileptic baboons suggest dysfunction mainly in the GABAergic system but the involvement of the monoaminergic system has been highlighted as well (Meldrum and Horton, 1971; Horton and Meldrum, 1973; Meldrum and Horton, 1980; Meldrum, 1984; Naquet and Meldrum, 1986). The seizures seem to be initiated in the fronto-rolandic cortex with activation of reticular formation as the seizure progresses (Menini, 1976). The activation of the occipital cortex is rather associated with the photic flashes, although the highly sensitive animals show alterations such as amplitude decrease in the early evoked responses. The thalamus, especially the lateral thalamic nuclei group, is activated at the later stages, when the paroxysmal cortical discharges increase in amplitude (Naquet *et al.*, 1987; Menini, 1976). Spontaneous myoclonic as well as tonic-clonic seizures

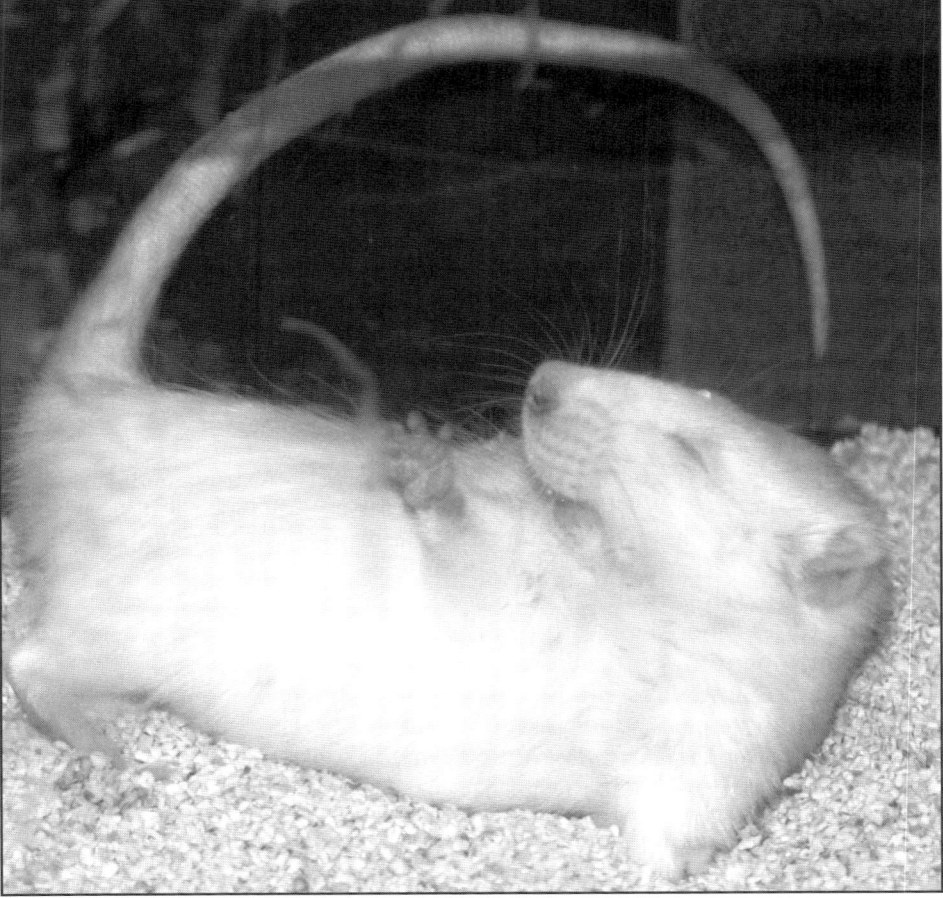

Figure 1. Generalized clonic seizure induced by pentylenetetrazol in the rat. The rat is still preserving upright position during a clonus of the right forelimb. Left forelimb on the floor along with a wide-base hindlimbs of the cage is stabilizing the rat during the torque of the torso. Note the clonus of face muscles here represented by closed eyelids. Additionally, a Straub tail is present. This presentation of clonic seizures is very common in chemically-induced clonic seizures.

have been observed in other baboon subspecies such as *Papio hamadryas anubis* and *cynocephalus/anubis* (Szabo et al., 2005). Photosensitivity is also present in these baboons (Szabo et al., 2005).

The tottering mouse is exhibiting intermittent focal myoclonic seizures with ataxia from the fourth postnatal week (Noebels, 1979; Noebels and Sidman, 1979; Noebels, 1986). In this model, the increase in the axonal projections originating from the locus coeruleus corresponds to overproduction of norepinephrine in the terminal fields, especially within the cortex (Levitt and Noebels, 1981; Noebels, 1986).

The Otx1-/- mouse is characterized by microcephaly with the reduction expressed preferentially in the neocortex (Acampora et al., 1996; Avanzini et al., 2000; Sancini et al., 2001; Cipelletti et al., 2002). Overall reduction of neurons involves mostly GABAergic interneurons. The seizures start occurring during the fourth postnatal week and are characterized by head nodding, forelimb clonus with rearing and falling.

In the flathead mutant rat, the myoclonic seizures develop in immature animals during the second postnatal week. The seizure phenotype is related to cortical malformations including microcephaly and cellular abnormalities such as cytomegalic neurons and abnormal neuronal death with preferential loss of GABAergic interneuons (Cogswell et al., 1998; Sarkisian et al., 1999; Roberts et al., 2000; Sarkisian et al., 2001). The seizures are myoclonic with loss of posture. Toward the third postnatal week, the seizures become rather tonic and lead to premature death. The main antiepileptic drugs effective against the myoclonic seizures in humans such as valproate, phenobarbital or ethosuximide are efficient only partially in block the seizures in these rats (Sarkisian et al., 1999).

Chemical models in rats

Systemic administration of chemical substances (convulsant drugs) can produce myoclonic seizures (Velíšek, 2006). The occurrence of this seizure type significantly depends on the drug used and on the dose and route of administration. Myoclonic seizures after convulsant drug administration do not occur isolated; they are always a part of a seizure syndrome. As a part of this syndrome, myoclonic seizures are usually simply called **clonic seizures**. Sometimes, when a large dose of the drug is used, the rapid progression in the syndrome development may preclude appearance of clonic seizures; they may be overlapped by tonic-clonic seizures. Similar situation may occur when a relatively low dose of the convulsant chemical is administered by a route allowing rapid absorption, such as i.v. instead of s.c. administration. Various chemical substances can be used, however generally only the substances affecting GABAergic inhibition are effective in producing generalized clonic seizures. It should be noted, however, that the clonic seizures are preceded by freezing behavior associated with rhythmic EEG activity with a high resemblance to absence seizures, which would preclude using these models in the strict sense as models for myoclonic seizures (Leppik, 2003).

Moderate doses of **pentylenetetrazol** induce clonic seizures (Swinyard et al., 1989). With higher doses, clonic seizures may occur just prior to the tonic-clonic seizures or can be completely masked by the tonic-clonic seizures. This is especially true in the immature rats. Here, PTZ elicits clonic seizures reliably from the third postnatal week

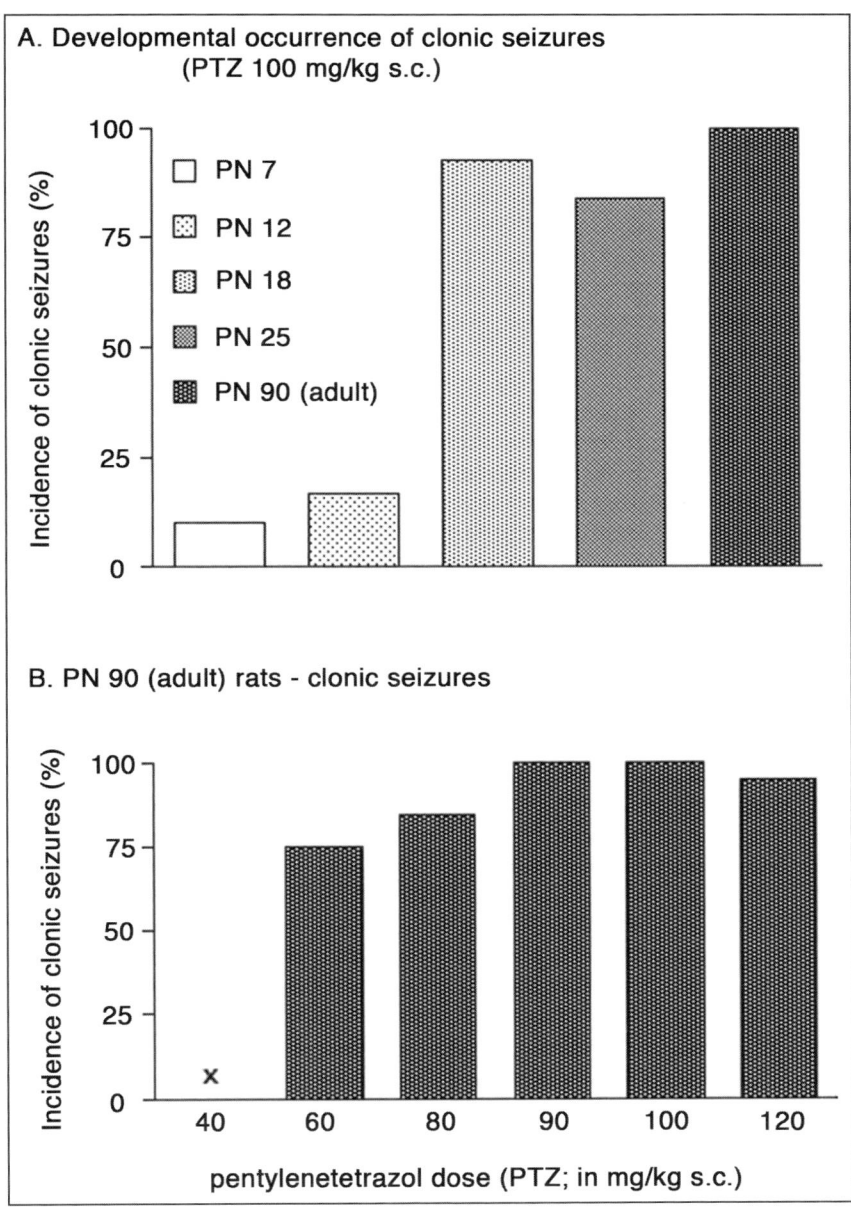

Figure 2. Incidence of pentylenetetrazol-induced seizures in the rat.
A. Developmental occurrence of pentylenetetrazol-induced clonic seizures in rats after an equal dose of pentylenetetrazol (100 mg/kg s.c.) In 7 and 12 day old rats (P7, P12), the occurrence of clonic seizures was negligible; these seizures regularly develop in P18 and older rats.
B. Dose-dependent occurrence of clonic seizures in the adult rats after the administration of pentylenetetrazol in doses from 40-120 mg/kg s.c. Dose of 40 mg/kg did not produce any clonic seizures, while the doses 60 mg/kg and more evoked clonic seizures in majority of tested rats (according to Velíšek et al., 1992).

of the rat (*Figure 2A*) and occurrence of clonic seizures cannot be easily titrated by decreasing the PTZ dose (*Figure 2B*) (Vernadakis and Woodbury, 1969; Velíšek et al., 1992). However, if a specific blocker, such as an NMDA receptor antagonist, blocks the tonic-clonic seizures, clonic seizures occur regularly (Velíšek et al., 1990; Velíšek et al., 1991).

Administration of **bicuculline** also produces clonic seizures in rats. Usually, intraperitoneal or intravenous administration is used, because bicuculline dissolved in weak acid and the subcutaneous injection is painful and stressful (Velíšek, 2006). The seizures are clinically similar to PTZ-induced clonic seizures. The difference in comparison to PTZ-induced clonic seizures is the developmental onset. Bicuculline-induced clonic seizures occur already during the second postnatal week of the rat (Velíšek, 2006).

Picrotoxin also produces clonic seizures. Usually, there is much longer latency to onset of picrotoxin-induced clonic seizures, compared to PTZ and bicuculline. Otherwise, the clinical symptoms are very similar if not identical. Developmentally, picrotoxin-induced clonic seizures, can be produced even earlier than bicuculline-induced clonic seizures occurrence of these seizures after picrotoxin has been reported already during the first postnatal week of the rat (Velíšková et al., 1990).

In the **flurothyl** model, clonic seizures always precede the tonic-clonic seizures. In our laboratory, the animals are tested in a flurothyl chamber (Lánský et al., 1997). This is an airtight chamber and flurothyl is delivered in a constant rate by a pump. The advantages of this model are that the seizures always occur, the onset of seizures can be modulated by changing the flurothyl infusion rate, seizures terminate within a short time after the animal is removed from the chamber, and the survival of the animals is very high allowing thus several re-testing (Sperber et al., 1999). The mechanism of flurothyl seizures is not well known but it involves both GABAA receptor-mediated and cholinergic neurotransmission (Wakamori et al., 1991; Eger et al., 2002). Thus, the seizures are slightly more violent than it is typical for GABAA receptor acting convulsants. In adult rats, a tonic component with body twisting is a part of the clonic forebrain seizure occurring just prior to the progression into the brainstem type (tonic-clonic) seizures (Velíšková, 2006). Clonic seizures can be elicited from the day of birth. During the first two postnatal weeks, clonic seizures consist of head tremor with tail erection and tapping or swimming like movements of forelimbs. The hindlimbs may also be involved, usually unilaterally.

Drugs inhibiting GABA synthesis at various levels, such as 3-mercaptopropionic acid (Mareš et al., 1993), allylglycine (the GAD inhibitors) (Horton et al., 1978), and isonicotinehydrazide (Mareš and Trojan, 1991), **as well as** the inverse agonists at the benzodiazepine receptors, the **beta-carbolines** (Braestrup et al., 1980; Braestrup et al., 1982; Braestrup et al., 1983), produce clonic seizures with a similar semiology as the above mentioned drugs. In the isonicotinehydrazide model especially in developing rats, clonic seizures immediately progress in the tonic-clonic seizures similarly as in the flurothyl model (Mareš and Trojan, 1991; Velíšková, 2006). The onset of seizures in isonicotinehydrazide and allylglycine models is relatively slow.

■ Focal myoclonus models

As generalized myoclonus can be elicited by a systemic administration of a stimulus (drug, electrical stimulation), focal myoclonus can be produced by focal irritation of the appropriate brain regions. The origin of this irritation may be various, focal electrical stimulation, topical administration of convulsant drugs, penicillin or conjugated estrogens will create an epileptic focus. If this focus is localized in the sensorimotor cortex, its activation will produce myoclonus of corresponding contralateral muscle groups.

Two paradigms of **electrical stimulation** have been developed, which can represent a focal or multifocal type of myoclonus by stimulation of one or both hemispheres (Voskuyl et al., 1989; Kubová et al., 1996). Low-frequency stimuli with increasing current intensity are used inducing myoclonic movements. Both models have been tested for efficacy of different anticonvulsant drugs. Mareš et al. used successfully the unilateral stimulation of the cortex in developing rats (Mareš et al., 2002). The low-frequency stimulation can be used consistently in 12-day old and older animals, with the highest sensitivity at the end of the third postnatal week (Mareš et al., 2002).

Almost all generally used **convulsant drugs** can be utilized to produce a focus in the motor cortex resulting in the development of clonic seizures initially in the contralateral side with possible generalization. Thus, pentylenetetrazol, bicuculline, picrotoxin, cholinergics, and strychnine, to name a few, can elicit clonic seizures from the motor cortex focus (Soukupová et al., 1993; Velíšek et al., 1993). Clonic seizures are usually preceded by myoclonic twitches. EEG usually shows individual discharges (*Figure 3*) associated with those myoclonic twitches, which over time develop into the ictal activity usually associated with a clonic seizure. There are several exceptions. If kainic acid, a glutamate analogue, is administered upon the cortex, seizures will highly likely occur first remotely in limbic structures due to high density of KA receptors. Therefore, myoclonus here may be secondary to a limbic focus with

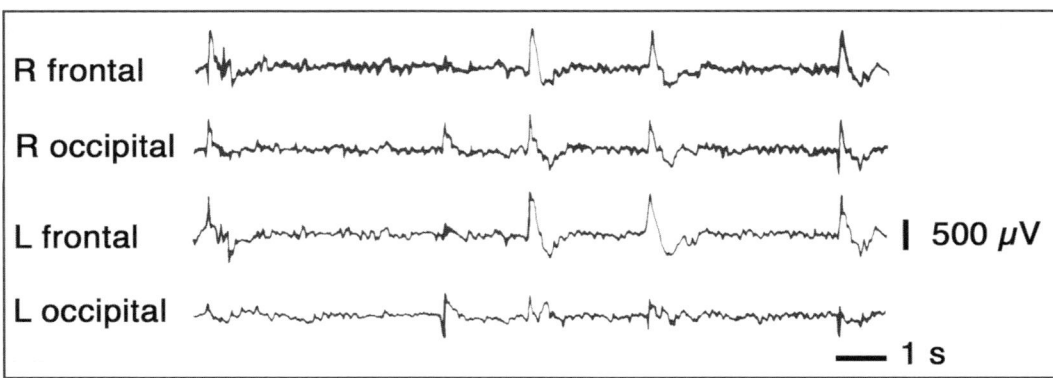

Figure 3. EEG activity after focal administration of pentylenetetrazol on the neocortex of a freely moving rat corresponding behaviorally to myoclonic twitches.
Pentylenetetrazol solution (2.5 µl of 200 mg/ml) was administered upon the right sensorimotor cortex *via* a chronically implanted canulla. The metallic canulla also served as an EEG electrode with additional silver electrodes on the left sensorimotor and left and right occipital cortices. Reference recording *versus* a screw electrode in the nasal bone. Time mark 1 s, calibration 500 µV.

automatisms. Second, N-methyl-D-aspartic acid, a prototypic agonist at NMDA receptors may not provide focal activation after topical administration since it has a significant propensity to create a spreading depression (Somjen, 2001).

Locally administered **penicillins and cephalosporins** (especially the first cephalosporine generation) are potent convulsant drugs and produce an epileptic focus (for review see (Velíšek and Moshé, 2000b, a)). If the administration is aimed in the motor cortex, it produces focal myoclonus. Individual discharges recorded on the EEG are usually associated with individual myoclonic twitches while ictal activity is associated with a clonic seizure. Sodium salts of the antibioiotics are preferred to the potassium salts as potassium excess may produce a spreading depression and mask the focus.

Topical application of **conjugated equine estrogens** on cerebral cortex has proepileptogenic properties (Marcus et al., 1963; Marcus et al., 1966). This model has been developed in cats and rabbits but not used for antiepileptic drug testing. Similar application of β-estradiol, however does not produce any epileptogenic focus (Marcus et al., 1966).

Similarly, **intraparenchymal administration of metals** and their compounds such as $CoCl_2$, $AlOH_3$, $NiCl_2$, $FeCl_3$ produce epileptic foci [for review see (Velíšek, 2006)]. The foci become activated within hours to days. If properly localized in the motor cortex, the metal implants produce myoclonic seizures in contralateral limbs. Generally, these models are more complicated and more expensive to prepare. Except for the alumina cream in monkeys, there is a spontaneous deactivation of the focus, *ergo* seizures, within days to weeks probably related to focal necrosis.

■ The role of the substantia nigra and the basal ganglia circuitry in myoclonic seizure control

One of the structures involved in regulation of the myoclonic seizures is the substantia nigra pars reticulata (SNR). The seizure-modulating effects are mediated especially *via* the GABAA receptors. The SNR has a strategic position allowing the communication with the output structures of the basal ganglia network – the thalamus, superior colliculus, and reticular formation and back to the striatum.

Metabolic studies in adult rats show increased 2-deoxyglucose utilization within the SNR during seizure activity (Engel et al., 1978; Pazdernik et al., 1985; Nehlig et al., 1998; Eells et al., 2000; Sawamura et al., 2001; Velíšková et al., 2005) or during forelimb movements induced by electrical stimulation of motor cortex (Collins et al., 1986).

The SNR seizure-controlling network has age-, sex-, and region-specific features. Within the adult SNR, two functionally distinct regions can be discriminated, the $SNR_{anterior}$ and the $SNR_{posterior}$ (Moshé et al., 1994; Shehab et al., 1996; Fan et al., 1997; Thompson et al., 2000; Velíšková and Moshé, 2001). These two regions differentially regulate the seizure onset and exist in both male and female rats. In adult male rats, activation of the GABAA receptor system, *i.e.* by muscimol in the

$SNR_{anterior}$ has anticonvulsant effects while it is proconvulsant in the $SNR_{posterior}$ (Velíšková and Moshé, 2001). In females, muscimol in the $SNR_{anterior}$ has anticonvulsant effects as well, but no effect in the $SNR_{posterior}$ (Velíšková and Moshé, 2001).

Using the flurothyl seizure model of generalized myoclonic seizures, we determined the changes in the 2-deoxyglucose (2DG) uptake during the pre-clonic, clonic and post-clonic state in male rats (Velíšková et al., 2005). During the pre-clonic state, we found increase in the 2DG uptake in the $SNR_{posterior}$. This selective alteration in neuronal activity most likely represents the involvement of the $SNR_{posterior}$ during the initiation/propagation of a seizure. A study of nigral electrophysiological activity during a clonic seizure induced by kindling shows that neuronal discharge rate increases selectively in the $SNR_{posterior}$ but not the $SNR_{anterior}$ (Gernert et al., 2004). Thus, these findings seem to be consistent with an interpretation that the $SNR_{posterior}$ would act as a "gateway" for seizure propagation (Velíšková et al., 2005). There was also co-activation of the ventromedial thalamic nucleus (VM) during the pre-clonic state, probably reflecting changes in the $SNR_{posterior}$ and resulting in GABA or acetylcholine release through the rich GABAergic and cholinergic projections (Di Chiara et al., 1979; Kha et al., 2001). However, pharmacological and lesion studies do not support the involvement of VM in seizure control (Moshé et al., 1985; Garant et al., 1993).

The $SNR_{anterior}$ becomes involved during the myoclonic seizure. The increase in glucose utilization within the $SNR_{anterior}$, is accompanied by a decrease in the glucose uptake in the superior colliculus (SC). Keeping in mind that the 2DG uptake reflects the changes at the pre-synaptic terminals (Ackermann et al., 1984; Sokoloff, 1999), the data suggest that the $SNR_{anterior}$ seizure controlling network involves the following events: The increased 2DG uptake in the $SNR_{anterior}$ is a result of increased GABA release from the striato-nigral projection, which inhibits the SNR GABAergic neuron firing. This leads to decrease of GABA release in the SC, which seems to correspond to a decrease in 2DG uptake. Pharmacological studies are in agreement with this conclusion. Thus, local injections of GABA receptor agonists in the SNR (Depaulis et al., 1989) have anticonvulsant effects while in the SC anticonvulsant effects are achieved by local infusions of a GABAA receptor antagonist bicuculline (Depaulis et al., 1990; Redgrave et al., 1992).

The post-clonic seizure events comprise a decrease in glucose metabolism in the pedunculopontine nucleaus (PPTg) and an increase in the subthalamic nucleus (STN). Both, the PPTg and STN play and important role in movement and behavioral arrest (Klemm, 2001). Postictal state following a myoclonic seizure is a type of movement arrest, using similar mechanisms during a seizure cessation. As the SNR represents an influential afferent projection of the PPTg (Rye et al., 1987; Spann and Grófová, 1991), the decreased 2DG uptake in the PPTg is consistent with decreased activity at the nigro-pontine GABAergic terminals and leading to increase of cholinergic and glutamatergic activity within the PPTg. This seems to be reflected by increased activity in the STN, the main ascending projection of the PPTg (Nakano et al., 2000).

During development, metabolic studies show no change in glucose uptake in the SNR in two-week old animals, which is in contrast to the dramatic increase in adult rats (Albala et al., 1984; Ackermann et al., 1989; Sperber et al., 1992). This, however, does not mean that the SNR is not involved in seizure regulation in developing animals but rather suggests playing a different role than in adult rats. This is supported by numerous pharmacological studies, which show that infusions of GABAergic agents lead to a change in the myoclonic seizure threshold (Sperber *et al.*, 1987; Xu *et al.*, 1992; Velíšková, 1999; Velíšková and Moshé, 2001). In contrast to adults, infusion studies show that in the two-week old rats, only one functional region exists (Moshé *et al.*, 1994; Velíšková and Moshé, 2001). Muscimol infusions in the SNR at this age have proconvulsant effects in males and no effect in females (Velíšková and Moshé, 2001). This seems to be related to developmentally regulated local features of the GABAergic system in the SNR, which is different in males and in females. In the SNR of a male rat, the GABA content per neuron and $GABA_A$ receptor $\alpha 1$ subunit mRNA expression is lower compared to females at the same age (Ravizza *et al.*, 2003). The male SNR neurons express lower levels of the neuronal specific potassium chloride contransporter KCC2 mRNA than females, which is associated with depolarization as a response to muscimol application or synaptically released GABA, while female neurons respond by hyperpolarization (Galanopoulou *et al.*, 2003; Kyrozis *et al.*, 2006).

■ Conclusion

Generalized models, except for minimal electroshock and some genetic models, are part of a seizure syndrome, which cannot be divided from absence-like behavior (often identified only with EEG recordings) and thus, according to classification do not constitute a good model of myoclonic seizures. However, since these models are readily available and easy to produce, they are widely used. This indicates that it is necessary to search for new, more suitable models of myoclonic seizures, which would better fit to human epileptic myoclonus.

Identification and characterization of structures involved in control of myoclonic seizures may allow using new therapeutical approaches such as deep brain stimulation of focal drug administration (Vercueil *et al.*, 1998; Loddenkemper *et al.*, 2001; Velíšek *et al.*, 2002).

Acknowledgements: Supported by the NINDS research grants NS-20253, NS-41366, a CURE Foundation grant, and a Heffer Family Medical Research Foundation.

References

Acampora D, Mazan S, Avantaggiato V, Barone P, Tuorto F, Lallemand Y, Brulet P, Simeone A. Epilepsy and brain abnormalities in mice lacking the Otx1 gene. *Nat Genet* 1996; 14: 218-22.

Ackermann RF, Moshé SL, Albala BJ. Restriction of enhanced 14C-2-deoxyglucose utilization to rhinencephalic structures in immature amygdala-kindled rats. *Exp Neurol* 1989; 104: 73-81.

Ackermann RF, Finch DM, Babb TL, Engel J, Jr. Increased glucose metabolism during long-duration recurrent inhibition of hippocampal pyramidal cells. *J Neurosci* 1984; 4: 251-64.

Albala BJ, Moshé SL, Okada R. Kainic-acid-induced seizures: a developmental study. *Dev Brain Res* 1984; 13: 139-48.

Avanzini G, Spreafico R, Cipelletti B, Sancini G, Frassoni C, Franceschetti S, Lavazza T, Panzica F, Acampora D, Simeone A. Synaptic properties of neocortical neurons in epileptic mice lacking the Otx1 gene. *Epilepsia* 2000; 41 (Suppl 6): S200-205.

Braestrup C, Nielsen M, Olsen CE. Urinary and brain beta-carboline-3-carboxylates as potent inhibitors of brain benzodiazepine receptors. *Proc Natl Acad Sci USA* 1980; 77: 2288-92.

Braestrup C, Schmiechen R, Neef G, Nielsen M, Petersen EN. Interaction of convulsive ligands with benzodiazepine receptors. *Science* 1982; 216: 1241-3.

Braestrup C, Nielsen M, Honore T, Jensen LH, Petersen EN. Benzodiazepine receptor ligands with positive and negative efficacy. *Neuropharmacology* 1983; 22: 1451-7.

Burgess DL. Transgenic and gene replacement models of epilepsy: Targeting ion channel and neurotransmission pathways in mice. In: Pitkanen A, Schwartzkroin PA, Moshé SL, eds. *Models of seizures and epilepsy*. San Diego: Elsevier, 2006: 199-222.

Cipelletti B, Avanzini G, Vitellaro-Zuccarello L, Franceschetti S, Sancini G, Lavazza T, Acampora D, Simeone A, Spreafico R, Frassoni C. Morphological organization of somatosensory cortex in Otx1(-/-) mice. *Neuroscience* 2002; 115: 657-67.

Cogswell CA, Sarkisian MR, Leung V, Patel R, D'Mello SR, LoTurco JJ. A gene essential to brain growth and development maps to the distal arm of rat chromosome 12. *Neurosci Lett* 1998; 251: 5-8.

Collins RC, Santori EM, Der T, Toga AW, Lothman EW. Functional metabolic mapping during forelimb movement in rat. I. Stimulation of motor cortex. *J Neurosci* 1986; 6: 448-62.

Commission on Pediatric Epilepsy of the International League Against Epilepsy. Myoclonus and epilepsy in childhood. *Epilepsia* 1997; 38: 1251-4.

Depaulis A, Snead OCI, Marescaux C, Vergnes M. Suppressive effects of intranigral injection of muscimol in three models of generalized non-convulsive epilepsy induced by chemical agents. *Brain Res* 1989; 498: 64-72.

Depaulis A, Liu Z, Vergnes M, Marescaux C, Micheletti G, Warter JM. Suppression of spontaneous generalized non-convulsive seizures in the rat by microinjection of GABA antagonists into the superior colliculus. *Epilepsy Res* 1990; 5: 192-8.

Di Chiara G, Porceddu ML, Morelli M, Mulas ML, Gessa GL. Evidence for a GABAergic projection from the substantia nigra to the ventromedial thalamus and to the superior colliculus of the rat. *Brain Res* 1979; 176: 273-84.

Eells JB, Clough RW, Miller JW, Jobe PC, Browning RA. Fos expression and 2-deoxyglucose uptake following seizures in developing genetically epilepsy-prone rats. *Brain Res Bull* 2000; 52: 379-89.

Eger EI, 2nd, Gong D, Xing Y, Raines DE, Flood P. Acetylcholine receptors and thresholds for convulsions from flurothyl and 1,2-dichlorohexafluorocyclobutane. *Anesth Analg* 2002; 95: 1611-5, table of contents.

Engel J, Jr., Wolfson L, Brown L. Anatomical correlates of electrical and behavioral events related to amygdaloid kindling. *Ann Neurol* 1978; 3: 538-44.

Fan XD, Zhang X, Yu PH, Li XM, Juorio AV. Induction of preconvulsive behavior and Fos expression by dopamine- induced nigral lesion in the rat. *Brain Res* 1997; 751: 31-6.

Galanopoulou AS, Kyrozis A, Claudio OI, Stanton PK, Moshé SL. Sex-specific KCC2 expression and GABA(A) receptor function in rat substantia nigra. *Exp Neurol* 2003; 183: 628-37.

Garant DS, Xu SG, Sperber EF, Moshé SL. The influence of thalamic GABA transmission on the susceptibility of adult rats to flurothyl induced seizures. *Epilepsy Res* 1993; 15: 185-92.

Gernert M, Fedrowitz M, Wlaz P, Loscher W. Subregional changes in discharge rate, pattern, and drug sensitivity of putative GABAergic nigral neurons in the kindling model of epilepsy. *Eur J Neurosci* 2004; 20: 2377-86.

Horton RW, Meldrum BS. Seizures induced by allylglycine, 3-mercaptopropionic acid and 4-deoxypyridoxine in mice and photosensitive baboons, and different modes of inhibition of cerebral glutamic acid decarboxylase. *Br J Pharmacol* 1973; 49: 52-63.

Horton RW, Jenner P, Marsden CD, Meldrum BS, Reavill C. Behavioural effects of allylglycine (2-amino-4-pentenoic acid) and 2- keto-4-pentenoic acid following focal injection into the rat cerebellum and caudate nucleus [proceedings]. *Br J Pharmacol* 1978; 63: 381.

Kha HT, Finkelstein DI, Tomas D, Drago J, Pow DV, Home MK. Projections from the substantia nigra pars reticulata to the motor thalamus of the rat: single axon reconstructions and immunohistochemical study. *J Comp Neurol* 2001; 440: 20-30.

Killam KF, Killam EK, Naquet R. An animal model of light sensitive epilepsy. *Electroencephalogr Clin Neurophysiol* 1967; 22: 497-513.

Klemm WR. Behavioral arrest: in search of the neural control system. *Prog Neurobiol* 2001; 65: 453-71.

Kubová H, Lanštiaková M, Mocková M, Mareš P, Vorlíšek J. Pharmacology of cortical epileptic afterdischarges in rats. *Epilepsia* 1996; 37: 336-41.

Kyrozis A, Chudomel O, Moshé SL, Galanopoulou AS. Sex-dependent maturation of GABAA receptor-mediated synaptic events in rat substantia nigra reticulata. *Neurosci Lett* 2006; 398: 1-5.

Lánský P, Velíšková J, Velíšek L. An indirect method for absorption rate estimation: Flurothyl-induced seizures. *Bull Math Biol* 1997; 59: 569-79.

Leppik IE. Classification of the myoclonic epilepsies. *Epilepsia* 2003; 44 (Suppl 11): 2-6.

Levitt P, Noebels JL. Mutant mouse tottering: selective increase of locus ceruleus axons in a defined single-locus mutation. *Proc Natl Acad Sci USA* 1981; 78: 4630-4.

Loddenkemper T, Pan A, Neme S, Baker KB, Rezai AR, Dinner DS, Montgomery EB, Jr., Luders HO. Deep brain stimulation in epilepsy. *J Clin Neurophysiol* 2001; 18: 514-32.

Marcus E, Watson C, DeLuca A. Factors influencing the epileptogenic effects of conjugated equine estrogens (Premarin) on cerebral electrical activity in cat and man. *Electroenceph Clin Neurophysiol* 1963; 15: 150-1.

Marcus EM, Watson CW, Goldman PL. Effects of steroids on cerebral electrical activity. Epileptogenic effects of conjugated estrogens and related compounds in the cat and rabbit. *Arch Neurol* 1966; 15: 521-32.

Mareš P, Trojan S. Ontogenetic development of isonicotinehydrazide-induced seizures in rats. *Brain Dev* 1991; 13: 121-5.

Mareš P, Kubová H. Electrical stimulation-induced models of seizures. In: Pitkanen A, Schwartzkroin PA, Moshé SL, eds. *Models of seizures and epilepsy*. San Diego: Elsevier, 2006: 153-9.

Mareš P, Haugvicová R, Kubová H. Unequal development of thresholds for various phenomena induced by cortical stimulation in rats. *Epilepsy Res* 2002; 49: 35-43.

Mareš P, Kubová H, Zouhar A, Folbergrova J, Koryntova H, Stankova L. Motor and electrocorticographic epileptic activity induced by 3-mercaptopropionic acid in immature rats. *Epilepsy Res* 1993; 16: 11-8.

Meldrum B. GABAergic agents as anticonvulsants in baboons with photosensitive epilepsy. *Neurosci Lett* 1984; 47: 345-9.

Meldrum B, Horton R. Effects of the bicyclic GABA agonist, THIP, on myoclonic and seizure responses in mice and baboons with reflex epilepsy. *Eur J Pharmacol* 1980; 61: 231-7.

Meldrum BS, Horton RW. Convulsive effects of 4-deoxypyridoxine and of bicuculline in in photosensitive baboons (Papio papio) and in rhesus monkeys (Maccaca mulatta). *Brain Res* 1971; 35: 419-36.

Meldrum BS, Balzano E, Gadea M, Naquet R. Photic and drug-induced epilepsy in the baboon (Papio papio): the effects of isoniazid, thiosemicarbazide, pyridoxine and amino-oxyacetic acid. *Electroencephalogr Clin Neurophysiol* 1970; 29: 333-47.

Menini C. Frontal cerebral cortex and photic epilepsy of the baboon Papio papio. *J Physiol* 1976; 72: 5-44.

Moshé SL, Okada R, Albala BJ. Ventromedial thalamic lesions and seizure susceptibility. *Brain Res* 1985; 337: 368-72.

Moshé SL, Brown LL, Kubová H, Velíšková J, Zukin RS, Sperber EF. Maturation and segregation of brain networks that modify seizures. *Brain Res* 1994; 665: 141-6.

Nakano K, Kayahara T, Tsutsumi T, Ushiro H. Neural circuits and functional organization of the striatum. *J Neurol* 2000; 247 (Suppl 5): V1-15.

Naquet R, Meldrum BS. Myoclonus induced by intermittent light stimulation in the baboon: neurophysiological and neuropharmacological approaches. *Adv Neurol* 1986; 43: 611-27.

Naquet R, Menini C, Riche D, Silva-Barrat C, Valin A. Photic epilepsy problems raised in man and animals. *Ital J Neurol Sci* 1987; 8: 437-47.

Naquet R, Menini C, Riche D, Silva-Barrat C, Valin A. Photic Epilepsy in Man and in the Baboon, Papio papio. In: Meldrum BS, Ferrendelli JA, Wieser HG, eds. *Anatomy of Epileptogenesis*. London-Paris: John Libbey, 1988: 107-26.

Nehlig A, Vergnes M, Boyet S, Marescaux C. Metabolic activity is increased in discrete brain regions before the occurence of spike-and-wave discharges in weanling rats with genetic absence epilepsy. *Dev Brain Res* 1998; 108: 69-75.

Noebels JL. Analysis of inherited epilepsy using single locus mutations in mice. *Fed Proc* 1979; 38: 2405-10.

Noebels JL. Mutational analysis of inherited epilepsies. *Adv Neurol* 1986; 44: 97-113.

Noebels JL. Exploring new gene discoveries in idiopathic generalized epilepsy. *Epilepsia* 2003a; 44 (Suppl 2): 16-21.

Noebels JL. The biology of epilepsy genes. *Annu Rev Neurosci* 2003b; 26: 599-625.

Noebels JL. Spontaneous epileptic mutations in the mouse. In: Pitkanen A, Schwartzkroin PA, Moshé SL, eds. *Models of seizures and epilepsy*. San Diego, 2006: 223-32.

Noebels JL, Sidman RL. Inherited epilepsy: spike-wave and focal motor seizures in the mutant mouse tottering. *Science* 1979; 204: 1334-6.

Pazdernik TL, Cross RS, Giesler M, Samson FE, Nelson SR. Changes in local cerebral glucose utilization induced by convulsants. *Neuroscience* 1985; 14: 823-35.

Racine RJ. Modification of seizure activity by electrical stimulation: II. Motor seizures. *Electroencephal Clin Neurophysiol* 1972; 32: 281-94.

Ravizza T, Friedman LK, Moshé SL, Velíšková J. Sex differences in GABA(A)ergic system in rat substantia nigra pars reticulata. *Int J Dev Neurosci* 2003; 21: 245-54.

Redgrave P, Simkins M, Overton P, Dean P. Anticonvulsant role of nigrotectal projection in the maximal electroshock model of epilepsy – I. Mapping of dorsal midbrain with bicuculline. *Neuroscience* 1992; 46: 379-90.

Roberts MR, Bittman K, Li WW, French R, Mitchell B, LoTurco JJ, D'Mello SR. The flathead mutation causes CNS-specific developmental abnormalities and apoptosis. *J Neurosci* 2000; 20: 2295-306.

Rye DB, Saper CB, Lee HJ, Wainer BH. Pedunculopontine tegmental nucleus of the rat: cytoarchitecture, cytochemistry, and some extrapyramidal connections of the mesopontine tegmentum. *J Comp Neurol* 1987; 259: 483-528.

Sancini G, Franceschetti S, Lavazza T, Panzica F, Cipelletti B, Frassoni C, Spreafico R, Acampora D, Avanzini G. Potentially epileptogenic dysfunction of cortical NMDA- and GABA-mediated neurotransmission in Otx1-/- mice. *Eur J Neurosci* 2001; 14: 1065-74.

Sarkisian MR, Rattan S, D'Mello SR, LoTurco JJ. Characterization of seizures in the flathead rat: a new genetic model of epilepsy in early postnatal development. *Epilepsia* 1999; 40: 394-400.

Sarkisian MR, Frenkel M, Li W, Oborski JA, LoTurco JJ. Altered interneuron development in the cerebral cortex of the flathead mutant. *Cereb Cortex* 2001; 11: 734-43.

Sawamura A, Hashizume K, Yoshida K, Tanaka T. Kainic acid-induced substantia nigra seizure in rats: behavior, EEG and metabolism. *Brain Res* 2001; 911: 89-95.

Shehab S, Simkins M, Dean P, Redgrave P. Regional distribution of the anticonvulsant and behavioural effects of muscimol injected into the substantia nigra of rats. *Eur J Neurosci* 1996; 8: 749-57.

Sokoloff L. Energetics of functional activation in neural tissues. *Neurochem Res* 1999; 24: 321-9.

Somjen GG. Mechanisms of spreading depression and hypoxic spreading depression-like depolarization. *Physiol Rev* 2001; 81: 1065-96.

Soukupová S, Mikolášová R, Kubová H, Mareš P. New model of cortical foci in freely moving developing rats. *Epilepsy Res* 1993; 15: 27-34.

Spann BM, Grofova I. Nigropedunculopontine projection in the rat: an anterograde tracing study with phaseolus vulgaris-leucoagglutinin (PHA-L). *J Comp Neurol* 1991; 311: 375-88.

Sperber EF, Brown LL, Moshé SL. Functional mapping of different seizure states in the immature rat using 14C-2-deoxyglucose. *Epilepsia* 1992; 33: 44.

Sperber EF, Wong BY, Wurpel JN, Moshé SL. Nigral infusions of muscimol or bicuculline facilitate seizures in developing rats. *Brain Res* 1987; 465: 243-50.

Sperber EF, Haas KZ, Romero MT, Stanton PK. Flurothyl status epilepticus in developing rats: behavioral, electrographic histological and electrophysiological studies. *Brain Res Dev Brain Res* 1999; 116: 59-68.

Swinyard EA, Woodhead JH, White HS, Franklin MR. Experimental selection, quantification, and evaluation of anticonvulsants. In: Levy RH, Dreifuss FE, Mattson RH, Meldrum BS, Penry JK, eds. *Antiepileptic Drugs, 3rd Edition*. New York: Raven Press, 1989; 85-102.

Szabo CA, Leland MM, Knape K, Elliott JJ, Haines V, Williams JT. Clinical and EEG phenotypes of epilepsy in the baboon (Papio hamadryas spp.). *Epilepsy Res* 2005; 65: 71-80.

Thompson K, Anantharam V, Behrstock S, Bongarzone E, Campagnoni A, Tobin AJ. Conditionally Immortalized Cell Lines, Engineered to Produce and Release GABA, Modulate the Development of Behavioral Seizures. *ExpNeurol* 2000; 161: 481-9.

Velíšek L, Kusá R, Kulovaná M, Mareš P. Excitatory amino acid antagonists and pentylenetetrazol-induced seizures during ontogenesis. I. The effects of 2-amino-7-phosphonoheptanoate. *Life Sci* 1990; 46: 1349-57.

Velíšek L, Verešová S, Pôbišová H, Mareš P. Excitatory amino acid antagonists and pentylenetetrazol-induced seizures during ontogenesis. II. The effects of MK-801. *Psychopharmacology (Berl)* 1991; 104: 510-4.

Velíšek L. Model of chemically-induced acute seizures. In: Pitkanen A, Schwartzkroin PA, Moshé SL, eds. *Models of seizures and epilepsy* San Diego: Elsevier, 2006: 127-52.

Velíšek L, Vondřičková R, Mareš P. Models of simple partial and absence seizures in freely moving rats: Action of ketamine. *Pharmacol Biochem Behav* 1993; 45: 889-96.

Velíšek L, Velíšková J, Moshé SL. Electrical stimulation of substantia nigra pars reticulata is anticonvulsant in adult and young male rats. *Exp Neurol* 2002; 173: 145-52.

Velíšek L, Kubová H, Pohl M, Staňková L, Mareš P, Schickerová R. Pentylenetetrazol-induced seizures in rats: An ontogenetic study. *Naunyn-Schmiedeberg's Arch Pharmacol* 1992; 346: 588-91.

Velíšek L, Moshé SL. Cephalosporins. In: Spencer PS, Schaumburg HH, eds. *Experimental and Clinical Neurotoxicology*. New York: Oxford University Press, 2000a: 345-8.

Velíšek L, Moshé SL. Penicillins. In: Spencer PS, Schaumburg HH, eds. *Experimental and Clinical Neurotoxicology*. New York: Oxford University Press, 2000b: 948-51.

Velíšková J. Age related mechanisms involved in the control of seizures. In: Nehlig A, Motte J, Moshé SL, Plouin P, eds. *Childhood Epilepsies and Brain Development*. London Sydney: John Libbey, 1999: 39-51.

Velíšková J. Behavioral characterization of seizures in rats. In: Pitkanen A, Schwartzkroin PA, Moshé SL, eds. *Models of seizures and epilepsy*. San Diego: Elsevier, 2006: 601-11.

Velíšková J, Moshé SL. Sexual dimorphism and developmental regulation of substantia nigra function. *Ann Neurol* 2001; 50: 596-601.

Velíšková J, Velíšek L, Mareš P, Rokyta R. Ketamine suppresses both bicuculline- and picrotoxin-induced generalized tonic-clonic seizures during ontogenesis. *Pharmacol Biochem Behav* 1990; 37: 667-74.

Velíšková J, Miller AM, Nunes ML, Brown LL. Regional neural activity within the substantia nigra during peri-ictal flurothyl generalized seizure stages. *Neurobiol Dis* 2005.

Vercueil L, Benazzouz A, Deransart C, Bressand K, Marescaux C, Depaulis A, Benabid AL. High-frequency stimulation of the subthalamic nucleus suppresses absence seizures in the rat: comparison with neurotoxic lesions. *Epilepsy Res* 1998; 31: 39-46.

Vernadakis A, Woodbury DM. The developing animal as a model. *Epilepsia* 1969; 10: 163-78.

Voskuyl RA, Dingemanse J, Danhof M. Determination of the threshold for convulsions by direct cortical stimulation. *Epilepsy Res* 1989; 3: 120-9.

Wakamori M, Ikemoto Y, Akaike N. Effects of two volatile anesthetics and a volatile convulsant on the excitatory and inhibitory amino acid responses in dissociated CNS neurons of the rat. *J Neurophysiol* 1991; 66: 2014-21.

Xu SG, Garant DS, Sperber EF, Moshé SL. The proconvulsant effect of nigral infusions of THIP on flurothyl-induced seizures in rat pups. *Dev Brain Res* 1992; 68: 275-7.

Systems and networks in myoclonic seizures and epilepsies

Matthias J. Koepp, Khalid Hamandi

Department of Clinical and Experimental Epilepsy, Institute of Neurology, University College London, Queen Square, London WC1N 3BG

"Epilepsy is a sudden, excessive, and rapid discharge of grey matter of some part of the brain... in a case of epilepsy grey matter is so abnormally nourished that it occasionally reaches very high tension and very unstable equilibrium, and therefore occasionally 'explodes'... symptoms of such instability in disease are, I suppose, an exaggeration or caricature of the effects of healthy discharges: on awakening from refreshing sleep, there commonly occurs and involuntary stretching of the muscles of the whole body, showing an immense undirected motor discharge... a sneeze is a sort of healthy epilepsy... I believe, then, that the highly unstable nervous matter of disease (in a discharging lesion) differs in composition, but not in constitution, from the comparatively stable grey matter of health."

John Hughlings Jackson

Myoclonus consist of brief, shock-like muscle jerks, similar to those provoked by stimulating the muscle's nerve with single electric shock. Myoclonic jerks may occur irregularly or rhythmically, and they often appear repetitively in the same muscles. They are of variable amplitude and force, ranging from mild and inconspicuous to violent – they may make the patient fall on the ground, drop or throw things or kick. Myoclonic jerks predominantly affect eyelids, facial and neck muscles, upper more than lower limbs and body. Myoclonic jerks of idiopathic generalized epilepsies (IGE) mainly occur on awakening. Precipitating factors are sleep deprivation, fatigue, excitement or distress and often photic stimulation. The patient is fully aware of myoclonic jerks except when they occur during absence seizures. Polyspikes are the electro-encephalogram (EEG) accompaniment of myoclonic jerks.

Negative myoclonus is defined as brief, jerky, involuntary movements due to interruption of muscular activity causing a sudden postural pause. This motor disturbance can be observed in various clinical conditions, ranging from physiological negative myoclonus to asterixis, a form of negative myoclonus observed in patients with toxic-metabolic encephalopathies, or as a paroxysmal phenomenon, labeled epileptic negative myoclonus, in patients with epilepsy (Tassinari 1995). Although cortical or subcortical origin of the epileptic negative myoclonus has been demonstrated, the exact neuronal pathway is not clear (Tassinari 1996) *(Table I)*.

Myoclonus can develop at any age. Irregular myoclonic jerking is common in syncope (Lempert, 1971) and is often mistaken for epilepsy, it occurs as whole body (hypnic) jerk in normal subjects on falling asleep (fragmentary physiological myoclonus), in the progressive myoclonic epilepsies (not discussed here), patients with mental retardation as a reflection of diffuse cerebral damage, or in a number of generalised epilepsies of infancy, childhood and adolescents *(Table II)*.

Table I. Clinical features of myoclonic seizures.

Brief jerk, singly or in series, may be induced by stimulus
Intensity varies from slight tremor to massive jerk
Distribution varies from single muscle to generalised jerking
Consciousness usually not altered
Rapid onset and cessation
Associated features depend on the clinical context of the myoclonus

■ Epilepsy syndromes with myoclonic seizures

As a seizure type, **myoclonic absences** consist of rhythmic jerks of the upper limbs, which mainly involve the shoulders and arms, and less frequently the lower limbs (Roger, 1992). Perioral jerks are frequent, but eyelid myoclonus is very unusual. Impairment of consciousness is variable and the patient remains aware of the limb movements. Jerks may be asymmetrical or unilateral, and are often precipitated by hyperventilation, although photosensitivity is rare. Polygraphic recording shows bilateral and symmetrical spike and slow-wave discharges, which, at first sight, look like pyknoleptic absence. However, the recoding most often comprises a series of polyspikes, each followed by a slow wave. The myographic recording shows that the jerk is linked to the first negative component of the polyspike, whereas the second component of the polyspike is linked to an inhibitory motor phenomenon that produces negative myoclonus. Thus, myoclonic jerk comprise a brief jerk followed by a drop of the affected limb (Tassinari, 1998).

As a specific epilepsy syndrome, **myoclonic absences** are the predominant seizure type of **myoclonic absence epilepsy**, although 2/3 years of patients exhibit other kinds of generalised seizures, including typical absences, tonic-clonic seizures and drop attacks. Onset ranges from 1-12 years (mean 7), and myoclonic absence epilepsy is more frequent than childhood absence epilepsy during the second year of life. Neurological examination is normal, but 45% of the patients are mentally disabled at onset and antoher 25% develop mental disability during the course of the disease; most of these are patients with intractable myoclonic absence epilepsy. Almost 10% of myoclonic absence epilepsy may evolve to Lennox-Gastaut syndrome (Tassinari, 1992).

Table II. Conditions with myoclonus as a prominent feature.

Idiopathic generalised epilepsies
    Childhood absence epilepsy
    Juvenile absence epilepsy
    Juvenile myoclonic epilepsy
    Epilepsy with generalised tonic-clonic seizures in awakening
    Epilepsy with myoclonic absences
    Benign myoclonus of infancy

Childhood myoclonic epilepsies
    Infantile spasms
    Lennox-Gastaut Syndrome
    Cryptogenic myoclonic epilepsy

Progressive myoclonic epilepsies
    Unverricht-Lundborg disease
    Lafora Body disease
    Sialidoses
    Mitochondiral cytopathy
    Ceroid lipofuscinosis
    GM1 and GM2 gangliosidoses
    Gaucher's disease
    Dentato-rubro-pallido-luysian atrophy
    Hallervorden Spatz disease
    Huntington's disease
    Juvenile neuroaxonal dystrophy
    Alper's disease
    Menkes disease
    Phenylketonuria
    Biotin-responsive progressive myoclonus

Infective
    Subacute sclerosing panencephalitis
    Acute viral encephalitis
    Creutzfeldt-Jakob disease

Other symptomative or systemic causes
    Postanoxic myoclonic epilepsy
    Toxic: lead and other poisons, drugs
    Metabolic: renal disease, hepatic disease
    Respiratory disease with hypercapnia

Withdrawal of sedative drugs
    Barbiturates, benzodiazepines, alcohol

Myoclonic-astatic epilepsy is particularly difficult to distinguish from **myoclonic absence epilepsy** because of the overlapping age of onset – between 2 and 5 years – and the combination of absences with myoclonus. However, mental development is normal before the first seizures in myoclonic astatic epilepsy and there are generalise tonic-clonic seizures (GTCS) over a few weeks or months before the occurrence of absences (Doose, 1970). In addition, there are drop attacks, caused by massive myoclonus, by the time the patient exhibits absences.

Typical absences with motor symptoms of perioral myoclonia are a non-specific symptom in **perioral mycoclonus with absences**. However, this often combines with a clustering of other clinical and EEG features, suggesting that this is an interesting syndrome with onset in childhood and adolescence (Panayiotopoulos, 1989).

Benign myoclonic epilepsy in infancy is a rare cause of myoclonus with onset between 16-24 months of life, without other neurological features, and with a normal interictal EEG. The myoclonus may be initially imperceptible but frequent, most attacks lasting 1-3 seconds and being accompanied by spikewave or polyspike discharges on the EEG. Other seizure types do not develop, but there is often a family history of IGE. The prognosis is good, most cases remitting spontaneously, but other seizure types may develop later in life.

Benign familial myoclonus is a rare condition that develops in childhood or early adult life (average onset 10 years), inherited as an autosomal dominant trait. The myoclonus is massive and symmetrical and involves the axial and proximal limb muscles initially, becoming more widespread. The myoclonus is often stimulus-sensitive and worsened by stress or fatigue. There are no other neurological abnormalities, the EEG is normal and other seizure types do not develop.

In **continuous spike wave in slow wave sleep** syndrome, myoclonic jerks primarily of the upper limbs are the result of atonia and therefore negative myoclonus (Patry, 1971). As soon as the patient falls asleep, in slow-wave sleep, the tracing shows continuous spikes and slow-wave activity. It has been shown that, when the focus affect the rolandic area, there is negative myoclonus as a results of intermittent loss of tone, which looks like clusters of jerks.

Jerks in the eyes and upper eylids are a common event in **childhood or juvenile absence epilepsies**, affecting over 80% of patients studied with video-EEG, but it does rarely affect the upper limbs (Stefan, 1982). The latency to involvements of the eyelids was the shortest, followed by the face and then the limbs. In juvenile absence epilepsy, one fifth of patients suffer from mild myoclonic jerks of random distribution. They usually occur in the afternoon hours when the patient is tired rather than in the morning after awakening (Panayiotopoulos, 1997).

Juvenile myoclonic epilepsy (JME) is one of the most important IGE syndromes that is genetically determined. The triad of absences, myoclonic jerks and GTCS shows a characteristic age-related onset. Myoclonic jerks occurring after awakening are the most prominent and pathognomonic seizure type. The myoclonic jerks are rhythmic and occur in clusters, although the clusters are brief, lasting 1-2 s without loss of consciousness. They may be violent enough to cause falls, but are often inconspicuous, restricted to the fingers, making the patient prone to drop things or look clumsy. The EEG shows variable amount of spike activity within a burst, and frequent photosensitivity (Janz, 1985).

■ Reflex Epilepsies

Epileptic seizures can arise in a spontaneous unpredictable fashion without detectable precipitant factors, or they can be provoked by certain recognisable stimuli. Reflex epilepsies are determined by the specific precipitant stimulus and the clinical-EEG response. The precipitating stimulus evoking an epileptic seizure is specific for a given patients and may be simple (flashes of light or tactile) or complex (reading or eating), or elaborate (higher brain function, emotions). The response to the stimulus consists of clinical and EEG manifestations, alone or in combinations. EEG activation may be subclinical only. Conversely, ictal clinical manifestations may be triggered without conspicuous surface EEG changes. Despite their regionally specific triggers, reflex seizures are often generalised (absences, myoclonic jerks, GTCS) with myoclonic seizures being by far the most common, manifested in the limbs and trunk or regionally, such as in the jaw muscles (**reading epilepsy**) or the eye lids (as in **eyelid myoclonia with absences**). GTCS may follow a cluster of myoclonic jerks *(Table III)*.

Neuroimaging studies in IGE

The development of highly sensitive neuroimaging techniques has allowed the identification of subtle functional and structural abnormalities, providing a means of elucidating the underlying mechanisms of myoclonic jerks and epilepsies, and the relative contribution of focal *versus* generalised dysfunction. The majority of neuroimaging studies are performed in patients with symptomatic partial epilepsies, as part of presurgical evaluasation. Patients with IGE are rarely studied, and if so, they are studied during adulthood rather than as children or adolescents during the "statu nascendi" of their condition. This often leads to the inclusion of either wrongly diagnosed or wrongly treated patients or those who did not respond to treatment or in other abnormal way presented in adulthood. Another major concern in respect of neuroimaging studies is that often various IGE syndromes are lumped together to generate enough numbers to allow meaningful statistical conclusions for the group of patients studied. At best, these group studies provide information about particular

Table III. Reflex seizures, related reflex mechanisms and the precipitating stimuli (see Panayiotopoulos 2002).

Somatosensory stimuli
- Benign childhood epilepsy with somatosensory evoked spikes
- Sensory evoked idiopathic myoclonic seizures in infancy
- Tooth-brushing epilepsy
- Hot water epilepsy
- Seizures induced by movements
- Seizures induced by eye-closure and/or eye movements
- Eating Epilepsy

Visual Stimuli
- Photosensitive epilepsies
- Pattern-sensitive epilepsies
- Fixation-off sensitive epilepsies

Auditory, vestibular and olfactory stimuli
- Seizures induced by sounds
- Musicogenic epilepsy
- Olfactorhinencephalic epilepsy
- Seizures triggered by vestibular and auditory stimuli

Complex stimuli
- Reading Epilepsy
- Thinking (noogenic epilepsy)
- Reflex decision making epilepsy
- Emotional epilepsies
- Startle epilepsy

seizure phenomenology, but there is not a single inter-ictal neuro-imaging study, which differentiates between the effects of generalised tonic-clonic, absence or myoclonic seizures on the observed imaging parameter. There are few ictal positron-emission tomography studies investigating haemodynamic and metabolic changes during hyperventilation-induced absences.

In the following part of this chapter, we will first present evidence from positron emission tomography (PET) and magnetic resonance imaging (MRI) studies for the involvement of the thalamus and the frontal lobe in various IGE syndromes. Secondly, we will summarise both PET and very recent functional MRI (fMRI) studies in reading epilepsy and other reflex epilepsies, which are the only studies investigating the metabholic or haemodynamic effects of myoclonic seizures directly.

■ Evidence for Thalamic involvement in IGE

The pathophysiological substrate of generalized spine-wave (GSW) remains enigmatic. The debate between a subcortical origin "the centrencephalic hypothesis" (Jasper and Drooglever-Fortuyn, 1947) *versus* a cortical origin (Marcus, 1968) was reconciled to an extent by the corticoreticular hypothesis. This proposed a role for both cortex and subcortical structures (Gloor, 1968), with aberrant oscillatory rhythms in reciprocally connected thalamocortical loops normally involved in the generation of sleep spindles (Gloor, 1968), leading to GSW. The primary neuroanatomical and neurochemical abnormality in IGE remains undetermined with evidence and arguments for onset in either cortex (Timofeev, 2004) or thalamus (Avoli, 2001).

Much of the evidence pertaining to the pathophysiology of GSW comes from invasive electrophysiological and neurochemical recordings in animals (Avoli, 2001). A small number of intracranial studies have been reported in man in which spike wave activity was recorded in both thalamus and cortex (Williams, 1953; Niedermeyer, 1969; Velasco, 1989). The spatial sampling of depth studies is limited to the immediate vicinity of the implanted electrodes, and their invasiveness, in the absence of clinical benefit precludes their current use in IGE.

Positron-Emission-Tomography (PET)

PET allows the tomographic delineation of cerebral structures and the measurement of tissue concentrations of injected radioactive tracers at the molecular level, and may be performed when the subject is at rest, or during or following the occurrence of a seizure, the undertaking of a cognitive or motor task, or the administration of a drug. A study using PET and bolus injections of $H_2^{15}O$ was used to measure cerebral blood flow in patients with IGE and a history of absence seizures (Prevett, 1995). It showed that, in addition to a global increase in cerebral blood flow during absence seizures, there was a significant focal increase in thalamic blood flow, providing evidence that the thalamus plays a key role in the pathogenesis of typical absence seizures (Gloor, 1968).

Quantitative magnetic resonance imaging (MRI) studies

Although visual inspection of routine MRI in patients with IGE appears normal, neuropathological autopsy studies have provided evidence of grey and white matter microdysgenesis (Meencke, 1984, 1985). Quantitative MRI can elucidate subtle changes not apparent on visual inspection.

Only one MRI-based volumetric study limited to the thalamus, found no difference in a heterogeneous group of patients with IGE, *versus* normal controls (Natsume, 2003). This finding contrasts with another MRI-based study in patients with IGE, in which subcortical structures (without further differentiation) appeared to be smaller in IGE patients as compared with healthy controls (Woermann, 1998). In a more recent study, the volumes of the caudate nucleus, putamen, pallidum as well as the thalamus were each determined in both hemispheres in 11 patients with various IGE syndromes, normalized for whole-brain volumes and then compared with 15 age-matched controls (Seeck, 2005). No differences were noted in thalamic volumes, confirming previous reports. However, smaller subcortical volumes were noted in the IGE patients ($p < 0.009$), mainly due to smaller putamen bilaterally ($p = 0.015$). Larger studies with more homogeneous patient populations are needed to determine the robustness of these findings and whether they are specific for particular IGE syndromes.

Magnetic resonance spectroscopy (MRS)

Whereas conventional MRI provides structural information based on signals from water protons, proton magnetic resonance spectroscopy (^{1}H-MRS) provides information on the chemical composition of the brain. Since N-acetyl aspartate (NAA) is found exclusively in neurons and neuronal processes (Simmons, 1991; Moffet, 1991), a reduction in the level of NAA can be an indication of neuronal damage or dysfunction (Savic, 2000). ^{1}H-MRS measurement of NAA provides a means of detecting neuronal damage when structural MRI is unable to do so (Hugg, 1993; Garcia, 1995; Stanley, 1998).

Using this technique, thalamic NAA concentrations were found to be significantly lower in IGE patients than in controls (Berasconi, 2003). Volumetric MRI did not identify a significant loss in thalamic volume in these patients, indicating thalamic neuronal dysfunction, rather than loss, in agreement with previous neuropathological studies (Meencke, 1984; Mouritzen, 1996). Moreover, a negative correlation was found between NAA levels and duration of epilepsy, indicating that thalamic dysfunction in IGE may be progressive (Bernasconi, 2003).

Functional MRI (fMRI)

EEG-correlated functional MRI (EEG-fMRI) provides a means of identifying and studying the neural correlates of spontaneously occurring GSW. This technique has been used to study a patient with IGE and frequent absences, demonstrating the reciprocal participation of focal thalamic blood flow increases (Salek-Haddadi, 2003).

Subsequently, two EEG-fMRI series, conducted in Australia (Archer, 2003) and Canada (Aghakani, 2004), have replicated these findings of altered thalamic and cortical blood flow, in larger groups of patients with IGE.

The British patient showed a 3% increase in BOLD signal bilaterally within the thalami, which was time-locked with the prolonged runs of GSW. In the Canadian patients, bilateral thalamic activations were more frequent than deactivation (eight vs. two) with two patients showing both activation and deactivations in adjacent thalamic regions. The differences in the amount and length of GSW studied and methodological differences (continuous versus triggered EEG-fMRI) might explain some of the commonalities (predominantly de-activations in cortical areas) and discrepancies (thalamic activations) in the human findings. The predominantly positive BOLD changes occurring in the thalamus and mixed positive and negative cortical BOLD changes are in keeping with a recent fMRI study during sustained absence seizures in an awake animal model (Tenney, 2003). The BOLD signal in the ventrobasal thalamus and sensory cortex increased with the onset of absence seizures, whilst there was a BOLD signal decrease in the temporal and motor cortices.

The predominant finding in individual subject and group analyses was of thalamic activation and cortical BOLD negative response. Thalamic signal change was seen in less than half of patients with IGE, but in almost all patients with secondarily generalized tonic-clonic seizures (SGE) (Hamandi, 2006). This may be due to the greater occurrence of GSW events in SGE cases compared to IGE (median SGE 44.5 versus IGE 8), and tended to be seen in those individual IGE cases with a higher number or longer duration of GSW. At the single subject level similar BOLD responses were seen across IGE syndromes and in SGE, suggesting that the predominant BOLD findings represent generic changes associated with GSW per se rather than syndrome specific patterns. This is unlikely due to syndrome misclassification (Berkovic, 1987) given the similarity of our findings in cases with very clear syndromic differences.

It is not possible to infer causality of the BOLD changes relative to our modeled covariate, GSW; they may represent areas generating GSW, or alternatively reflect areas secondarily affected by GSW. This difficulty in inferring causality is in contrast to paradigm driven fMRI where it is generally safe to assume a primary association between the task or stimulus and the observed fMRI changes; in addition a prior hypothesis about a relatively well defined location of expected neural activity usually exits. In EEG-fMRI of GSW, however, we have little prior anatomical hypothesis regarding the spatial extent of BOLD changes. We propose that thalamic activation seen here represents subcortical activity necessary for the maintenance of GSW (Avoli, 2001). The lack of thalamic activation in a number of our cases may reflect low sensitivity of our model at 1.5 T (Laufs, 2006).

Experiments comparing patients with primary and secondary GTCS are required to further elucidate whether the observed neurochemical and CBF changes in the thalamus reflect cause or effect of generalised seizures. A recent HMPAO-single photon emission computed tomography study (Blumenfeld, 2003) indirectly addressed this issue by investigating CBF changes after termination of either spontaneously occurring secondary GTCS or following induced GTCS. These were induced by electro-convulsive therapy (ECT) either bilateral fronto-parietal (resembling primary generalised seizures), or unilateral ECT (resembling secondary GTCS). Selective frontal, parietal and temporal networks were activated after both spontaneous and induced GTCS, but thalamic CBF was only increased following bilateral ECT.

■ Evidence for frontal lobe involvement in IGE

The early observation by Dieter Janz of the association of a particular personality profile with JME has been corroborated by anecdotal reports documenting behavioural disturbances in JME patients that are similar to those usually associated with frontal lobe injury (Janz, 1957; Beech, 1976; Devinsky, 1997). Furthermore, neuropsychological studies have demonstrated that patients with JME exhibit impaired performance in tests measuring frontal lobe functions (Swartz, 1994). These impairments were found most frequently in tests of concept formation, mental flexibility, preservative tendencies, planning and cognitive speed, whereas fine motor speed and coordination were normal (Devinsky, 1997). In tests measuring cognitive performance, patients with JME were shown to have significantly impaired verbal and visual memory, and impaired frontal and visuospatial function, compared with normal controls (Sonmez, 2004). During tasks involving working memory, patients with JME exhibited deficits in performance that were almost as severe as in patients with known frontal lobe epilepsy (Swartz, 1997).

JME is associated with normal intelligence (Delgado-Escueta, 1984). However, it has been noted that JME is associated with a particular personality profile (Janz, 1957; Devinskly, 1997), and behavioural and neuropsychological studies have suggested subtle frontal lobe dysfunction (Beech, 1976; Savic, 2000; Swartz, 1994). Moreover, neuropathological studies have provided evidence of microdysgenesis in IGE, in the form of cortical and subcortical dystopic neurons and other microscopic structural abnormalities (Meencke, 1984, 1985).

PET studies

Flumazenil (FMZ), a specific, reversibly bound, high-affinity neutral antagonist of cBZR (Olsen 1990), can be ^{11}C-labelled and used with PET to provide a marker for the integrity of γ-amino butyric acid (GABA) – the principal inhibitory neurotransmitter in the brain. A study using ^{11}C-FMZ-PET demonstrated that $GABA_A$-cBZR binding is globally increased in the cerebral cortex of patients with JME and other forms of IGE (Koepp, 1997). Frontal lobe $GABA_A$-cBZR binding was particularly elevated in patients with JME, but not in patients with other forms of IGE (Koepp, 2000).

Similarly, a study using PET to measure the uptake of ^{18}F-fluoro-2-deoxyglucose (^{18}FDG) demonstrated that in JME frontal lobe abnormalities subtle may affect epileptogenic potential and cognitive functioning (Swartz, 1996). Correlating with impaired performance during a visual working memory test, JME patients were shown to have reduced ^{18}FDG uptake in the dorsolateral prefrontal cortex, premotor and basal frontal cortex.

Quantitative MRI

Quantitative MRI can elucidate subtle changes in the ratio of cortical and subcortical matter in specified volumes of interest, providing a means of detecting structural changes not normally visible using high-resolution MRI. This technique has been used to demonstrate subtle, but widespread cerebral structural changes in patients with IGE (Woermann, 1998). Of the patients with JME included in this study, 40% (8/20) had a significant abnormality of cerebral structure.

When voxel-based statistical parametric mapping was used to analyse structural MRI data, patients with JME were shown to have an increase in cortical grey matter in the mesial frontal lobes compared with normal subjects (Woermann, 1999). This objective technique revealed significant abnormalities in the cortical grey matter of a quarter (5/20) of the JME patients studied, four of whom had previously been shown to have widespread abnormalities using quantitative MRI (Woermann, 1998). Two patients had bilateral areas of increased grey matter volume, one in the temporoposterial and the other in the mesioparietal region, whilst three had areas of decreased grey matter volume, two in the frontopolar area and one in the frontomesial region (Woermann, 1999). For the correct interpretation of these voxel-based techniques, it has to be emphasised that uni- or bilateral findings very much depend on the level of thresholding chosen for the analysis.

Smaller subcortical volumes were noted in a recent comparison of IGE patients ($p < 0.009$) with healthy controls, mainly due to smaller putamen bilaterally ($p = 0.015$). The putamen has close connections with the caudate nucleus and sends and receives projections from the subthalamic nucleus, substantia nigra, pallidum, various thalamic nuclei, and motor and premotor cortex (Niewenhuys, 1988). If the frontal cortex has privileged connections to the putamen, structural changes of the putamen should therefore result in frontal lobe deficits.

MRS pectroscopy

^{1}H-MRS has also demonstrated that patients with JME have significantly reduced prefrontal concentrations of NAA, compared with controls, demonstrating that prefrontal cerebral changes – neuronal in origin – exist in JME (Savic, 2000, 2004; Simister, 2003a). This finding seems to be specific to JME, compared with other forms of IGE, such as pure primarily generalized tonic clonic epilepsy (Savic, 2004).

In addition, ^{1}H-MRS revealed frontal lobe metabolite changes in IGE, with increased levels of glutamate plus glutamine (GLX), an indication of increased neuronal excitability in this region (Simister, 2003a). ^{1}H-MRS has also demonstrated elevated levels of GLX and GABA in the occipital lobes of patients with IGE (Simister, 2003b).

fMRI

Cortical BOLD signal changes were detected in about 3/4 of sessions across studies (Hamandi, 2006; Salek-Haddadi, 2003; Archer, 2003; Aghakhani, 2004; Laufs, 2006). Those with no BOLD response had only very few events, all of which were of less than 2 seconds duration. There is a striking lack of changes in the primary cortices, except in a few cases, the primary visual cortex. Cortical BOLD changes are found predominantly in a frontal and posterior, often symmetrical distribution and primarily comprise negative changes in cortex.

Widespread but symmetrical cortical deactivation with a frontal maximum (~8%) was reported in a (British) case with prolonged runs of GSW (Salek-Haddadi, 2003). In the Australian series, signal reductions in the posterior cingulate were observed in four out of five patients (Archer, 2003), while the Canadian series reported a variable, but in the majority of patients symmetrical deactivation in the cortex of both hemispheres, involving the anterior as much as posterior brain regions (Aghakani, 2004).

The cortical distribution of signal change in frontal, posterior-parietal and precuneus comprises areas of association cortex that are hypothesized, at rest, to be involved in an organized, baseline level of activity, a "default mode" of brain function (Raichle, 2001; Mazoyer, 2001). The default mode concept came from observations of consistent deactivations in meta analyses of different task related paradigms in fMRI, in addition to independent PET measurements of increased blood flow to these areas during awake conscious rest (Raichle, 2001). Activity in these areas as measured by PET is also altered during sleep, coma and anesthesia (Laureys, 2004). Default mode areas likely represent part of a neural network subserving human awareness (Laureys, 2004). All fMRI studies (Hamandi, 2006; Archer, 2003; Aghakhani, 2004; Laufs, 2006) show alteration of activity in these regions during GSW, which would be consistent with the clinical manifestation of absence seizures. These findings are also consistent with PET findings of opioid release in association neocortex, most marked in parietal cortex and posterior cingulate, following absence seizures (Bartenstein, 1993).

The majority of cortical BOLD responses were negative, in keeping with transcranial Doppler (TCD) (Sanada, 1988; Klingelhofer, 1991; Bode, 1992; Nehlig, 1996; De Simone, 1998; Diehl, 1998) and near infrared spectroscopy studies (Buchheim, 2004; Haginoya et al., 2002). A number of lines of evidence suggest that BOLD negative responses represent a reduction in neural activity. In visual cortex, a reduction of BOLD signal, elicited by stimulating part of the visual field is due, primarily, to a reduction of neuronal activity (Shmuel, 2002). A decrease in BOLD signal is seen in the occipital cortex during auditory induced saccades (Wenzel, 2000), a manipulation known to suppress neuronal activity (Duffy, 1975). BOLD decreases have also been observed in the context of neuronal synchronization, modulated by sub-cortical structures (Parkes, 2004).

Visual stimulation during sleep leads to occipital BOLD negative responses, confirmed as a decrease in rCBF with $H_2^{15}O$ PET (Born, 2002). Similarly auditory BOLD negative responses occur on auditory stimulation during sleep, the amplitude and extent of which correlate positively with measures of EEG synchronization in sleep (Czisch, 2004).

Evidence for thalamo-cortical networks in relation to myoclonic seizures

Reflex epilepsies provide the potential to study neuroanatomical correlates of myoclonic seizures with improved experimental efficiency as they may be induced during the neuroimaging session by known provoking stimuli. Induced seizure activity is more conducive to neuroimaging: reading epilepsy (RE), a frequently un-diagnosed idiopathic focal epilepsy syndrome, and reflex epilepsies, such as musicogenic epilepsy, may provide unique opportunities to image induced seizure activity within the brain scanner, which could allow differentiation between generators of interictal activity and propagation of ictal activity.

Reading epilepsy, typically presents with orofacial reflex myoclonus (ORM) on reading silently or aloud, associated with spikes or sharp waves on the EEG. Patients with jaw jerks occurring on silent reading are most suitable for neuroimaging studies, given that the reading-induced ORM would only cause minor motion artefacts compared to those caused by reading aloud.

PET studies

Using paired ^{11}C-diprenorphine PET studies in healthy controls and patients with RE, we studied dynamic neurotransmitter changes in specific brain areas in relation to myoclonic seizures. We found evidence for the release of endogenous opioids during and following reading-induced orofacial reflex myoclonus in areas of the brain involved in normal reading (Koepp, 1998a). This led to the hypothesis that there are networks of cortical areas concurrently subserving both cognitive functions and epileptic activity.

fMRI studies

Archer et al. (Archer, 2003b) were the first to report EEG/fMRI findings in one patient in a cortical and subcortical distribution. These involved cortical and subcortical structures, seen bilaterally in the precentral gyrus and central sulcus and basal ganglia. This was compared to activations from a block design reading task. There was overlap of spike activity with that of the reading task, namely the posterior aspect of the left dorsolateral prefrontal cortex (DLPFC). The authors suggest that in their patient epileptiform discharges arose from spread of reading induced activity in working memory (the DLPFC) areas to adjacent motor areas and a cortical/subcortical circuit. This does not take account of the limitations of the temporal resolution of fMRI. Inferences cannot be made about the onset or spread of neural spread of activity form statistical maps, only that certain areas correlate with this activity. A greater number patients with a well defined electro clinical RE need to be studied before comment can be made about the typical patterns of fMRI activation on RE and possible pathophysiological substrates or classification categories.

We performed simultaneous EEG, EMG, and functional MRI in nine patients with RE. In six of nine patients, typical reading-induced ORM were induced either by silent reading associated with a clear EEG spikes or only whilst reading aloud. Ictal fMRI revealed consistent patterns of BOLD activations within cortical and subcortical areas: three patients showed activations in the language dominant motor cortex for hand and face; two patients showed additional BOLD increases in BA 47 on the left; five patients showed subcortical BOLD responses either within the striatum (n = 4) or the thalami (2). Most of the cortical areas were either in close proximity or directly overlapping with areas activated by cognitive and motor functions.

These cortical and subcortical areas may represent both, hyperexcitable cortex, and constitute part of the normal reading network or are involved in physiological motor function. Recruitment of a "critical mass" of such an area with synchronisation and subsequent spreading of excitation in response to the epileptogenic stimulus could precipitate epileptiform EEG activity or a clinical seizure. Increasing the complexity of epileptogenic stimuli may facilitate such a recruitment (Koepp, 1998b). This recruitment may involve the participation and interaction of several cortical and subcortical structures activated by reading, and need not be confined to physically contiguous brain sites or established neuronal links. It may rely on both exisiting and re-organised functional links between brain regions. The reported observations are consistent with this concept of variable hyperexcitability at multiple cortical and subcortical levels allowing for any asymmetric or symmetric generalised ictal EEG discharge, regional and focal discharges. This theory can also explain the heterogeneity of clinical phenomena encountered and efficacy of various linguistic stimuli as seizure triggers (Koutroumanidis, 1998).

The thalamus and a complex reciprocal thalamo-cortical network are thought to be critically important in generalised seizures (Norden, 2002). Interestingly, a recent nonlinear association signal analyses of multiple spike-wave discharges showed a consistent focus within the perioral region of the somatosensory cortex (Meeren, 2005). From this focus, seizure activity generalised rapidly over the cortex with initially the cortex driving the thalamus, while thereafter cortex and thalamus drove each other, thus amplifying and maintaining the rhythmic discharge.

Similar to the initial finding in Archer et al's single case (2003) of subcortical BOLD changes, we have now observed changes in the putamen and pallidum in five of our six patients with ORM-associated BOLD changes. BOLD changes (increases and decreases) in the globus pallidum were also reported in association with interictal discharges in 2 out of 6 patients with malformations of cortical development, which are thought to be intrinsically epileptogenic (Federico, 2005). We detected a network of cortical and subcortical areas of significant BOLD changes time-locked with seizure activity in five patients. These areas of potential cortical hyperexcitability were in close proximity or overlapping with functional areas relevant for verbal and motor functions. There were no gross abnormalities in cognitive or motor organisation. We conclude that a network of cortical areas involved in language and motor function, subserved by subcortical structures, is involved in ictogenesis in reading-epilepsy.

Morocz et al. (Morocz, 2003) reported fMRI findings in a patient with musicogenic epilepsy. The patient had music induced complex partial seizures with aurae, triggered by specific songs. fMRI "tasks" consisted of music in a block design of 39 seconds each of music known trigger followed by control music (not associated with seizure provocation). There was no concurrent EEG recording. Seizure activity was identified by patient button press at onset of aura. Differential activation during the aura session (during epileptogenic music) was seen in the left anterior temporal lobe, consistent with previous EEG recording and previous SPECT results showing ictal hyperperfusion and interictal hypoperfusion in the left temporal lobe. BOLD activation was also seen in the right gyrus rectus earlier during exposure to epileptogenic music. Emotional processing of music was suggested as a possible trigger for seizure activity.

■ Evidence for thalamo-cortical networks in relation to negative myoclous

Abnormal firing in association with myoclonus generation was observed in a similar cortical localisation of the neck and orofacial division of the primary motor cortex pointing to the importance of the somatosensory/motor cortex for the generation of myoclonus and GSW (Kubota, 2004). To clarify the neurophysiological mechanism of epileptic negative myoclonus in a patient with atypical benign partial epilepsy whose myoclonus was completely suppressed with ethosuximide, polygraphic recordings of whole-head type magnetoencephalography (MEG), EEG and electromyography were made during negative myoclonus of the bilateral hands. The silent period of 200-400 ms duration in the bilateral biceps muscles was associated with paroxysmal spikes on EEG and MEG. Single equivalent current dipoles (ECD) were calculated for each spike component associated with negative myoclonus and the estimated generator sources of spikes were superimposed on the patient's head MRI. The magnetic fields of each peak associated with negative myoclonus showed clear single dipole pattern and ECDs of each peak were located in the neck and orofacial division of the primary motor cortex. Taking the beneficial effect of ethosuximide (a T-type Ca^{2+} channel blocker in thalamic neurons and the corresponding cortex) and the MEG result together, the authors suggested that abnormal interaction of the thalamo-cortical network might be closely related to the pathogenesis of negative myoclonus.

The main finding of this study was that the current source of the spikes associated with negative myoclonus of the bilateral hands or neck was localized mainly in the lower precentral area including the neck and orofacial division of the primary motor cortex. This was an area closely related to the areas obtained by the RE study. Some functional alteration of the cortex or thalamocortical circuit should be considered when discussing the pathophysiology of negative myoclonus. As Tassinari *et al.* indicated (1995, 1996) negative myoclonus can occur in heterogenous epileptic disorder, ranging from benign syndromic conditions such as RE to focal static lesional epilepsy, and even to progressive myoclonic encephalopathies. They demonstrated that epileptic negative myoclonus originated in the cortex including the centroparietal and frontal supplementary motor areas, and that a cortical inhibitory active mechanism plays an important role in the genesis of epileptic negative myoclonus.

■ Evidence for thalamo-cortical connectivity in IGE

The importance of interactions between cortical and subcortical structures for the generation of generalised epilepsies has long been acknowledged. Numerous animal model systems have demonstrated that these types of interactions occur within and between cortical and subcortical structures. On the molecular level, perturbations in neurotransmitters as their receptors as assessed using MRS and PET *in vivo* can also contribute to generalised seizures. Elucidating the subtle mechanisms involved in communication between the networks during the generation of these seizures may help to explain how epileptic activity occurring in one region of the brain, such as the cortex, can be transmitted to structures such as the thalamus and subsequently result in a massive, synchronous epileptic discharge involving widespread brain regions. Functional MRI may help to ascertain whether this activity homogenously occurs throughout the entire brain or whether there are selective brain regions that are more important than other for the generation of these seizures. PET and MRS may identify regional variation of neurotransmitter synthesis, which may be responsible for restricted and heterogenous seizure activity. Such heterogeneity may indicate that there are crucial nodes in the network that may provide useful therapeutic targets for the modification or elimination of seizure discharge.

Even though fMRI and PET provide the location of functionally defined cortical regions, but offers rather less insight into how these regions are connected together. Investigating the influence of brain circuitry on function has been hindered by the lack of a technique for exploring brain connectivity *in vivo*. Understanding brain function in terms of connectional architecture is a major goal of neuroimaging. There is good reason to expect a strong correspondence between regional brain function and the underlying connectional architecture. Anatomical connections constrain the nature of the information available to a region and the influence that it can exert over other regions in a distributed network. An analogy can be made with a modern computer network: the amount of data that can be transferred between any two workstations is limited by the conformation of connections between them (whether they are directly linked or are connected through intermediary computer(s)), and by the data capacity of the link between them, and this connectivity can affect the way the two computers interact.

In the brain, local structural organization of connectivity can similarly be expected to influence local functional specialization. However, this relationship between circuitry and function has proved difficult to test directly in the absence of a mechanism for investigating connectivity in the functioning brain. Conventional MRI can easily distinguish between white and grey matter but it cannot be used to distinguish between the different bundles of white matter tracts that have been observed in gross anatomical studies. Direct investigation of the influence of brain circuitry on function has been hindered by the lack of a technique for exploring anatomical connectivity in the brain *in vivo*.

Using a novel probabilistic tractography algorithm with diffusion tensor imaging data, Johansen-Berg and colleagues (Johansen-Berg, 2005) explored anatomical connectivity in the human brain testing the hypothesis that connectivity-defined regions in thalamus co-localise with functional activations during tasks expected to involve specific thalamic nuclei and their cortical connectivity targets. They performed probabilistic diffusion tensor imaging (DTI) tractography from voxels within the thalamus demonstrating the success of this technique in tracing pathways into gray matter. DTI is an MRI application that utilizes sequences sensitive to the diffusion properties of water molecules *in vivo* (LeBihan, 2003; Basser, 1994). This has led to the development of diffusion tensor tractography, in which white matter tracts may be reconstructed in three dimensions by sequentially piecing together discrete and shortly spaced estimates of fibre orientation to form continuous trajectories. Although these tracts are "virtual" (the connectivity maps produced usually demonstrate the likelihood of connection to a defined start region rather than the true axonal pathway itself), the technique has been used successfully in the living human brain to define thalamic (Behrens, 2003), occipitotemporal (Catani, 2003), parahippocampal (Powell, 2005) and other white matter tracts consistent with known anatomical structures.

In future work, the combined use of different imaging modalities will serve to overcome important limitations of the latter (Friston, 1994). The connectivity of the cerebral cortex is immensely complex. Understanding myoclonic seizures in terms of connectional architecture and understanding the connectivity of the human cerebral cortex and its relevance for physiological as well as pathological processes are the major goals and challenges.

References

Aghakhani Y, Bagshaw AP, Benar CG, *et al*. fMRI activation during spike and wave discharges in idiopathic generalized epilepsy. *Brain* 2004; 127: 1127-44.

Archer JS, Abbott DF, Waites AB, Jackson GD. fMRI "deactivation" of the posterior cingulate during generalized spike and wave. *NeuroImage* 2003a; 20: 1915-22.

Archer JS, Briellmann RS, Syngeniotis A, Abbott DF, Jackson GD. Spike-triggered fMRI in reading epilepsy: involvement of left frontal cortex working memory area. *Neurology* 2003b, 60: 415-21.

Avoli M, Rogawski MA, Avanzini G. Generalized epileptic disorders: an update. *Epilepsia* 2001; 42: 445-57.

Bartenstein PA, Duncan JS, Prevett MC, *et al*. Investigation of the opioid system in absence seizures with positron emission tomography. *J Neurol Neurosurg Psychiatry* 1993; 56: 1295-302.

Basser PJ, Mattiello J, LeBihan D. MR diffusion tensor spectroscopy and imaging. *Biophys J* 1994; 66: 259-67

Bech P, Pedersen K, Simonsen N, Lund M. A multidimensional study of personality traits ad modum Sjobring. *Acta Neurol Scand* 1976; 54: 348-58.

Behrens TE, Johansen-Berg H, Woolrich MW, *et al*. Non-invasive mapping of connections between human thalamus and cortex using diffusion imaging. *Nat Neurosci* 2003; 6: 750-7.

Berkovic SF, Andermann F, Andermann E, Gloor P. Concepts of absence epilepsies: discrete syndromes or biological continuum? *Neurology* 1987; 37: 993-1000.

Bernasconi A, Bernasconi N, Natsume J, Antel SB, Andermann F, Arnold DL. Magnetic resonance spectroscopy and imaging of the thalamus in idiopathic generalized epilepsy. *Brain* 2003; 126: 2447-54.

Blumenfeld H, Westerveld M, Ostroff RB, *et al*. Selective frontal, parietal, and temporal networks in generalized seizures. *Neuroimage* 2003; 19: 1556-6.

Bode H. Intracranial blood flow velocities during seizures and generalized epileptic discharges. *Eur J Pediatr* 1992; 151: 706-9.

Born AP, Law I, Lund TE, Rostrup E, Hanson LG, Wildschiodtz G, Lou HC, Paulson OB. Cortical deactivation induced by visual stimulation in human slowwave sleep. *NeuroImage* 2002; 17: 1325-35.

Buchheim K, Obrig H, Pannwitz W, Muller A, Heekeren H, Villringer A, Meierkord H. Decrease in haemoglobin oxygenation during absence seizures in adult humans. *Neurosci Lett* 2004; 354: 119-22.

Catani M, Jones DK, Donato R, Ffytche DH. Occipito-temporal connections in the human brain. *Brain* 2003; 126: 2093-107.

Commission on Classification and Terminology of the International League Against Epilepsy. Proposal for revised classification of epilepsies and epileptic syndromes. Commission on Classification and Terminology of the International League Against Epilepsy. *Epilepsia* 1989; 30: 389-99.

Czisch M, Wehrle R, Kaufmann C, Wetter TC, Holsboer F, Pollmacher T, Auer DP. Functional MRI during sleep: BOLD signal decreases and their electrophysiological correlates. *Eur J Neurosci* 2004; 20: 566-74.

De Simone R, Silvestrini M, Marciani MG, Curatolo P. Changes in cerebral blood flow velocities during childhood absence seizures. *Pediatr Neurol* 1998; 18: 132-5.

Delgado-Escueta AV, Enrile-Bacsal F. Juvenile myoclonic epilepsy of Janz. *Neurology* 1984; 34: 285-94.

Devinsky O, Gershengorn J, Brown E, Perrine K, Vazquez B, Luciano D. Frontal functions in juvenile myoclonic epilepsy. *Neuropsychiatry Neuropsychol Behav Neurol* 1997; 10: 243-6.

Diehl B, Knecht S, Deppe M, Young C, Stodieck SR. Cerebral hemodynamic response to generalized spike-wave discharges. *Epilepsia* 1998; 39: 1284-9.

Doose H, Gerken H, Leonhardt R, Voltzke E, Colz C. Centrencephalic myoclonic-astatic petit-mal. *Neuropediatrics* 1970: 2; 59-78.

Duffy FH, Burchfiel JL. Eye movement-related inhibition of primate visual neurons. *Brain Res* 1975; 89: 121-32.

Federico P, Archer JS, Abbott DF, Jackson GD. Cortical/subcortical BOLD changes associated with epileptic discharges: an EEG-fMRI study at 3 T. *Neurology* 2005; 64 (7): 1125-30.

Friston KJ. Functional and effective connectivity in neuroimaging: A synthesis. *Hum Brain Map* 1994; 2: 56-78.

Garcia PA, Laxer KD, van der Grond J, Hugg JW, Matson GB, Weiner MW. Proton magnetic resonance spectroscopic imaging in patients with frontal lobe epilepsy. *Ann Neurol* 1995; 37: 279-81.

Gloor P. Generalized cortico-reticular epilepsies. Some considerations on the pathophysiology of generalized bilaterally synchronous spike and wave discharge. *Epilepsia* 1968; 9: 249-63.

Haginoya K, Munakata M, Kato R, Yokoyama H, Ishizuka M, Iinuma K. Ictal cerebral haemodynamics of childhood epilepsy measured with near-infrared spectrophotometry. *Brain* 2002; 125: 1960-71.

Hamandi K, Salek-Haddadi A, Laufs H, Liston A, Friston KJ, Fish DR, Duncan JS, Lemieux L. EEG-fMRI of Idiopathic and Secondarily Generalized Epilepsies. *Neuroimage* 2006 submitted.

Hugg JW, Laxer KD, Matson GB, Maudsley AA, Weiner MW. Neuron loss localizes human temporal lobe epilepsy by *in vivo* proton magnetic resonance spectroscopic imaging. *Ann Neurol* 1993; 34: 788-94.

Janz D. Epilepsy with impulsive petit mal (juvenile myoclonic epilepsy). *Acta Neurol Scand* 1985; 72: 449-59.

Johansen-Berg H, Behrens TEJ, Sillery E, *et al*. Functional-Anatomical Validation and Individual Variation of Diffusion Tractography-based Segmentation of the Human Thalamus. *Cerebral Cortex* 2005; 15: 31-9.

Klingelhofer J, Bischoff C, Sander D, Wittich I, Conrad B. Do brief bursts of spike and wave activity cause a cerebral hyper- or hypoperfusion in man? *Neurosci Lett* 1991; 127: 77-81.

Koepp MJ, Richardson MP, Brooks DJ, Duncan JS. Focal cortical release of endogenous opioids during reading-induced seizures. *Lancet* 1998a; 19 (352): 952-5.

Koepp MJ, Hansen ML, Pressler RM, *et al.* Comparison of EEG, MRI and PET in reading epilepsy: a case report. *Epilepsy Research* 1998b; 29 (3): 251-7.

Koepp MJ, Duncan JS. Positron emission tomography in idiopathic generalized epilepsy: imaging beyond structure. In: Schmitz B, Sander T, eds. *Juvenile Myoclonic Epilepsy: The Janz Syndrome*. London: Wrightson, 2000: 91-9.

Koepp MJ, Richardson MP, Brooks DJ, Cunningham VJ, Duncan JS. Central benzodiazepine/gamma-aminobutyric acid A receptors in idiopathic generalized epilepsy: an [11C]flumazenil positron emission tomography study. *Epilepsia* 1997; 38: 1089-97.

Koutroumanidis M, Koepp MJ, Richardson MP, *et al.* The variants of reading epilepsy. A clinical and video-EEG study of 17 patients with reading-induced seizures. *Brain* 1998; 121: 1409-27.

Kubota M, Nakura M, Hirose H, Kimura I, Sakakihara Y. A magnetoencephalographic study of negative myoclonus in a patient with atypical benign partial epilepsy. *Seizure* 2005; 14: 28-32.

Laufs H, Lengler U, Hamandi K, Kleinschmidt A, Krakow K. Linking generalized spike and wave discharges and resting state brain activity using EEG/fMRI in a patient with absence seizures. Epilepsia in press. 2006.

Laureys S, Owen AM, Schiff ND. Brain function in coma, vegetative state, and related disorders. *The Lancet Neurology* 2004; 3: 537-46.

LeBihan D. Looking into the functional architecture of the brain with diffusion MRI. *Nature Reviews Neuroscience* 2003; 4: 469-80.

Lempert T, Bauer M, Schmidt DSyncope: a videometric analysis of 56 episodes of transient cerebral hypoxia. *Ann Neurol* 1994; 36 (2): 233-7.

Marcus EM, Watson CW, Simon SA. An experimental model of some varieties of petit mal epilepsy. Electrical-behavioral correlations of acute bilateral epileptogenic foci in cerebral cortex. *Epilepsia* 1968; (9): 233-48.

Mazoyer B, Zago L, Mellet E, *et al.* Cortical networks for working memory and executive functions sustain the conscious resting state in man. *Brain Res Bull* 2001; (54): 287-98.

Meencke HJ, Janz D. Neuropathological findings in primary generalized epilepsy: a study of eight cases. *Epilepsia* 1984; 25: 8-21.

Meencke HJ. Neuron density in the molecular layer of the frontal cortex in primary generalized epilepsy. *Epilepsia* 1985; 26: 450-4.

Meeren H, van Luijtelaar G, Lopes da Silva F, Coenen A Evolving concepts on the pathophysiology of absence seizures: the cortical focus theory. *Arch Neurol* 2005; 62: 371-6.

Moffett JR, Namboodiri MA, Cangro CB, Neale JH. Immunohistochemical localization of N-acetylaspartate in rat brain. *Neuroreport* 1991; 2: 131-4.

Morocz IA, Karni A, Haut S, Lantos G, Liu G. fMRI of triggerable aurae in musicogenic epilepsy. *Neurology* 2003; 60: 705-9.

Mouritzen-Dam A, Moller A, Scheel-Kruger J, Jensen LH, Marescaux C, Vergnes M. Total number of neurons in the ventro-lateral/posterior thalamic nuclei in a genetic petit mal-like rat strain. *Epilepsy Res Suppl* 1996; 12: 303-7.

Natsume J, Bernasconi N, Andermann F, *et al.* MRI volumetry of the thalamus in temporal, extratemporal, and idiopathic generalized epilepsy. *Neurology* 2003; 60: 1296-300.

Nehlig A, Vergnes M, Waydelich R, *et al.* Absence seizures induce a decrease in cerebral blood flow: human and animal data. *J Cereb Blood Flow Metab* 1996; 16: 147-55.

Niedermeyer E, Laws ER, Jr., Walker EA. Depth EEG findings in epileptics with generalized spike-wave complexes. *Arch Neurol* 1969; 21: 51-8.

Niewenhuys R, Voogd J, van Huijzen C. The human central nervous system. 3rd ed. New York: 1988.

Norden AD, Blumenfeld H. The role of subcortical structures in human epilepsy. *Epilepsy Behav* 2002; 3: 219-31.

Olsen RW, McCabe RT, Wamsley JK. GABAA receptor subtypes: autoradiographic comparison of GABA, benzodiazepine, and convulsant binding sites in the rat central nervous system. *J Chem Neuroanat* 1990; 3: 59-76.

Panayiotopoulos CP. A Clinical Guide to Epileptic Syndromes and their Treatment. Bladon Medical Publishing, 2002.

Panayiotopoulos CP, Obeid T, Waheed G. Differentiation of typical absences in epileptic syndromes: a video-EEG study of 224 seizures in 20 patients. *Brain* 1989; 112: 1039-56.

Panayiotopoulos CP. Absence epilepsies. In: Engel J Jr, Pedley TA, eds. *Epilepsy: A comprehensive textbook*. Philadelphia: Lippincott-Raven, 1997: 2327-46.

Panayiotopoulos CP. A clinical guide to Epileptic Syndromes and Their Treatment. *Bladon Med Publ Chipping Norton*, 2002; 217.

Parkes LM, Fries P, Kerskens CM, Norris DG. Reduced BOLD response to periodic visual stimulation. *NeuroImage* 2004; 21: 236-43.

Patry G, Lyagoubi S, Tassinari CA. Subclinical electric status epilepticus induced by sleep in children. *Arch Neurol* 1971; 4: 242-52.

Powell R, Guye M, Parker GJM, Symms MR, Koepp MJ, Duncan JS. Non-Invasive in vivo Demonstration Of The Connections Of The Human Parahippocampal Gyrus. *NeuroImage* 2005; 22: 740-7.

Prevett MC, Duncan JS, Jones T, Fish DR, Brooks DJ. Demonstration of thalamic activation during typical absence seizures using H2(15)O and PET. *Neurology* 1995; 45: 1396-1402.

Raichle ME, MacLeod AM, Snyder AZ, Powers WJ, Gusnard DA, Shulman GL. A default mode of brain function. *Proc Natl Acad Sci* 2001; 98: 676-82.

Salek-Haddadi A, Lemieux L, Merschhemke M, Friston KJ, Duncan JS, Fish DR. Functional magnetic resonance imaging of human absence seizures. *Ann Neurol* 2003; 53: 663-7.

Sanada S, Murakami N, Ohtahara S. Changes in blood flow of the middle cerebral artery during absence seizures. *Pediatr Neurol* 1988; 4: 158-61.

Savic I, Lekvall A, Greitz D, Helms G. MR spectroscopy shows reduced frontal lobe concentrations of N-acetyl aspartate in patients with juvenile myoclonic epilepsy. *Epilepsia* 2000; 41: 290-6.

Savic I, Osterman Y, Helms G. MRS shows syndrome differentiated metabolite changes in human-generalized epilepsies. *Neuroimage* 2004; 21: 163-72.

Seeck M, Dreifuss S, Lantz G, Jallon P, Foletti G, Despland PA, Delavelle J, Lazeyras F. Subcortical Nuclei Volumetry in Idiopathic Generalized Epilepsy. *Epilepsia* 2005; 46: 1642-5

Seeck M, Lazeyras F, Michel CM, *et al*. Non-invasive epileptic focus localization using EEG-triggered functional MRI and electromagnetic tomography. *Electroencephalogr Clin Neurophysiol* 1998; 106: 508-12.

Shmuel A, Yacoub E, Pfeuffer J, Van de Moortele PF, Adriany G, Hu X, Ugurbil K. Sustained negative BOLD, blood flow and oxygen consumption response and its coupling to the positive response in the human brain. *Neuron* 2002; 36: 1195-210.

Simister RJ, McLean MA, Barker GJ, Duncan JS. Proton MRS reveals frontal lobe metabolite abnormalities in idiopathic generalized epilepsy. *Neurology* 2003a; 61: 897-902.

Simister RJ, McLean MA, Barker GJ, Duncan JS. A proton magnetic resonance spectroscopy study of metabolites in the occipital lobes in epilepsy. *Epilepsia* 2003b; 44: 550-8.

Simmons ML, Frondoza CG, Coyle JT. Immunocytochemical localization of N-acetyl-aspartate with monoclonal antibodies. *Neuroscience* 1991; 45: 37-45.

Sonmez F, Atakli D, Sari H, Atay T, Arpaci B. Cognitive function in juvenile myoclonic epilepsy. *Epilepsy Behav* 2004; 5: 329-36.

Stanley JA, Cendes F, Dubeau F, Andermann F, Arnold DL. Proton magnetic resonance spectroscopic imaging in patients with extratemporal epilepsy. *Epilepsia* 1998; 39: 267-73.

Stefan H, Burr W, Hildenbrand K, Penin H. Basic temporal structure of absence symptoms. In: Akimoto H, Kazamatsuri H, Seino MD, Ward A, eds. *Advances in epileptology: the XIIIth Epilepsy International Symposium*. New York: Raven Press, 1982: 55-60.

Swartz BE, Halgren E, Simpkins F, Syndulko K. Primary memory in patients with frontal and primary generalized epilepsy. *J Epilepsy* 1994; 7: 232-41.

Swartz BE, Simpkins F, Halgren E, *et al.* Visual working memory in primary generalized epilepsy: an 18FDG-PET study. *Neurology* 1996; 47: 1203-12.

Tassinari CA, Bureau M, Thomas P. Epilepsy with myoclonic absences. IN: Roger J, *et al.*, ed. *Epileptic syndromes in infancy, childhood and adolescence*. London: J. Libbey, 1992: 151-60.

Tassinari CA, Rubboli G, Gardella E. Negative myoclonus. *Clin Neurosci* 1996; 3: 209-13.

Tassinari CA, Rubboli G, Parmeggiani L, *et al*. Epileptic negative myoclonus. In: Fahn S, Hallet M, Luders HO, Marsden CD, eds. *Negative motor phenomena: advance in neurology*, vol. 67. Philadelphia: Lippincott-Raven, 1995: 181-97.

Tassinari CA. Myoclonus and epilepsy in childhood 1996 Royaumont meeting. *Epilepsy Research* 1998; 30: 91-106.

Tenney JR, Duong TQ, King JA, Ludwig R, Ferris CF. Corticothalamic modulation during absence seizures in rats: a functional MRI assessment. *Epilepsia* 2003; 44: 1133-40.

Timofeev I, Steriade M. Neocortical seizures: initiation, development and cessation. *Neuroscience* 2004; 123: 299-336.

Velasco M, Velasco F, Velasco AL, Lujan M, Vazquez DM. Epileptiform EEG activities of the centro-median thalamic nuclei in patients with intractable partial motor, complex partial, and generalized seizures. *Epilepsia* 1989; 30: 295-306.

Wenzel R, Wobst P, Heekeren HH, Kwong KK, Brandt SA, Kohl M, Obrig H, Dirnagl U, Villringer A. Saccadic suppression induces focal hypooxygenation in the occipital cortex. *J Cereb Blood Flow Metab* 2000; 20: 1103-10.

Williams D. A study of thalamic and cortical rhythms in petit mal. *Brain* 1953; 76: 50-69.

Woermann FG, Free SL, Koepp MJ, Sisodiya SM, Duncan JS. Abnormal cerebral structure in juvenile myoclonic epilepsy demonstrated with voxel-based analysis of MRI. *Brain* 1999; 122: 2101-8.

Woermann FG, Sisodiya SM, Free SL, *et al.* Quantitative MRI in patients with idiopathic generalized epilepsy. *Brain* 1998; 121: 1661-7.

Connections between primary reading epilepsy and Juvenile Myoclonic Epilepsy

Thomas A. Mayer*, Peter T. Wolf**, Frauke Schroeder***, Theodor W. May ****

*Kleinwachau – Saxonian Epilepsy Centre Radeberg
**Epilepsihospitalet, Dianalund
***Department for Neurology, Bielefeld
****Department for Epilepsy Research, Bielefeld, Germany

Reading epilepsy (RE) is a rare syndrome with a male preponderance and a strong genetic component (Wolf, 1992, Mayer, Wolf, 1999). According to the International Classification of Epilepsies and Epileptic Syndromes "all or almost all seizures in the syndrome of RE are precipitated by reading (especially aloud) and are independent of the content of the text. They are simple focal motor – involving masticatory muscles, or visual, and if the stimulus is not interrupted, generalized tonic-clonic seizures (GTCS) may occur". Seizures usually start in late puberty, the course is benign with little tendency to spontaneous seizures. Physical examination and imaging studies are normal.

The seizures in RE are myoclonic, seldom tonic or tonic-clonic seizures, the consciousness is clear in myoclonic or tonic seizures. Myoclonic seizures are defined as short, isolated or repetitive arrhythmic jerks in a part of the body or in the whole body. For some epileptic syndromes they are the namegiving features, *e.g.* Juvenile Myoclonic Epilepsy (JME) or Progressive Myoclonus Epilepsy (PME). In other syndromes like primary, the main seizure type are myoclonic jerks involving the perioral muscles, triggered by reading (aloud and silently), in 25-30% of the patients also talking. Reading induced perioral myoclonias were considered to be a more or less exclusive seizure type in primary RE (Wolf, 1992). However, since we could observe perioral myoclonias increasingly frequently in JME where they are triggered by talking and less frequently by reading (Mayer, Wolf, 1999), but do not occur spontaneously, we questioned the specificity of perioral reflex myoclonias (PORM, Wolf, Mayer, 2000). PORM are short, sometimes repetitive, abrupt myoclonias around the mouth which will clearly be noticed by the patients, sometimes with interruption of reading and speaking. Most of these jerks appear strongly localized and do not change the side in individual patients. In some cases, PORM are bilateral.

Bickford et al. (1956) distinguished primary and secondary RE. The primary form, in which only reading induced seizures occur, belongs to the idiopathic localisation-related epilepsy syndromes. Secondary reading epilepsies, in which spontaneous and reading induced seizures (e.g. psychomotor seizures) occur, belong to different epilepsy syndromes (e.g. symptomatic focal epilepsies). Another proposal by Bickford (1973) was to distinguish a specific (= "primary") form from a non-specific (= "secondary") form. Since several patients were published with the co-occurrence of RE and JME (Radhakrishnan et al., 1995), there is also a discussion whether RE should be considered as an idiopathic generalized epilepsy syndrome.

EEG findings in reading epilepsy

In Routine EEG-recordings, nearly 80% of the findings are negative (Wolf, 1992), infrequently bilateral spike and waves or temporal sharp waves are seen. Photic stimulation is negative in more than 90% of the cases (Wolf, 1992). Ictal findings are not specific. Paroxymal discharges were found in 76,8% of the investigations, 30,1% of them focal, 38,4% bilateral lateralized and 31,5% bilateral symmetric. If there is a focal discharge, in 75% of the cases it is temporal, in 25% of the cases frontal. There is a left predominance of 78% of the cases with a focal discharge (Wolf, 1992).

Pathophysiology of perioral reflex myoclonias

The clinical symptoms of perioral reflex myoclonias (PORM) bear the characteristics of cortical reflex myoclonias (CRM): The CRM is related to a small area of the sensorimotor cortex; it typically involves only a few adjacent muscles (Hallett, 1985).

In RE the common precipitating mechanism of PORM, best investigated is the formal act in reading, i.e. the transformation of graphemes into phonemes (Wolf, 1992). In patients with RE, the sensorimotor cortex is not hyperexcitable per se, because spontaneous seizures never occur. A hypothesis exists that the hyperexcitable neuronal network that subserves speech may drive the relative motor cortex effectively through a direct transcortical pathway (Hallett et al. 1979, Obeso et al. 1985). This assumed bilaterally hyperexcitable speech network, under reading provocation, would give rise to bilateral myoclonic jerks, which need not be necessarily symmetric (Koutoumanidis et al. 1998).

MR-Imaging is unspecific in primary RE, variable lesions were seen in patients with secondary RE (Koutroumainidis et al., 1998).

Functional imaging in reading epilepsy

Only patients with secondary RE and localized lesions were investigated by interictal HMPAO-SPECT or PET. In all cases the authors (Koepp 1998, Miyamoto, 1995) found hypometabolism in the area of the lesion.

Ictal PET-findings were investigated by Koepp and coworkers (1998). They found a significant reduced binding of 11 C-DPN with opioid rezeptors in different regions:
- left parieto-temporo-okzipital (Brodmann area 37)
- left gyrus temporalis medialis (Brodmann area 21)
- parieto-occipital posterior bilateral (Brodmann area 40)

They did not find any significant opioid release at the Wernicke area.

Ictal HMPAO-SPECT – findings shows focal hyperperfusion frontal bilateral and left temporal (Miyamoto, 1995).

Juvenile myoclonic epilepsy (JME)

"JME appears around puberty and is characterized by seizures with bilateral, single or repetitive, arrhythmic, irregular myoclonic jerks, predominantly in the arms. No disturbance of consciousness is noticeable" (Commission, 1989). Seizure triggers are sudden awakening, sleep deprivation, stress and alcohol. Valproic acid (VPA) is the antiepileptic drug (AED) of choice. The prognosis is good, but some authors believe that in 90% of all cases a lifelong AED therapy is required (Calleja et al., 2001). The age at onset is typically between 12 and 18 years. The typical EEG features are generalized spike waves and polyspike waves, but also focal epileptic discharges appear in up to 36% (Lancman et al., 1997). At least one third of the patients are photosensitive (Wolf, Goosses, 1986).

Panzica and coworkers (2001) investigated the cortical myoclonus in JME with jerk-related back averaging on ictal epochs. They concluded that the ultimate mechanism responsible for ictal myoclonic jerks in JME is largely similar to that sustaining cortical myoclonus in more severe pathological conditions such as progressive myoclonus epilepsy.

■ Methods

In a pilot phase we looked for the frequency of PORM in general. Systematic questioning of all new outpatients seen by the first author between 1994 and 1998 (n=600) identified 17 patients with PORM. In the same period, another seven cases of PORM were detected among the inpatients of our hospital. Of these 24 patients, ten had symptomatic focal epilepsies, two idiopathic generalized epilepsy (IGE) with Grand mal on awakening and twelve JME. Patients who were newly diagnosed with RE in the same period were not included in this study. Since JME appeared to be the syndrome in which PORM are most frequent, we began to investigate this co-occurrence systematically. We conducted a questionnaire survey for all our ambulatory patients with the diagnosis JME to search for PORM and other reflex epileptic traits. The questionnaire was sent to 86 patients with a well-established diagnosis of JME.

The diagnosis of JME was given based upon a case history including a description, by the patients and their relatives, of typical myoclonic seizures and, possibly, generalised tonic-clonic seizures and absences, and the presence of generalised Spike-Waves or Poly-SW in the interictal EEG. All patients were investigated with MRI, which was normal in all cases. 65 (75%) of the patients responded to the questionnaire. Not considering non-specific facilitating factors of seizures like lack of sleep, 33 patients answered "yes" to questions about specific precipitating stimuli. 25 of these 33 patients were available for a prolonged polygraphic video-EEG-recording and were compared with a group of patients with focal epilepsies.

Comparison group

The comparison group consisted of 25 matched consecutive patients of our epilepsy centre with different types of focal epilepsies, i.e. epilepsies without known propensity for reflex epileptic mechanisms. 19 patients in this group suffered from temporal lobe epilepsy, four from frontal lobe epilepsy, two from parieto-occipital epilepsy. They were collected during one year. Seizure frequency in this group ranged from 3 seizures per week to one seizure per month.

We performed a standardized interview with all patients and a Video-EEG investigation lasting three hours as a minimum, including five min hyperventilation, intermittent light stimulation and complex neuropsychological tests. For the latter, we used the protocol of Matsuoka *et al.* (19) with some modifications as follows.

- Reading silently (modification: 15 min., standardised unknown difficult text)
- Reading aloud (modification: 15 min., standardised unknown English text)
- Speaking (modification: Speaking in a stressful manner to the camera about epilepsy and medical history)
- Mental calculations, 10 tasks: *e.g.*: 11x11, 125 / 5
- Written calculation: 10 tasks: e.g. 15x67x23x48
- Writing of standardised texts (modification: duration minimum 15 min.)
- Spatial constructions, to build up a tower (the Jenga tower), drawing figures (people, dog, cow,), block design test.
- Modification: Rubik's cube: to arrange one side of the cube in one colour.

Between two tests, there always was a period of rest. The total investigation lasted 3 hours or more including a total of 1 hour or more of interspersed rest. Interictal spikes were rated as induced if there was an increase in number of more than 200% compared to the baseline resting condition. The results were statistically investigated with Fisher's exact test (extended version).

■ Results

Video-EEG investigation

Twenty-five patients with JME were compared with 25 matched (1:1, age and sex) patients with different types of focal epilepsies. The mean age of the JME patients was 29,8 ± 7,2 years (range: 17-42), the mean age of the comparison group was 30,0 ± 10,4 years (range: 17-52). Sex ratio was identical: 13 males *vs.* 12 females in both groups. No seizures, especially no perioral myoclonias were seen at rest *(Table I)*.

Table I. General patient data

	JME patients	Comparison group
Number	25	25
Mean Age in years (range)	29,8 ± 7,2 (17-42)	30,0 ± 10,4 (17-56)
Sex Ratio men: women	13:12	13:12
Syndromes	JME	Focal epilepsies: TLE: 19, FLE: 4; POLE: 2
Age at onset	14,0 ± 3,5 (5-28)	16,0 ± 11,7 (1-47)
Positive family history (epilepsy)	9	8

TLE: temporal lobe epilepsy, FLE: frontal lobe epilepsy, POLE: parieto-occipital lobe epilepsy.

Interictal EEG

Normal interictal EEG recordings were seen in 10 patients with JME and in 13 patients with focal epilepsies (all patients were on AED medication). We saw a statistical significant difference (Fishers exact test, two-tailed), in two items of the EEG-recording *(Figure 1)*: Generalized epileptic discharges were seen in the JME group in 16 patients (Fisher's exact test, two-tailed $p<0,001$) and in five patients in the focal group (not clearly focal, but bilateral synchronous with frontal maximum), whereas none patients with JME but 11 patients in the comparison group had focal discharges (Fisher's exact test, two-tailed $p<0,001$). Special attention was paid to possible local onset of epileptiform discharges in the polygraphic EEG-recording.

EEG activation

Activation induced by hyperventilation shows a difference in both groups: HV provoked generalized spikes and poly spike waves in 7 patients with JME, but also in two patients of the focal group with a frontal maximum (probably as an expression of rapid secondary synchrony) *(Figure 2)*. This difference was only marginally significant (two-tailed Fisher exact test: $p=0,074$) Photosensitivity was seen in 5 patients with JME but never in the focal group (two- tailed Fisher exact test: $p=0,022$). There was also a significant difference between the JME patients and the comparison group (Fisher's exact test two-tailed, $p<0.01$) comparing the precipitation of epileptiform discharges with different triggers during the EEG recording (ten patients with JME, 2 patients of the focal patients). 5 patients of the JME-group (20%) showed epileptic discharges during reading, 4 during speaking. These discharges were spikes and rapid spike waves, and they were generalised or centrally. Only one of the comparison patients showed epileptiform discharges during reading with spikes related to the left parieto-central region. This difference is statistically significant, whereas the subanalysis of reading and speaking induced epileptic discharges was not significant probably due to small numbers of patients (Fisher's exact test, $p=0,189$ two- tailed; $p=0,095$ one- tailed). Four patients showed epileptiform discharges during speaking, none of the comparison group (two-tailed Fisher's exact test $p=0,055$). Praxis-induced (manipulating with Rubik's cube) EEG-discharges were seen in 4 Patients with JME, but in none of the

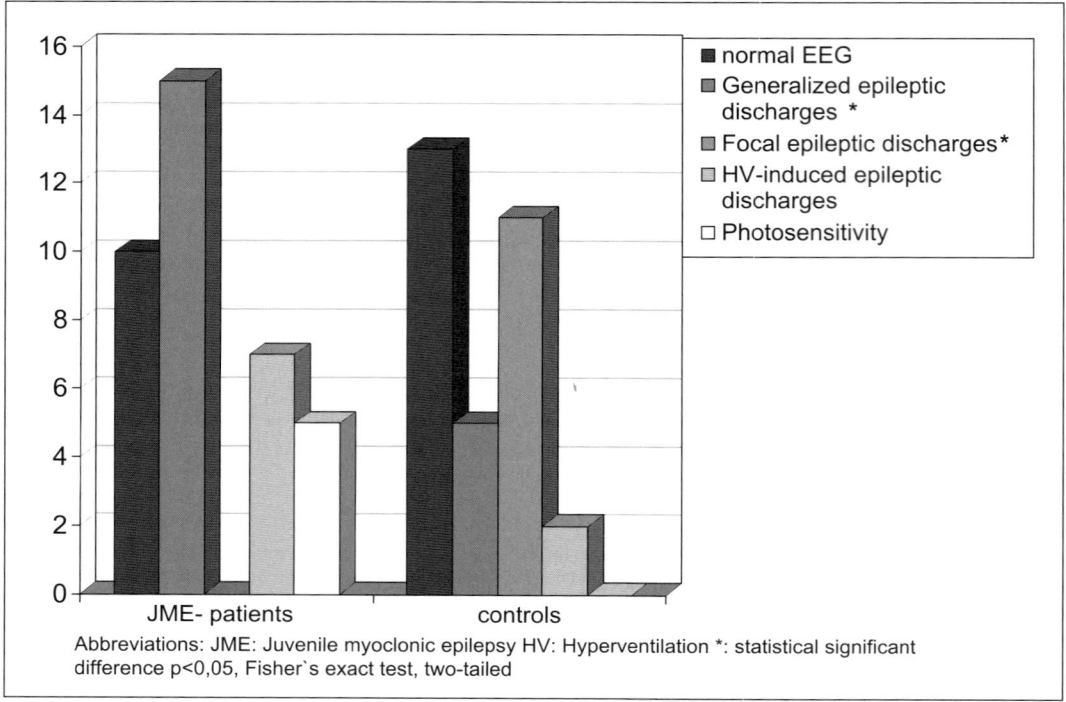

Figure 1. Interictal EEG recording.
Abbreviations: JME: Juvenile myoclonic epilepsy HV: Hyperventilation
*: statistical significant difference p<0,05, Fisher's exact test, two-tailed.

comparison group (two-tailed Fisher's exact test p=0,05). Calculating (n=1) and writing (n=2) were only little provocative in the JME group, and none of the patients in the focal group showed epileptic EEG-discharges with this kind of precipitation.

Ictal EEG

The ictal characteristics are in most cases rapid spike waves with frontal maximum, whereas in one patient with focal epilepsy left parieto-central spike wave activity appeared during silent reading. Sometimes, myoclonic jerks made EEG analysis impossible. There was no overlap of focal and generalised discharges in individual patients. The EEG pattern was not different in PORM and in praxis – induced seizures.

Precipitation of perioral reflex myoclonias (PORM)

In nine of the patients with JME (36%) we recorded PORMs induced by reading, speaking, and other neuropsychological activation. Only one comparison patient (4%) showed seizures induced by reading. The difference was statistically significant (two-tailed Fisher-exact-Test: p=0,037). This result can be explained by the selection of patients with the questionnaire. PORMs were not found in all patients with JME who had reported them in the questionnaire.

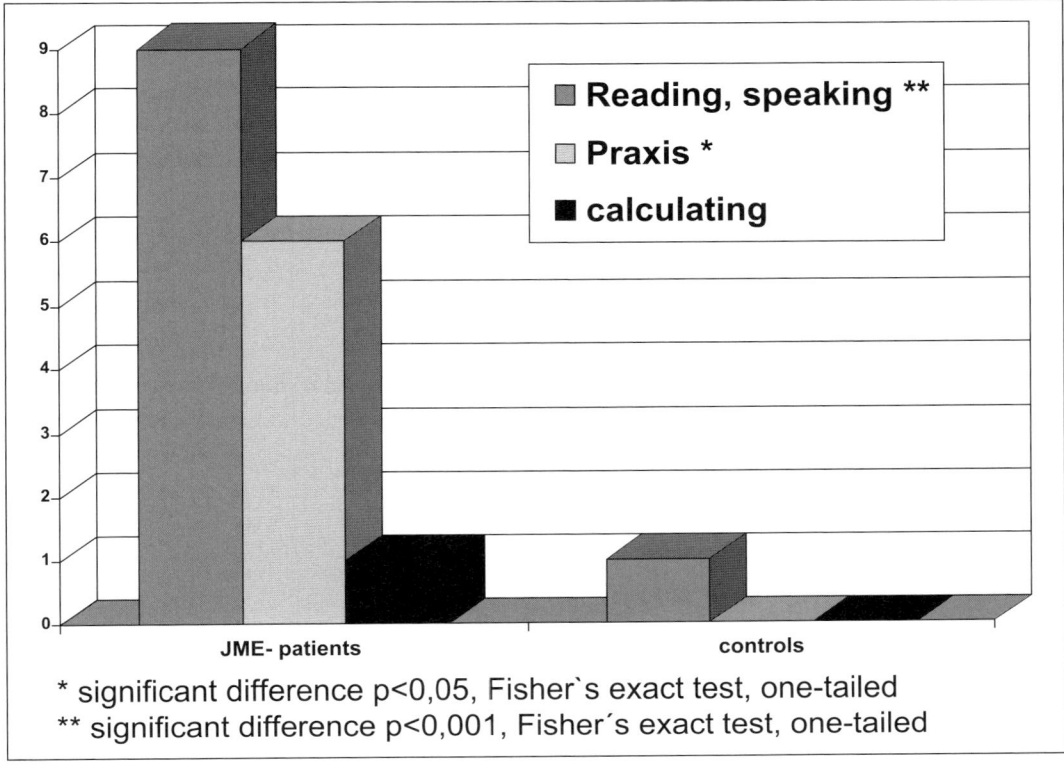

Figure 2. Induced epileptic discharges.
Induction of epileptic discharges by reading/speaking/praxis of more than 200% per time unit in comparison to baseline EEG recording at rest.

Precipitation of Praxis-induced seizures

Six of the JME patients had praxis-induced epileptiform EEG discharges (generalised spike waves), and two of them had praxis-induced seizures. One patient from the comparison group with induced seizures showed atypical myoclonias around the mouth and a complex partial seizure with impairment of consciousness as the main symptomatology.

The group of JME patients with PORMs and/or praxis-induction was not different from the group of JME patients without these. In terms of sex, age, seizure-types, age of onset or specific details of the medical history we found no differences. In both groups photosensitivity appeared frequently (e.g. 3/6 patients with praxis-induced epileptic discharges were photosensitive)

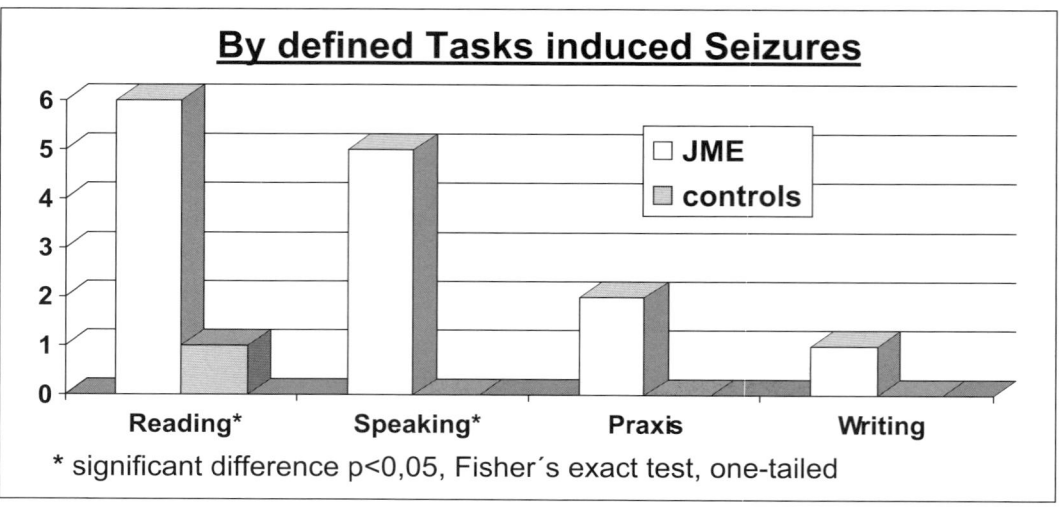

Figure 3. Induced epileptic seizures.

Treatment

All 25 patients with JME but two were on antiepileptic medication, 18 with valproic acid (VPA), 9 in monotherapy, 9 in combination therapy. Two patients received lamotrigine, two topiramate and one phenytoin in monotherapy. Combination therapies involved lamotrigine, primidone, carbamazepine, levetiracetam, phenobarbitone and ethosuximide...

Three of the patients with JME and PORM were not seizure-free with VPA, only one did not respond at all, the other patients were seizure-free with VPA. Polymedication reflects that these were patients of a tertiary referral centre and include a selection of patients who are more difficult to treat.

Two patients in the comparison group did not take any medication, 12 were treated with VPA, 9 with carbamazepine, and 7 with lamotrigine, all in combination with VPA. Other medications were oxcarbazepine (3), levetiracetam (2), gabapentin (2), topiramate, phenytoin, clonazepam and clobazam (n=1).

■ Discussion

In the database Medline we found 525 published papers between 1950 and 2005 dealing with JME. Only a few papers are dealing with special investigations on reflex epileptic traits (Matsuoka, 2000, Inoue, 1994, 2000). We found 378 papers about the combination of reading and epilepsy, few of them were dealing in detail with RE, and only one paper was dealing with PORMs in patients with JME (Radhakrishnan et al, 1995). In this paper 18 patients with RE are described, four of whom also had a diagnosis of JME. Three of them were females. The age of onset was between 14 and 17, one patient was 46 years old at the onset of RE. The seizure trigger in all patients was reading, in three patients also calculations. Listening to conservation, playing chess or speaking were triggers in individual cases. The interictal and ictal

EEG showed generalized epileptic discharges in all patients; none of the patients was photosensitive. Two of them responded to VPA, partial control was seen in two patients treated with phenytoin and primidone.

Matsuoka et al. (2000) investigated 480 patients with different epileptic syndromes with a specially designed neuropsychological EEG activation program. This program consisted of different tasks including reading and speaking (both very brief), arithmetics, writing, drawing and a block design test. In 133 patients an inhibitory effect of the activation was seen in the EEG. In 38 patients, activation induced epileptic discharges, most of them in response to mental or written calculation (n=21), writing of special standardized sentences (n=26) or spatial constructions (n= 24). Only in two of the 38 patients reading was a specific trigger, in none of them speaking induced seizures.

Concerning the relation of these findings to epilepsy syndromes, Matsuoka and coworkers (2000) found that all but two of the patients who responded to activation had idiopathic generalized syndromes. Most of them (n=22) had JME. Two patients had temporal lobe seizures. Considering the semiology of precipitated seizures they found in most cases (n=32) myoclonic seizures in both arms, 23 patients had GTCS, 19 had absence seizures, two patients had secondarily GTCS and two had partial seizures. PORM were not described in any of the patients, probably because the patients read and talked too briefly in this protocol. Another reason for missing PORM could be that patients and investigators were not aware of the probability of brief PORM. Ictally often no EEG correlate but only a EMG artefact was seen.

Inoue and coworkers (2000) investigated patients with JME with a special test battery to search for praxis-induced seizures (PIS). Such seizures are triggered by a complex interaction of thinking with a manual task. More than one fifth of the investigated 213 patients were photosensitive (n=47). In 20 patients typing or writing was provocative. In 16 patients playing cards or chess precipitated myoclonic jerks in the active arm. Mental or written calculation was provocative in 15 patients, complicated finger manipulation in eleven patients. Only a few patients responded to playing video games (n=6) or playing musical instruments (n=4). PORM were reported in none of the patients.

All these patients have in common that some local motor performance, with which the patients are active, provokes local myoclonic phenomena or, as Bickford (1956) put it in his first description of RE, that "proprioceptive bombardment" results in "reflex firing through the same motor segment". It is thought-provoking that these minimal focal motor seizures occur both in a condition which is considered a "generalized epilepsy syndrome" (JME) and a "localisation-related epilepsy syndrome" (RE). Furthermore, the reflex-like phenomena we observed here look substantially different from the typical bilateral brachial jerks of JME. The reflex epileptic seizure symptoms remain restricted to rather circumscribed areas. It is an intriguing question how rather direct, local reflex-like sensorimotor interactions fit into a "generalized" syndrome.

In our study we investigated JME patients who in response to a questionnaire concerning specific reflex epileptic traits had described such traits in their history. We tried to document these traits with video-EEG. This was not possible in all patients and this may be due to the situation of investigation where some patients are not sufficiently relaxed but also to other reasons. Some patients may have been mistaken when they reported trigger mechanisms. Almost all were on antiepileptic medication, which was not interrupted for the investigation and may have suppressed the triggered responses. In addition it seems that in many patients these reflex epileptic traits, just as photosensitivity, are only present temporarily in a certain period of age. In fact, quite a few patients had warned us that they had known PORM or praxis induction earlier but didn't believe they still had it. So we cannot in absolute terms answer the question how frequent these traits are in JME.

Interestingly, reflex epileptic traits were occasionally seen also in the comparison group, so that their specifity seems not to be very high. The control group were matched in age and sex and all of them had focal epilepsies. Frontal lobe epilepsies especially have similiarities in semiology to JME, which may have something to do with the positive results in the control group. An optimal design for this study would have been to investigate consecutively both untreated JME patients and matched controls, but such patients are seen too rarely to make such a study feasible.

VPA is the treatment of choice in JME (and also for PORMs in RE), but not all investigated JME-patients responded to VPA. Three of these non-responders had the combination of PORMs and JME, which could support the results of the investigation of Genton and coworkers (2001), who found that significant more patients with the combination of different seizure types in JME (absences, myoclonic jerks, generalized tonic clonic seizures) were therapy resistant. It is possible that in some patients inappropriate treatment could have had a facilitating effect to the occurrence of PORM. Two patients were without any treatment, three had carbamazepine and three oxcarbazepine in combination, both antiepileptic drugs are ineffective in JME and can increase the frequency of myoclonic jerks.

An ongoing discussion (Wolf, 1994) considers the relationship of supposed "generalized" widespread bilateral discharges to bilateral or unilateral regional expression of clinical symptoms. This discussion needs perhaps to be pursued. One of the open questions in this respect is, in photosensitive JME patients, by what intermediaries the occipital cortical input of intermittent lights produces myoclonic jerks of the extremities. Still, these are bilateral and roughly symmetric. New patients, especially with the association of different epilepsy syndromes will give more information in pathophysiology of epileptic seizures with bilateral symmetric expression (1998).

These observations seem to indicate that the distinction between focal and generalized epileptic phenomena may to some extent be artificial. The closer we look at the prototype of an idiopathic generalized epilepsy syndrome, JME, the more we have to realise, so it seems, that it is indeed a syndrome that challenges our syndromic concepts.

For better understanding of the pathophysiology of RE, Koepp and coworkers (2001) investigated EEG, MRI and PET in a patient with RE. MRI was normal, whereas (11C)-diprenorphine PET revealed peri-ictal opoid binding decreased in both temporal lobes and the left frontal lobe, maybe due to an abnormal activity in the network subserving reading.

Archer and coworkers (2003) investigated 2 patients with reading epilepsy using fMRI. Spike activity overlapped with reading activity in the left middle frontal gyrus, a structure recruited during working memory cognitive tasks. The authors postulate that, because of a local structural anomaly, the spikes of reading epilepsy spread from working memory areas into adjacent motor cortex, activating a cortical subcortical circuit. It would be necessary for understanding the pathophysiology of PORM to investigate all patients with PORM during reading provocation to look for the brain activity in comparison to normal controls more patients (Price, 1994). The next step to show differences between both groups was investigated in a recent study and failed, probably because all seven investigated patients had an effective treatment before fMRI was done (Salek-Haddadi et al., 2004). None of our patients showed a structural abnormality as Archer (2003) had shown.

■ Conclusion

PORM may represent a frequent but often unobserved focal seizure-type in different epileptic syndromes, not only in RE, with a restricted local epileptic activity. They are more frequent in JME compared to focal epilepsy syndromes. The three reflex epileptic traits, i.e., photosensitivity, praxis and reading in JME may be found alone or coexist in one patient. They thus seem to be genetically independent. The semiology of PORM is not fundamentally different in various epileptic syndromes. These observations seem to indicate that the distinction between focal and generalized epileptic ictogenesis may be less clear than is traditionally believed. VPA seems to be the AED of choice in most cases of both primary RE and of PORM in JME. The response of PORM in other epilepsy syndromes to AED remains to be investigated.

References

Archer JS, Briellmann RS, Syngeniotis A, Abbott DF, Jackson GD. Spike-triggered fMRI in reading epilepsy: involvement of left frontal cortex working memory area. *Neurology* 2003; 11; 60 (3): 415-21.

Bartolomei F, Farnarier G, Elias Z, Bronsard G, Soulayrol S, Bonnet A, Chave B, Gastaut JL. Facial reflex myoclonus induced by language: a neuropsychological and neurophysiological study. *Neurophysiol Clin* 1999; 29: 263-70.

Bickford RG. Discussion. *Trans Am Neurol Ass* 1973; 98: 187-8.

Bickford RG, Whelan JL, Klass DW, Corbin KB. Reading epilepsy: clinical and electroencephalographic studies of a new syndrome. *Trans Am Neurol Ass* 1956; 81: 100-2.

Calleja S, Salas-Puig J, Ribacoba R, Lahoz CH: Evolution of juvenile myoclonic epilepsy treated from the outset with sodium valproate. *Seizure* 2001; 10 (6): 424-7.

Commission on Classification and Terminology of the International League against Epilepsy. Proposal for revised classification of epilepsies and epileptic syndromes. *Epilepsia* 1989; 30: 389-99.

Gelisse P, Genton P, Thomas M, Rey JC, Samuelian, Dravet C. Clinical factors of drug resistance in juvenile myoclonic epilepsy. *J Neurol Neurosurg Psychiatry* 2001; 70: 240-3.

Hallett M, Chadwick D, Marsden CD. Cortical reflex myoclonus. *Neurology* 1979; 8: 1107-25.

Hallett M. Myoclonus: relation to epilepsy. *Epilepsia* 1985; 26 (Suppl 1): S67-77.

Inoue Y, Kubota H. Juvenile myoclonic epilepsy with praxis induced seizures In: Schmitz B, Sander T, eds. *Juvenile Myoclonic Epilepsy: the Janz Syndrome*. Whrightson Biomedical Publishing Ltd. Petersfield, UK, Philadelphia, USA, 2000: 73-81.

Inoue Y, Seino M, Kubota H, Yamakaku K, Tanaka M, Yagi K. Epilepsy with praxis-induced seizures. In: Wolf P, ed. *Epileptic Seizures and Syndromes*. London: J. Libbey, 1994: 81-91.

Koepp MJ, Hansen ML, Pressler R, Brooks, DJ, Brandl U, Guldin B, Duncan JS, Ried S. Comparison of EEG, MRI and PET in reading epilepsy: a case report. *Epil Res* 1998: 29: 251-7.

Koutroumanidis M, Koepp MJ, Richardson MP, Camfield C, Agathonikou A, Ried S, Papadimitriou A, Plant GT, Duncan JS, Panayiatopoulos CP. The variants of reading epilepsy. *Brain* 1998; 121: 1409-27.

Lancman ME, Asconape JJ, Penry JK. Clinical and EEG asymmetries in juvenile myoclonic epilepsy. *Epilepsia* 1997; 38 (2): 258.

Matsuoka H, Takahashi T, Sasaki M, Matsumoto K, Yoshida S, Numachi Y, Saito H, Ueno T, Sato M. Neuropsychological EEG activation in patients with epilepsy. *Brain* 2000; 123: 318-30.

Mayer T, Wolf P. Reading epilepsy: Related to Juvenile Myoclonic epilepsy? *Epilepsia* 1997; 38 (Suppl. 3): 18-9.

Mayer T, Wolf P. Reading epilepsy: clinical and genetic background. In: Berkovic S, Genton P, Marescaux C, Picard F, eds. *Genetics of Focal Epilepsies: Clinical Aspects and Molecular Biology*. London: John Libbey & Company Ltd, 1999: 159-67.

Miyamoto A, Takahashi S, Tokumitsu A, Oku J. Ictal HMPAO-single photon emission computed tomography findings in reading epilepsy in a Japanese boy. *Epilepsia* 1995; 36 (11): 1161-3.

Obeso JA, Rothwell JC, Marden CD. The spectrum of cortical myoclonus. From focal reflex jerks to spontaneous motor epilepsy. *Brain* 1985; 108 (Pt 1): 193-24.

Panzica F, Rubboli G, Franceschetti S, Avanzini G, Meletti S, Pozzi A, Tassinari CA. Cortical myoclonus in Janz Syndrome. *Clin Neurophysiol* 2001; 112: 1803-9.

Price CJ, WIse RJS, Watson JDG, Patterson G, Howard D, Frackowiak K. Brain activity during reading. *Brain* 1994; 117; 1255-69.

Radhakrishnan K, Silbert PL, Klass DW. Reading epilepsy. An appraisal of 20 patients diagnosed at the Mayo Clinic, Rochester, Minnesota, between 1949 and1989, and delineation of the epileptic syndrome. *Brain* 1995; 118: 75-89.

Salek-Haddadi A, Hamandi K, Woermann FG, Mayer T, Wolf P, Koepp MJ. Functional MRI activation in reading epilepsy assessment. *Epilepsia* 2004; 45 (suppl 3): 64.

Valenti MP, Tinuper P, Cerullo A, Carcangiu R, Marini C. Reading epilepsy in a patient with previous idiopathic focal epilepsy with centrotemporal spikes. *Epileptic Disord* 1999; 1 (3): 167-71.

Wolf P, Goosses R. Relation of photosensitivity to epileptic syndromes. *J Neurol Neurosurg Psychiatry* 1986; 49: 1386-91.

Wolf, P. Reading epilepsy. In: Roger J, Bureau M, Dravet Ch, Dreyfuss FE, Perret A, Wolf P, eds. *Epileptic syndromes in infancy, childhood and adolescence*. 2nd. Edition, 1992: 281-98.

Wolf, P. *Epileptic seizures and Syndromes*. London: J. Libbey, 1994.

Wolf P, Mayer T, Reker M. Reading epilepsy: Report of five new cases and further considerations on the pathophysiology. *Seizure* 1998; 7: 271-9.

Wolf P, Mayer Th. Juvenile Myoclonic Epilepsy: A Syndrome Challenging Syndromic Concepts. In: Schmitz B, Sander T, eds. *Juvenile Myoclonic Epilepsy: the Janz Syndrome*. Whrightson Biomedical Publishing Ltd. Petersfield, UK, Philedelphia, USA, 2000: 33-40.

Wolf P, Inoue Y. Complex reflex epilepsies: reading epilepsy and praxis induction. In: Roger J, Bureau M, Dravet Ch, Genton P, Tassinari CA, Wolf P, eds. *Epileptic syndromes in infancy, childhood and adolescence*. 3nd. Edition. 2002: 315-25.

Section V:
Primary versus Secondary Tonic-clonic seizures

Behavior, neural circuits and plasticity in acute and chronic models of generalized tonic-clonic seizures

Norberto Garcia-Cairasco

Neurophysiology and Experimental Neuroethology Laboratory, Physiology Department, Ribeirão Preto School of Medicine, University of São Paulo, Brazil

---

"It seems reasonable to assume, therefore, that generalization of the motor seizure does not take place by spread of excitation through cortical circuits. It must spread through the more closely interrelated neuronal network of the higher brainstem, in a centrencephalic system with symmetrical functional relationships to both sides of the body."

Penfield and Jasper (1954)

In the present chapter we aim to critically review models of generalized tonic-clonic seizures (GTCS) that include, besides the traditional maximal electroshock (MES) and high doses of pentylenetetrazol (PTZ) models, usually applied to drug screening, acute and chronic audiogenic seizures (AS) mostly in the genetically developed Wistar Audiogenic Rat (WAR) strain.

Furthermore, the chapter considers the integration of behavioral, EEG, cellular and molecular approaches to the study of AS and AS kindling in combination with models such as MES, PTZ, amygdala kindling and pilocarpine-induced seizures (*Status Epilepticus*/spontaneous recurrent seizures). This comparative, multidisciplinary and multilayer approach reveals how important is the combination of predisposition to epilepsy with seizure experience in different epilepsy models.

Finally, it will be discussed, in the context of GTCS models, critical questions such as endogenous anticonvulsant systems, post-ictal phenomena, differential diagnostic, e.g. seizure versus fear/flight related behaviors.

■ Primary and secondary human generalized tonic-clonic seizures: behavior, EEG and prognosis at a glance

"Generalized tonic-clonic seizure or bilateral tonic-clonic seizure, are bilateral symmetrical tonic contraction then bilateral clonic contractions of somatic muscles usually associated with autonomic phenomena"
(Report of the ILAE Task Force on Classification and Terminology, Engel, 2001).

In clinical neurology, GTCS are considered the oldest and most feared of all seizures and the final common pathway in the ictal progression of other seizure types and the maximal behavioral and electrophysiological expression of epilepsy (Fisch, 1997). Not only for clinical purposes but for experimental modeling some of the features such as loss of consciousness and generalization are now challenged and may be altered in the ongoing revision of epileptic seizures and epileptic seizures syndromes classification (Engel, 2001; Engel and Schwartzkroin, 2006).

Although most of the time it is accepted that in GTCS there is a primary generalized EEG, the latter is not totally bisynchronous and might have a focal origin with rapid generalization. In the case of generalized absence (non-convulsive seizures) a model of that possibility is reported by Meeren et al. (2002, 2005). The so-called "cortical focus" theory, would bridge cortical and thalamic theories. Interestingly the animals from the WAG/Rij strain that were used in those experiments (Midzyanovskayaa et al., 2005) have concomitant absence seizures and AS, a model of GTCS that we will discuss below.

Abbreviations List

AP7: amino-phosphonoheptanoate
AS: Audiogenic Seizures
ASK: Audiogenic Seizures Kindling
BOLD: Blood Oxygenation Level Dependent
BrdU: 5-bromo2'-deoxy-uridine
2DG: 2-deoxy-D-glucose
ECT: electroconvulsive therapy
GAD: Glutamic acid Decarboxylase
GEPRs: Genetically Epilepsy-Prone Rats
GTCS: Generalized tonic-clonic seizures
IC: inferior colliculus
LL: lateral lemniscus
MES: maximal electroshock
MFS: Mossy Fiber Sprouting

MYOh= Head Myoclonus
MYO_1 = Forelimb myoclonus
NO: nitric oxide
NOS: nitric oxide synthase
PAG; periaqueductal gray
PRL: prolactin
PTZ: pentylenetetrazol
SC: superior colliculus
SE: Status Epilepticus
SNL: Substantia Nigra Lateralis
SNR: Substantia Nigra Reticulata
SRS: spontaneous recurrent seizures
WAR: Wistar Audiogenic Rat

Most of the GTCS are classified in one of two main groups: 1. *Symptomatic* generally associated to a known brain disturbance and 2. *Idiopathic* generally associated to unknown etiology and mostly of genetic background (Engel, 2001). A great number of GTCS are of the type subsequent to partial simple, partial complex and secondary generalization. As Fisch (1997) points out, the case of secondarily EEG epileptiform activity, already in the early times of epileptology (Tukel and Jasper, 1952), was associated to the "centrencephalic system", or to an epileptogenic pathway within which primary generalized seizures were initiated and propagated ("primary bilateral synchrony"). The main facts observed in the ictal EEG are the presence on routine analysis of generalized (symmetrical-bilateral) epileptiform ictal activity. However, on more dedicated computational analysis, both ictal and interictal EEG are rarely bisynchronous (Gotman, 1981). Thus, although primary GTCS are thought to be by definition always symmetrical, it is frequent the finding of GTCS with a focal origin (McNally and Rumenfeld, 2004) and sometimes partial and GTCS co-exist (Jeha *et al.*, 2005).

Additionally, secondary GTCS have poorer prognosis than idiopathic GTCS (Annegers *et al.*, 1979). Seizure repetition and seizure progression are facts that have called a lot of attention in situations such as limbic SE or limbic kindling (Post, 2002; Sutula, 2004), because of subsequent complex partial seizures and eventually spontaneous recurrent seizures (SRS). But, what happens with seizure repetition in GTCS? If GTCS are untreated, the chance of remission and the interval between seizures decreases, which gives support to a progression phenomenon (Fisch, 1997). Behavioral, EEG and anatomical changes could be a by-product of seizure repetition if GTCS are then secondary to temporal lobe epilepsy (TLE) and for example, become pharmaco-resistant. How do we model these alterations in experimental protocols? We will be able to discuss this issue below. Another typical feature of GTCS is the presence of a severe post-ictal phase, in general characterized by profound depression with a combination of postural, sensory (*e.g.* lack of response to nociceptive stimulation), memory disturbances, PET brain hypometabolism, hyperprolactinemia, among others (Fisch, 1997). How do we also model these features in experimental animals? Post-ictal prolactin and post-ictal analgesia are features clearly detected in experimental models and we will discuss them at the end of the chapter.

■ Basic questions and problems when modeling the human epilepsies and specifically GTCS

A myriad of the so-called experimental models of epilepsy has been developed and discussed over near 70 years with wider or restricted applications to human epileptology. This in fact depends on how each model is placed, whether in more semiological, electrophysiological, neurochemical, pharmacological, cellular or even molecular contexts. Actually, what characteristics should have a model to be considered a good one? What do we finally model? How do we do the modeling? The recent publication of the book "*Models of Seizures and of Epilepsy*" (Pitkanen *et al.*, 2006) has been a great addition to the classical books and literature reviews already published on experimental models of epilepsy. Basically the first (Engel and Schwartzkroin, 2006) and last (Schwartzkroin and Engel, 2006) chapters of that book synthesize the main goals of the experimental epileptology field, talk about the main advantages and restrictions of each one of the models, and challenge researchers to look critically at their specific experimental models and to express how distant they are from clinical questions, how close they are from explanations of mechanisms of hyperexcitability, how those models are useful for pharmacology of seizure treatment (AEDs development) and how they could be applied to other broader scientific and clinical needs.

In a recent example in the same line, Sarkisian (2001) revised a great deal of animal models of epilepsy and discussed the criteria that should be satisfied in order to model particular human epileptic conditions: similar EEG, etiologies, age of onset, pathological changes, response to AEDs and behavioral characteristics. Sarkisian (2001) then concludes: *"Despite the logical necessity of these criteria, most models fail to faithfully reproduce all aspects"*. We would like to comment that in addition to describing how current models are eventually restricted versions of human epilepsy, this author also shows many of the clinical epileptic conditions that do not have even a single animal model. In general his review contains the obvious invitation (as in the book by Pitkanen *et al.*, 2006) to work on the improvement of the existent models and the development of new ones, and to design and develop protocols for those human conditions that do not have models at all.

Following on Sarkisian (2001) and Pitkanen *et al.* (2006) discussions, indeed most of those experimental protocols have been considered models of convulsion or models of acute seizures rather than models of epilepsy or of epileptic syndromes. Obvious exceptions (not without restrictions) are those models, for example of TLE, the most common seizure disorder in humans, that display SRS and have several of the behavioral, EEG and structural alterations seen in humans (for reviews on kainic acid and pilocarpine models of TLE, see Cavalheiro *et al.*, 2006; Leite *et al.*, 2002).

However, our own obvious impression is that there is no viable way to produce a single animal model that totally mimics human epileptic conditions. We believe strongly that we can build ideal strategies, even with limited models, but also that we need multitask and integrated approaches to resolve this apparently insoluble issue. If experimental models are questioned because they are not similar to human epilepsies, what happen then when the patients are not humans? This is the case in Veterinary Medicine when the veterinary neurologist seeks for treatment or even cure for their patients. In a very interesting paper Chandler (2006) asks paradoxically: "Canine epilepsy: What we can learn from human seizure disorders?" and it is paradoxical because part of the criticism on our restricted knowledge on human epilepsy depends on the use of inappropriate animal models (see Sarkisian, 2001; Pitkanen *et al.*, 2006), however, when the patient is a dog or a cat, which animals will be the models? We do not think humans (exactly because of our restricted knowledge of their epilepsies) will be the best ones. Obviously this may not be the concern of clinical neurology in humans. Conversely, Loscher (1997) reports that within the few genetic animal models of epilepsy with SRS and that allows selection of animals with pharmacoresistant seizures are epileptic dogs, consequently a model of intractable epilepsies.

Models have been developed not only to increase our knowledge on epileptogenesis, but also to test potential AEDs. Discussions on the neuropharmacology of anticonvulsion (Loscher and Schmidt, 1994; Loscher, 1998) describe the preclinical strategies for development of new AEDS such as random screening, structural variations and mechanism-based drug development, and confirm that, with the exception of the bromides and phenobarbital, the anticonvulsant effect of all standard AEDs was first determined in animal models such as MES or PTZ. Additional up-to-date discussion on using multi-model strategies for AEDs development has been reported recently by White et al. (2006).

Furthermore, what if we consider multifactorial changes over time in a given experimental model? Shaw and Wilson (2003) had developed the concept of evaluation of neurological diseases in four dimensions (could be "n" dimensions depending on specific questions) using an animal model that combines Alzheimer disease, Parkinson disease and amyotrophic lateral sclerosis. This model is related to the known intoxication with cyca seeds of the Chamorro natives in Guam (Spencer et al., 1987; Shaw and Wilson, 2003). What is interesting is that the model incorporates behavioral (first dimension), cellular (second dimension) and biochemical (third dimension) evaluation over the fourth dimension "time". It is worth noting that in epilepsy and neuropsychiatric research concepts like this have gained already acceptance after the studies of Post (2002). This is particularly valid when studying the evolution of the epileptic process, altogether with the evolution of AEDs action and the progression and plasticity toward either pharmaco-resistance or pharmacological success, or in Post (2002) words: *the good guys against the bad guys.*

Obviously that all these primary considerations talk about the difficulties in modeling not only epilepsy but any neurological or neuropsyquiatric condition basically because of their multi-factorial features, dynamics, complexity and emergent properties appearance (see below). In fact, Post (1992) interpretation of kindling-like phenomena as common in neuropsyquiatric disorders talks about a more universal mechanism that extrapolates epilepsy. In that sense, Doman and Pelligra (2004) for example, defend that *"What leads to neuronal hyperexcitability and seizures is an inadequate mitochondrial energy production due to hypoxia and hypoxia-equivalent state"*. *"The seizure cascade"*, in their words, *"is a heroic effort to perfuse the brain when local mechanisms fail to restore energy production and ionic equilibrium"*. Their conclusion is that: *"A multilayered therapeutic approach may not be as convenient or appealing as a single pharmaceutical drug that can eliminate the visual offense of a seizure by inhibiting the CNS response"*. Contrast this view with Loscher (1998) "three" most common strategies to design antiepileptic drugs (AEDs) and White et al. (2006) on multi-models approach to AEDs research.

It is not our intention in this chapter to review all the experimental models of GTCS, but to contrast two of the classic ones: MES and PTZ with others from our own expertise: acute and chronic AS induced in the inbred Wistar audiogenic rat (WAR) strain, a genetic model of GTCS. We aim also to compare the acute expression of AS with ASK, a situation where the repetition of GTCS induces recruitment of the forebrain associated to behavioral and cellular changes similar to those found in classical models of TLE. In the process of discussing brain substrates for epileptogenesis, we would like to address the question of brainstem-forebrain and forebrain-brainstem interactions. Finally, we will discuss to what extent these models, alone or in combination with others such as amygdala kindling and SE induced by pilocarpine, had helped increasing our knowledge in behavioral semiology, in the characterization of Video-EEG correlations and in cellular and molecular correlates of primary and secondary GTCS.

■ Why maximal electroshock and pentylenetetrazol?

Pentylenetetrazol (PTZ) or metrazol, was first used by Von Meduna (1935) as convulsive therapy in psychiatry. Initial studies highlighted the role of PTZ in the so-called "generalizing system" correlated with spikes and waves, myoclonus and tonic-clonic seizures. More recently other studies demonstrated that cortex, medial thalamus, brainstem and spinal cord (Magistris et al., 1988; Miller and Ferrendelli, 1988) were also involved with PTZ pro-convulsant actions. In the case of MES this test was first used by Spiegel (1937) and was very important for the discovery of the antiepileptic effects of phenytoin by Merritt and Putnam (1938). Loscher (1998), Loscher and Schmidt (1988) and Fischer (1989) confirm that the most commonly employed animal models in the search for new anticonvulsant drugs are the MES test and the PTZ seizure test. Higher doses of PTZ induce generalized tonic-clonic seizures (Del Bel et al., 1997, 1998; Sarkisian, 2001). Sarkisian (2001) states that repeated injections of PTZ can be given to produce a type of chemical kindling that resembles electrical kindling. At high doses, PTZ reliably produces tonic-clonic convulsions in rats or mice and is a rapid and efficient measure of both seizure susceptibility and screening of new AEDs.

One of the strongest criticisms to the use of MES and PTZ to screen new AEDs is because of the fact that these models are executed in normal animals. In that sense, Meldrum (2002) highlights how levetiracetam, recently introduced to clinical use, is inactive in MES and PTZ but highly active in genetic models such as AS in mice and in acquired epilepsy models such as amygdala kindling.

For example, Ito et al. (2004) using the PTZ model but in a kindling protocol, have shown that when PTZ-kindled rats were challenged by a lower dose PTZ after withdrawal, severe GTCS developed and continued for at least 15 minutes even though nitric oxide (NO), surprisingly, was not induced by a challenge dose of PTZ. Consequently, these findings suggest that NO generation by neuronal nitric oxide synthase (NOS) plays an important role during PTZ kindling development, but not long-term kindling. The above mentioned study with PTZ kindling and NO neurotransmission was done with MRI combined to biochemical studies (Ito et al., 2004). In another study, the first published with fMRI of PTZ (65 mg/Kg) in a dose sufficient to induce generalized clonic or clonic-tonic seizures (Van Camp et al., 2003), an excellent correlation was detected between the hemodynamics (BOLD) and the epileptiform EEG associated with specific cortical and subcortical structures. Although of poorer spatial resolution when compared, for example, with Fos immuno-histochemistry after PTZ treatment (Del Bel et al., 1998), the temporal resolution is an advantage and in this case helped detecting an asymmetrical pattern of spreading of perfusion associated to the EEG epileptiform activity.

Besides this, it has been shown that PTZ is also useful to look at gene expression *in vivo* (Valente et al., 2004) and *in vitro* (Kajiwara et al., 1996). We used also PTZ to look for mechanisms of seizure modulation by nitric oxide (Del Bel et al., 1997) and brain mapping of seizure networks using Fos as a marker (Del Bel et al., 1998).

Why acute and chronic (kindled) audiogenic seizures?

Audiogenic seizures (AS) were first described in the thirties of the last century by former Soviet Union researchers (Krushinski, 1963). Although at that time AS were widely used as a model for psychiatric disorders, later studies demonstrated their value as a model of GTCS (Faingold, 1999) and nowadays we recognize that there is no contradiction on the fact that AS represent also a model of neurological and neuropsyquiatric co-morbidities (Garcia-Cairasco, 2002). The specific participation of brainstem areas in the origin of AS and the association of sensory areas with motor nuclei for the expression of AS semiology, gave place to studies of sensorimotor integration (Garcia-Cairasco, 2002; Faingold, 2004). With the advent of the ASK model (Kiesmann *et al.*, 1988; Naritoku *et al.*, 1992; Garcia-Cairasco *et al.*, 1996a; Hirsch *et al.*, 1997; Moraes *et al.*, 2000; Feng and Faingold, 2002; Romcy-Pereira and Garcia-Cairasco, 2003; Galvis-Alonso *et al.*, 2004; Moraes *et al.*, 2005), sensorimotor integration was coupled to sensorilimbic integration and data on plasticity and permanence associated to these substrates were soon available.

How do we evaluate behavior in these models?

One of the first concerns when studying an epilepsy model in freely-moving animals is about semiology or behavioral alterations. Usually seizures or epilepsies are studied based upon behavioral descriptions such as those contained in seizure severity scores, scales or indexes. One of the most known is the limbic scale of Racine (1972), extremely useful for characterization of TLE models and that has been extended by Pinel and Rovner (1978) to include brainstem-dependent behaviors typical of GTCS. Another is the Jobe *et al.* (1973) seizure severity scale that measures wild running and tonic-clonic seizures present in GEPRs, a genetic model of GTCS. We also developed a midbrain seizure severity index that measures also GTCS triggered by sound in the WAR strain (Garcia-Cairasco *et al.*, 1996a).

Scales, scores or indexes represent only an approximation of seizure severity, particularly because all of them are built on linear and arbitrary basis. These scales measure the behavior evolution over time and are also suitable for detection of any changes if a given pharmacological treatment has been applied to the animals. However, the study of sequences of behavior is more complex and ideally ethological methods rather than arbitrary indexes should be used (see below for details).

Behavioral characterization of audiogenic seizures in susceptible animals

In the early eighties, and using quantitative neuroethological techniques, we characterized AS susceptible and resistant animals based on the description of the presence of different behavioral clusters (Garcia-Cairasco and Sabbatini, 1983). Susceptible animals, taken from the general population of Wistar rats maintained in our Main Vivarium, display wild running composed of turning behavior followed by jumping and atonic falling, followed by a tonic-clonic seizure pattern with back arching tonus (opisthotonus) and generalized clonic seizures. The seizure ends with apnea and lack of postural and antinociceptive reflexes (post-ictal depression). Background behavioral clusters such as exploration and grooming, were distinguished from convulsive patterns. Before the genetic selection of the inbred strain we recorded after the wild running pattern only opisthotonus, generalized clonus and clonic spasms. Only with the beginning of our inbred audiogenic colony we recorded fore- and hindlimb hyperextensions, behavioral items frequently described in other genetically selected strains (Jobe et al., 1973). In the case of the resistant animals (our controls), they displayed two predominant behavioral clusters: exploration and grooming. During the sound stimulation, instead of the wild running pattern, typical of susceptible animals, resistant rats displayed oro-facial automatisms together with exaggerated grooming (see flowcharts in Garcia-Cairasco and Sabbatini, 1983). At the end of the stimulus, resistant rats froze. The statistical expression of the associations of behaviors in each normal or convulsive cluster was described previously (Garcia-Cairasco et al., 1992). Thus, using the method called *Ethomatic*, complex behavioral sequences typical of AS were detected (Garcia-Cairasco and Sabbatini, 1983).

Detailed behavioral descriptions are useful for the detection of sequences that can be markers of specific neural circuits' activity. The whole concept of neuroethology (Fentress et al., 1973; Garcia-Cairasco et al., 1992), or the search for neural substrates of behavior, is based on the correlation between behavior expression and brain circuitry activity (Garcia-Cairasco et al., 1996a). For example, it is very common to talk about limbic seizure activity when we detect the progression from immobility to behavioral classes such as those detected by the Racine (1972) limbic seizure scale: facial automatisms, head and forelimb clonus, rearing and falling. Also, when we talk about brainstem seizures, we think of wild running and tonic-clonic seizures or those detected, for example, by Jobe et al. (1973) scale in GEPRs. Obviously that in both cases, limbic and brainstem seizures would be only validated as such if we do concomitant EEG recordings, but the ethologically-based behavioral analysis signalizes the potential circuits to look for, as their neural substrates. We have done these types of Video-EEG recordings in AS and ASK protocols and used neuroethological behavioral sequences reconstructions in several models of epilepsy over the last 20 years. What is also interesting is that these behavioral recording and analysis models are now applied to sequences of patients with temporal TLE that present complex partial seizures and secondary GTCS (Dal-Cól et al., 2006).

■ Genetically selected sensitive rats as a first step to model epilepsy predisposition

Audiogenic seizures in rats, as well as similar events in mice, have been recognized as models of GTCS in different laboratories worldwide. Recently Ross and Coleman (2000) have compared the so-called developmental-derived models of AS and the genetic rats and mice strains, showing in detail their differences and similarities. Soviet researchers published the first descriptions of AS in the 1920s when they developed the Wistar-derived Krushinsky-Molodkina strain (Krushinski, 1963). In the 1950s, another strain derived from Sprague-Dawley rats was developed in the USA. By inbreeding they developed the GEPRs maintained until recently at the University of Illinois (Jobe et al., 1995). Currently this strain is maintained at the Southern Illinois University (Faingold, personal communication). In the 1980s, three additional Wistar-derived strains were described, one in Strasbourg, France (Marescaux et al. 1987), other in China, the so-called P77PMC (Zhao et al., 1985) and the other one in Brazil, the WAR strain (Garcia-Cairasco et al., 1990; Doretto et al., 2003), the latter selected in our Laboratory. Work from 20 generations of inbreeding (sister/brother mating) with near 1500 animals and more than 9000 behavioral observations of WARs demonstrated that the genetic selection produced a strain with a very short latency for the onset of seizures and a high seizure severity index. Although we still have not published data on the genetic determinants of the epilepsy susceptibility of the WARs, ongoing experiments are devoted to the molecular characterization of gene expression in different areas of the brain associated to either naive animals (endogenous expression), acute AS, the so-called brainstem dependent seizures, or to the limbic recruited networks, particularly after ASK.

■ Brainstem substrates of audiogenic-like seizures induced in normal audiogenic-resistant rats

The inferior colliculus (IC) has been shown as one of the most critical points for the initiation of AS. Bilateral IC lesions, as well as bilateral lesions of the lateral lemniscus (LL) or lesions reaching the transition between LL and IC, completely blocked AS (Kesner, 1966; Willot and Lu, 1980; Garcia-Cairasco and Sabbatini, 1991). Previous studies have shown that audiogenic-like seizures could be evoked by microinjections of bicuculline into the IC (Frye et al., 1983; Millan et al., 1986). In accordance with those data, we observed complex audiogenic-like responses when we applied bicuculline into the central nucleus of the IC. This behavior was generally explosive in resistant rats (Tsutsui et al., 1992; Terra and Garcia-Cairasco, 1992). The majority of responses happened before sound stimulation and never ended in tonic-clonic seizures. Additional experiments were performed with N-methyl-D-aspartate (NMDA) microinjections in IC subnuclei in resistant rats, The best NMDA dose, potentiated by sound, was $2.5 \mu g/0.2 \mu L$, even though we observed different responses when comparing both central and cortical dorsal IC subnuclei. When we pre-treated animals with the NMDA antagonist amino-phosphonoheptanoate (AP7; $0.3 \mu g/0.2 \mu L$), we blocked completely seizure patterns in both central and cortical IC subnuclei (Terra and Garcia-Cairasco, 1994). In susceptible animals, AP7 blocked totally audiogenic-like seizures when applied into the IC central nucleus and partially when applied into IC cortex (Terra and Garcia-Cairasco, 1994). Different from the so-called submaximal audiogenic-like seizures, because they never ended in tonic-clonic seizures, induced by bicuculline (Tsutsui et al., 1992; Terra and Garcia-Cairasco, 1992) the NMDA-evoked audiogenic-like seizures in resistant rats were more similar to the genetic ones. It is possible that the characteristic epileptogenicity of IC cortex may be necessary for the behavioral expression of AS, and the IC central nucleus is necessary for the sensory-dependent triggering of AS.

Behavioral reactions seen after applications of bicuculline (Brandão et al., 1988) or NMDA (Cardoso et al., 1994) to the IC are similar to flight patterns. For these reasons they have been characterized as aversive responses supporting that the IC is part of brain aversive systems (Brandão et al., 1994). In that direction, using the *switch-off* paradigm in which the animal is trained to disconnect the stimulation when its effect is aversive, Bagri et al. (1992) found that wild running induced by electrical stimulation of the IC is aversive, but the *switch-off* worked only when ventral central IC nucleus was stimulated, not the IC dorsal cortex. In the latter when the stimulus was *switched off*, epileptogenic activity was still evoked outlasting the electrical stimulation, and the behavior was blocked by conventional anticonvulsants (Bagri et al., 1991), thus confirming previous data from McCown et al. (1987) and Pierson et al. (1989) on the epileptogenicity of IC cortex stimulation (see below). Accordingly, an equivalent flight behavior evoked by electrical stimulation of the IC was also blocked by benzodiazepines (Mello et al., 1992). In our experience, higher doses of bicuculline (80 µg/0.2 µL) applied to the IC evoked overt flight behavior during which the animals were unresponsive to sound stimulation (Tsutsui et al., 1992). The obvious conclusion is that the IC activation expresses strong overlapping, or at least sequenced, aversive and convulsive behaviors. What would be then the relevance of a flight behavior preceding a seizure? In that direction, Plotnikoff (1963) noticed that animals exposed to acoustic stimuli avoided the seizures if they had the opportunity to escape. That author then suggested that tests of psychoactive drugs could be performed using as a model the flight component (wild running) of AS, whereas the tonic-clonic seizure phase could be used to test actual anticonvulsants such as barbiturates. These data might be in agreement with the theoretical proposition by Doman and Pelligra (2003) mentioned above in which the seizure response of a given animal can be seen as an adaptive defense response, although they think every seizure would be always triggered by hypoxia or hypoxic-similar states. Complementarily, it is important to recall at this point Post (2002) who suggests that epileptic seizures, pain syndromes and other neuropsyquiatric disorders have a kindling-like pattern, with similarity of mechanisms of progression in those, otherwise different neuropathological entities.

■ Sensory-motor transduction in the brainstem

Besides IC subnuclei (data with bicuculline and NMDA) other midbrain areas are needed to transduce sensory into motor information. Pierson et al. (1989) demonstrated the presence of an NMDA-dependent epileptiform activity in slices in the IC cortical nucleus. Furthermore, McCown et al. (1984, 1987) obtained audiogenic-like seizures after electrical stimulations of the IC and a concomitant 2-deoxyglucose metabolism pattern including the IC cortex, the deep layers of the superior colliculus (SC) and the periaqueductal gray (PAG), initially recruited in a partially asymmetrical and then generalized manner (McCown et al., 1991). In the same study it was highlighted that IC cortex nuclei displayed a stimulus-independent activity and the substantia nigra lateralis (SNL)/peripeduncular area displayed a stimulus-dependent activity. In view of the selective epileptogenicity of IC subnuclei, one of the greater paradoxes is related to cell number in IC of GEPRs and their expected inhibitory function. While Roberts et al. (1985) showed in GEPRs an increase in the number of Gamma-aminobutyric acid (GABA)-ergic neurons correlated with an increase in glutamic acid decarboxylase (GAD) mRNA-labeled neurons (Ribak et al., 1990), a parallel decrease in the inhibitory function of the IC of GEPRs was demonstrated (Faingold et al., 1991) Furthermore, Ribak et al. (1994) have shown that midcollicular knife cuts and separation of IC subnuclei (*e.g.* IC central from IC external subnuclei) blocked AS in GEPRs, confirming similar but previous data on the WAR strain from our laboratory (Tsutsui et al., 1992). Moreover, Ribak et al. (1993) found an increase in GAD mRNA in both central and in cortical IC nuclei and in dorsal SC. In an additional study, with in situ hybridization of c-fos, Ribak et al. (1997) showed the involvement of the SC in the propagation of seizure activity in GEPRs. In these neuroanatomical and functional experiments, the data pointed to the IC central nucleus as the critical area in the origin of AS. However, all the work done with other audiogenic-like responses, such as those evoked by in vivo and in vitro (slices) electrical stimulation of the IC in resistant rats, suggests intrinsic epileptogenicity of the IC cortex (McCown et al., 1987; 1991; McCown and Breese, 1991; Snyder-Keller and Pierson, 1992; Swann et al., 1999). Obvious discrepancies were derived from the use of genetic strains (Faingold's and Ribak's data) *versus* normal animals with acquired audiogenic responses (McCown's and Pierson's data). Additional work in rats, however, has shown that the SC deep layers participate in flight-orientation responses (Sahibzada et al., 1986; Dean et al., 1989) and flight behaviors (Coimbra and Brandão, 1993; Coimbra et al., 1996), all of them very similar to AS responses. Consequently the integrity of the IC-SC projections is important for the sensorimotor transduction needed, not only for adaptive responses such as flight but also for pathological conditions such as AS. In addition to IC cortex and SC deep layers, non-acoustic structures such as PAG and substantia nigra reticulata (SNR) and SNL have been shown to be critically involved in the AS network. Some of the most severe manifestations of AS are related to the appearance of tonic-clonic convulsive behavior, specifically apnea, vocalizations, barrel rolling and clonic spasms (Garcia-Cairasco and Sabbatini, 1983, 1989). It seems plausible that vocalizations are related to known morphological connections between IC and PAG matter (Herrera et al., 1988). However, data from Bagri et al. (1992) have indicated that bicuculline application to the IC evoked audiogenic-like seizures that were not modified by massive lesions of the PAG, thus suggesting that this structure is not necessary for the sensorimotor processing of these seizures. In contrast N'Gouemo and Faingold (1998, 1999) demonstrated that the ventrolateral PAG is involved in the modulation of AS in GEPRs through a complex mechanism mediated by NMDA, GABA and opiates. Complementarily, unitary activity of PAG neurons is also increased during wild running, tonus and hindlimb hyperextensions of GEPRs (Faingold, 1999).

■ Substantia nigra and nigro-tectal modulation of seizures

It is clear that AS are basically triggered by acoustic stimulation (Kesner, 1966; Willot and Lu, 1980; Garcia-Cairasco and Sabbatini, 1989, 1991). However, because AS are a model of GTCS, it is possible that they share some neuroanatomical and neurochemical substrates with other known seizure models. Iadarola and Gale (1982) demonstrated that MES-induced seizures are blocked by manipulations of the SNR in a GABA-dependent mechanism. Garant and Gale (1987) and Bonhaus et al. (1986) demonstrated that bilateral lesions in the SNR blocked midbrain seizures or slowed the onset of kindling development, respectively. These and subsequent studies have led investigators to propose the nigro-tectal pathway as an anticonvulsant circuit (Garant and Gale, 1987; Redgrave et al., 1992a,b). In the search for specific nigral-dependent anticonvulsant networks, we made selective nigral lesions that sensitized resistant animals to AS (Garcia-Cairasco and Sabbatini, 1983, 1991; Doretto and Garcia-Cairasco, 1995). We therefore suggested that antagonistic circuits or neurotransmitter systems are located in the SNR and that their differential regulation explains the expression of either convulsant or anticonvulsant states. Although we made that statement near 20 years ago, with the only available data of electrolytic SNR lesions and neuroethology, it is important to recall at this point that Velisek et al. (2002) demonstrated concordant results with another model of GTCS: flurothyl, where anterior and posterior SNR possesses age-dependent antagonistic, anticonvulsant and convulsant properties, respectively. Also in the same model were determined the effects of bilateral zolpidem (a BZD1 agonist) microinfusions in SNR (Veliskova et al., 1998). Briefly, in adults and in anterior SNR, zolpidem microinfusions were anticonvulsant but ineffective in posterior SNR. In 15 day old rats, the SNR microinfusions of zolpidem had anticonvulsant effects on clonic and tonic-clonic seizures, no matter which SNR region was microinjected. We are in the process of evaluating whether anterior and posterior portions of SNR as reported by Veliskova et al. (1998) have an equivalent pattern of anticonvulsant response in WARs.

Although we induced susceptibility in AS resistant rats by unilateral SNR lesions (see above), additional data have shown that bilateral SNR lesions do not produce any alteration in AS responses in WARs (Doretto and Garcia-Cairasco, 1995). Complementarily, it has been demonstrated that nigral muscimol application in ethanol-withdrawn rats partially (Frye et al., 1983) or totally (Gonzalez and Hettinger, 1984) blocked AS. Millan et al. (1986, 1988) also demonstrated that GEPRs displayed a greater sensitivity to bicuculline and NMDA applied to the IC, than normal controls. Additionally, they were able to induce blockade of AS by selective application of AP7 in IC and SNR of these animals. Further observations in the MES model of epilepsy (Redgrave et al., 1992a,b) have pointed at the SNL as the possible specific anticonvulsant projection (nigro-tectal pathway) rather than the one originating in the SNR. Since SNL-IC connections were already described (Tokunaga et al., 1984; Olazabal and Moore, 1989), we believe that this pathway may also be involved in the sensorimotor processing of AS. Furthermore, McCown et al. (1991) have shown that besides IC subnuclei, SNL displays metabolic activity, possibly indicative of modulation of IC-evoked seizures. Complementarily, we believe that nigrocollicular connections are relevant because AS susceptibility was induced in normal audiogenic-resistant rats submitted to combined (inter-hemispheric) SNR-IC lesions (Garcia-Cairasco and Sabbatini, 1991). However, because Depaulis et al. (1990) made microinjection of muscimol, a GABA-A agonist into SNR of Strasbourg audiogenic rats, and this treatment was not able to block AS, we think the participation of that nigro-tectal projection in the control of AS is, at minimum, arguable. Below we will do additional considerations on this issue.

Coimbra and Brandão (1993) and Coimbra et al. (1996) have shown that nigrotectal projections are crucial to the expression of fear. What is intriguing is that those circuits are well overlapped to the ones here discussed in the endogenous control of brainstem-dependent seizures (Redgrave et al., 1992a,b; Garcia-Cairasco, 2002). In addition to that, the neurobiological mechanisms associated to post-ictal analgesia after PTZ-induced seizures (Freitas et al., 2005) and after AS (unpublished observations in WARs) are also overlapped to those of seizure and fear controlling activity in these regions. Additionally, when pos-ictal chemo-architecture is evaluated after AS, a clear-cut surge of prolactin (PRL) accompanies the comatose behavior of the animal with post-ictal analgesia and all the postural sequela (lack of righting reflex). We have evaluated this post-ictal PRL peak and similarly to what has been shown in clinical neurology; it serves as a marker of genuine GTCS, in our case induced by AS (Garcia-Cairasco et al., 1996b; Doretto et al., 2003). Behavioral perturbations after seizures (Caldecott-Hazard et al., 1987) might be explained by the exaggerated release of compounds, some of them certainly potent endogenous anticonvulsants: adenosine, opiates, oxytocin, ACTH, PRL, among others. Exploring the correlation between endogenous substances, endogenous anticonvulsant systems and AED therapies is certainly a logical perspective. Curiously, most of the known AEDs have nothing to do with endogenous anticonvulsant systems, however a growing amount of data point, for example, to the SNR and subthalamic nucleus as good candidate sites, among others, for deep anti-epileptic electrical stimulation (Velisek et al., 2002; Theodore and Fisher, 2004). See below comments and our data on SNR as a participant in endogenous anticonvulsant systems.

■ Alterations of GABA release or GABA receptors in SNR in GEPRs and WARs and the endogenous substrates of anticonvulsion

The rationale for the use of GABAergic drugs and benzodiazepines microinjected to the SNR was based on data previously mentioned when muscimol applied to this site acted as anticonvulsant in normal animals submitted to biculline (Garant and Gale, 1986). Consequently, we demonstrated that bilateral SNR microinjections of clobazam completely blocked audiogenic-like seizures evoked by unilateral IC microinjection of bicuculline in AS resistant rats (Terra and Garcia-Cairasco, 1992). King et al. (1987) obtained equivalent data when nigral microinjection of clonazepam blocked amygdala kindling. Interestingly both types of seizures were evoked in animals that were normal and became epileptic after the electrical kindling or after chemical manipulations with bicuculline (AS-like seizures). However, we did not block genetic AS, by nigral application of clobazam in WARs (Terra and Garcia-Cairasco, 1992), probably reflecting a GABA defficiency in this strain. Also, although we were able to block AS in WARs after systemically applied phenobarbital (Rossetti et al., 2005) SNR microinjection of phenobarbital, as well as microinjection of muscimol into the SNR were not able to block AS (unpublished observations). Recall that Depaulis et al. (1990) were also unable to block AS in the Wistar audiogenic strain from Strasbourg, but although their conclusion was that the nigro-tectal pathway is not involved in the network controlling the expression of AS in rats, we think that their data are essentially similar to ours with clobazam and muscimol in WARs. In fact, their results match pretty well with binding data from the Strasbourg audiogenic rat, supportive also of an endogenous deficiency in the strain, where there is a 40% reduction in GABA receptor in SNR (Deransart et al., 2001).

Similarly, Hjeresen et al. (1987) have suggested a developmental alteration, which may be correlated with a decrease in GABA binding in the SNR of GEPRs (Franck and Schwartzkroin, 1987). Because possible endogenous biochemical alterations might occur also in WARs, one approach is to neurochemically characterize their whole brain and regional content, message/protein expression and functionality of both neurotransmitters and their receptors.

In addition to the known endogenous neurochemical alterations, among others: in raphe nuclei, IC, SC, locus coeruleus in GEPRs (Jobe et al., 1973; Jobe et al., 1991; Lasley, 1991; Ribak et al., 1988) we characterized the pattern of SNR amino acid release triggered by 100 mM KCl by means of microdialysis in GEPR-9s. Briefly, we demonstrated that GEPR-9s displayed a statistically significant decrease in SNR GABA release (Doretto et al., 1994), whereas release of aspartate, glycine, taurine and glutamate was not altered. Because the importance of SNR outputs for the expression of AS, as co-adjuvant networks to the IC key role in the afferent pathway, we believe the current SNR GABAergic alteration in GEPRs can be added as a critical factor in GEPRs AS predisposition. It is possible that common functional inhibitory disturbances are responsible for similar alterations in WARs. Consequently, ongoing experiments in our laboratory are designed to measure SNR GABA receptors, GABA release and up-take in naïve and seizing WARs.

With the rationale that structures responsible for the onset, propagation, and cessation of generalized seizures are not known, Velizkova et al. (2005) did experiments with SNR lesion and muscimol microinfusion and 2DG mapping after seizures induced by flurothyl, another model of generalized seizures. They demonstrated that caudal SNR was selectively active during the pre-clonic period and may represent an early gateway to seizure propagation. Rostral SNR and SC changed their activity during progression to tonic-clonic seizure, suggesting the involvement in coordinated regional activity that results in inhibitory effects on seizures. The postictal suppression state was correlated with changes in the SNR projection targets, specifically the pedunculopontine tegmental nucleus and SC.

As another set of data supporting brainstem control of GTCS, Rossetti et al. (2005) tested the possibility of AS blockade in WARs by systemic phenobarbital. Besides behavioral studies, these authors executed EEG recording and profiles (Morlet's wavelets transform) of the nuclei involved in endogenous control of seizures (SNR and SC). Briefly, phenobarbital (15 mg/Kg) exerted a dose-dependent behavioral and EEG anticonvulsant effect in WARs, without sedation or ataxia. SNR and SC exhibited high frequency episodes during seizures, mainly after forelimb hyperextension, with significant second frequency alterations both in the natural period of seizure recovery and during the anticonvulsant effect of phenobarbital. These data are in agreement with the eventual recruitment of SN-SC network as part of endogenous anticonvulsant systems (Redgrave, 1992a,b) challenged with AS. Previous data from our laboratory had shown that although SNR microinjection of clobazam could block AS-like seizures induced by IC bicuculline in normal audiogenic-resistant rats, this treatment has no effect on WARs (Terra and Garcia-Cairasco, 1992). In this group of experiments we were confirming the hypothesis that convulsant protocols in normal rats give different effects than seizures induced in genetically developed strains and this produce a unique chance to establish protocols to look for markers of seizure susceptibility either structural, neurochemical or molecular. This in fact is one of the recommended strategies for contemporary epilepsy research (Schwartzkroin and Engel, 2006).

Nehlig et al. (1994) have demonstrated that AS metabolic mapping of Strasbourg audiogenic sensitive animals by the autoradiographic [14C] iodoantipyrine technique of Sakurada (1978) shows an increase of more than 150% of the controls in IC, medullary, pontine and mesencephalic reticular formation and SNR. Also were recorded such large amounts of blood flux in monoaminergic cell groups of the brainstem and brainstem auditory relay nuclei, posterior vegetative areas and hypothalamic and thalamic regions. The lowest blood flux values appeared in cortical, forebrain areas and limbic areas including hippocampus, piriform and enthorinal cortex, among others. These data confirm that AS are dependent basically on brainstem substrates because blood flow results match well with behavioral and EEG information.

If we look also at the complementary data collected over the years by Browning's group (Browning, 1994), these authors tested the hypothesis that separate substrates are able to support specific types of seizures, for example: clonic seizures and tonic-clonic seizures. Browning and Nelson (1986) demonstrated that in animals that have pre-collicular transections, PTZ (50 mg/Kg) produced running-bouncing clonus which progressed to tonic forelimb extension. But facial forelimb clonus, that occurred in rats with sham-transection, was never observed in the transected animals. The same result was observed if rats were transected and submitted to transcorneal electroshock with the animals presenting running, bouncing and tonic convulsions but without facial and forelimb clonus. These authors confirmed these results in GEPRs (Browning et al., 1999) and also demonstrated that forebrain-evoked seizures induced by microinjection of bicuculline into deep pepiriform cortex (*area tempestas*; Browning et al., 1993) are present even without brainstem connections. Together with other studies (Garcia-Cairasco, 2002; Faingold, 2004; Moraes et al., 2005) these data highlight the participation of sub-regions of the reticular core, IC, SC and SNR in the generation, development and spreading of GTCS.

It is interesting to notice that a lot of data we have discussed on the value to characterize SNR role as part of an endogenous anticonvulsant system in experimental models (Redgrave, 1992a,b; Garcia-Cairasco, 2002; Faingold, 2004). The above mentioned GABA failures might be at least part of the neurochemical culprits of the hyperexcitable states of these strains. The following study uses, however, a model for network characterization in clinical setups. The model of cortical-subcortical and specifically brainstem substrates participation, not only in the initiation but also in the propagation and behavioral manifestations of generalized seizures, comes from the study by McNally and Blumenfeld (2004). They describe a new human model to investigate generalized seizures: single-photon emission computed tomography, ictal-interictal difference imaging of GTCS induced by electroconvulsive therapy (ECT). Briefly, if bitemporal ECT is used it activates focal bilateral fronto-temporal and parietal association cortex, whereas, if bifrontal ECT is used it activates mainly prefrontal cortex. Furthermore, if right unilateral ECT is used, left frontotemporal region is relatively spared and associated midline subcortical networks are also involved. They conclude that further studies of this kind may elucidate specific networks in GTCS, providing targets for new therapeutic interventions in epilepsy.

As a corollary, Lopes da Silva and Post (2002) highlight that data from the kindling model of epilepsy (and we think this can be extended to the GTCS and to other epilepsy models), such as alterations at the level of gene expression, are related to epileptogenesis, while others secondary and compensatory events are potentially associated to endogenous anticonvulsants. Thus, they suggest that for drug development we need to group neurobiological alterations into these two opposing categories of primary pathological and secondary adaptive, then alterations related to the primary pathophysiology can be targeted for inhibition or suppression, while those related to compensatory and adaptive changes can be facilitated by exogenous medications and other therapeutic procedures. May be, if we explore better all the information collected over the years on the endogenous anticonvulsant systems, the data on trophic factors (NGF, BDNF, ERF, FGF) and endogenous anti-epileptic molecules (enkephalins, endorphins, ACTH, NPY), a practical consequence will be the improvement in protocols for seizure control such as deep brain stimulation (Theodore and Fischer, 2004). Accordingly, several sets of new data have confirmed the importance of the participation of basal ganglia and brainstem nuclei in experimental and human epileptogenesis and even in seizure origin (Morimoto, Fehnestock and Racine, 2004; Norden and Blemenfeld, 2002).

■ Behavioral, electrophysiological and morphological characterization of acoustic-limbic interactions during the development of ASK

Acutely induced AS or AS-like responses induced by bicuculline or NMDA microinjections to the IC may represent only activation of midbrain systems, since massive ablation of the cortex and forebrain structures preserves AS integrity (Bagri et al., 1989). In addition to that, complete pre-collicular transections in GEPRs (Browning et al., 1999; Moraes et al., 2005) are unable to block AS, supporting the view that this is a brainstem-dependent model.

However, when chronic AS are evoked by sound or electrical stimulation, the newly displayed behavioral patterns may well represent the co-activation and recruiting of forebrain circuits. Marescaux et (1987) and Kiesmann et al. (1988) made the first description of the so-called ASK, by means of repeated sound stimulation. They demonstrated the onset of myoclonus after the 10-20th acoustic stimulation of their Wistar audiogenic rat strain, correlated with epileptiform cortical EEG. In some animals, the tonic-clonic component completely disappeared. McCown et al. (1987) made equivalent studies with electrical stimulation of the IC of normal rats, obtaining a similar pattern of limbic recruitment. Recent studies in our laboratory have shown that ASK paradigm with 30 daily trials or 60 stimulations (two per day) induced behavioral changes with oscillating and decreasing midbrain seizures, accompanied by growing limbic seizures (Garcia-Cairasco et al., 1996a). These results support a bidirectional midbrain-forebrain seizure interaction and modulation. Equivalent, although in opposite direction, interactions have been described in mice exposed to fluorothyl, where forebrain epileptogenesis seems to work, both decreasing the brainstem seizure threshold and facilitating the propagation of the forebrain seizures to the brainstem (Ferland and Applegate, 1998).

McCown et al. (1987) demonstrated that when ASK is induced by chronic electrical stimulation of the IC cortex, not only local afterdischarges appear but also amygdala and cortical post-ictal spiking, indicating a recruitment of these areas in the progression of IC kindling. Other studies have suggested that hippocampal kindling, as well as amygdala kindling, are indeed facilitated in ASK (Hirsch et al., 1992, 1997). In these protocols, made in the Wistar audiogenic strain from Strasbourg, hippocampus is not involved in the expression of the newly evoked limbic behaviors. Briefly, Hirsch et al. (1997) applied lidocaine locally in the hippocampus and amygdala, and observed the disappearance of the new limbic behaviors only when the local anesthetic was applied into amygdala. Although the transference from the brainstem to the forebrain was already suggested when cortical EEG was done in these protocols (Naritoku et al., 1992; Hirsch et al., 1997), and although there were some EEG recordings in hippocampus after the ASK ended (Hirsch et al., 1992), there was no chronic recording of either amygdala or hippocampus that demonstrated the sequential recruitment of either area during the ASK evolution. At the same time, Naritoku et al. (1992) have suggested that IC-medial geniculate body-amygdala connections are crucial to the manifestations of the ASK state in GEPRs. Thus, we developed ASK protocol with WARs (up to 28 and 40 acoustic stimulations, three stimulations/day) where IC, amygdala and cortical electrodes were implanted. Briefly, we found a clear-cut recruitment and growing synchronization of forebrain areas, concomitant with seizure repetition. At the same time amygdala and cortex were recruited, IC was either synchronized or not with these forebrain areas, depending on the behavioral outcome (Moraes et al., 2000). This was the first time that amygdala recruitment has been documented during the evolution of ASK. Obvious correlations appeared in the literature showing Fos expression when compared across a diversity of AS protocols. Simler et al. (1999) showed the expression of Fos in acute AS *versus* ASK in animals from the Strasbourg strain. Basically the pattern of Fos expression followed the one suggested by the behavioral studies and the one shown in the electrophysiology protocols. Other laboratories demonstrated in GEPRs a contrast between Fos expression in acute and chronic animals and between developing *versus* adult animals (Clough et al., 1997; Eells et al., 2000). Similar data was found by Klein et al. (2004) in the Frings strain, a mouse model of AS and GTCS.

Because with the ASK the new phenotype was similar to limbic kindled seizures (Marescaux et al., 1987; Naritoku et al., 1992; Garcia-Cairasco et al., 1994; Garcia-Cairasco et al., 1996a; Moraes et al., 2000) we also were looking for structural correlates associated to kindling progression. In the last 18 years, most studies have found evidence of collateral sprouting of the mossy fibers (axons of the hippocampal dentate granule cells) after animals have been exposed to either limbic kindling or status epilepticus (SE) induced by systemically applied drugs such as pilocarpine or kainic acid (Sutula et al., 1988; Leite et al., 2002; Cavalheiro et al., 2006). Using the Neo-Timm staining (Danscher, 1981) that stains zinc present in the mossy fibers, we were unable to detect the expected sprouting of the molecular layer of the dentate granule cells after ASK. In contrast, we found and described also for the first time, substantial Timm-positive alterations in the amygdaloid complex, perirhinal and piriform cortices of ASK animals (Garcia-Cairasco et al., 1996a). We replicated these data with additional seizures in WARs, even in a group of animals submitted subsequently to amygdala kindling (Galvis-Alonso et al., 2004). It is possible that the differences we found, when compared to the electrical kindling or to the SE models, are related to different cellular or molecular mechanisms or to recruitment of different circuitry. In that sense, in a very recent set of experiments (Romcy-Pereira and Garcia-Cairasco, 2003) we demonstrated that although mossy fiber sprouting is still absent in ASK WARs (28 stimulations; two per day) a clear pattern of increased dentate granule cells proliferation (neurogenesis) accompanies the severity of the limbic recruitment. Obvious differences will appear when we compare these animals for example, with those treated with pilocarpine and that also develop GTCS. That is the case on a recent report by Hagihara et al. (2005) where there is a huge detection of BrdU-positive cells after GTCS induced by pilocarpine, associated to the expression of several growth factors and neuronal degeneration.

These data altogether suggest that a combination of neuronal loss, cell proliferation and plastic rearrangement is present in selective regions of the ASK brain. In that direction, Holmes et al. (1990) suggested that chronic AS in GEPRs induce memory alterations, learning difficulties, and possible interictal disturbances, in agreement with other epilepsy models in which learning and memory problems seem to be a common feature (Leite et al., 1999; Sutula et al., 1995). Tracking midbrain-forebrain interactions in AS research has been enhanced by the work on acoustic-evoked emotional memories (Ledoux et al., 1990) that have demonstrated morphological and physiological connections between IC, medial geniculate body and lateral amygdala. We suggest that the fear-potentiated startle (Lee et al., 1996) and acoustic-evoked endocrine changes, such as the post-ictal prolactin peak after AS, a marker of generalized seizures (Garcia-Cairasco et al., 1996b), may use these pathways as their specific neural substrates. Studies in GEPRs, tracking with the same rationale that ours, the circuitry involved in AS and in GTCS, have found very similar results and added specific regions, among them the perirhinal cortex (Raisinghani and Faingold, 2005), in the acute AS and ASK protocol. The use of GEPRs as an epilepsy model not only contributed to the knowledge of the whole network here commented, but to the evaluation of classic and new AEDs. Additional and detailed data on GEPRs are discussed in this volume in the chapter by Phillip C. Jobe and Ronald Browning.

■ WARs are genetically predisposed to epilepsy: evidence from combination of audiogenic seizures and audiogenic seizures klinding with MES, PTZ, amygdala kindling and SE induced by pilocarpine

When we combine AS and ASK in WARs, a genetically selected strain with other electrical or chemical convulsants, we notice that we need sub-convulsant amounts of drugs or sub-threshold stimulations in order to observe the seizures. Specifically,

WARs need less amount of pilocarpine to entry into SE induced by this cholinergic muscarinic agonist applied systemically (Garcia-Cairasco et al. 2004). The neuroethological methodology captured the presence of secondary GTCS only during the development of SE in WARs and not in the Wistar controls. In addition to that, the SE and the SRS induced by pilocarpine in WARs are more severe and in the case of SRS they are both of the partial seizure type (measured with the Racine's scale) and of the brainstem type, as in the case of actual AS, which means that even in the SRS (unpublished observations), brainstem substrates are rapidly recruited.

Additional studies have shown that WARs respond with a decreased threshold to MES and PTZ (Scarlatelli-Lima e cols (2003) and display epileptiform amygdala activity, induced by transauricular MES, even in acute tests, before any kindling process has happened (Magalhães e cols, 2004). This makes WARs, originated from Wistar rats, comparable to other epilepsy-prone strains such as GEPRs, that are derived from Sprague-Dawley rats (Jobe et al., 1991; Lasley, 1991).

Hirsh et al. (1994, 1997) have shown that only after ASK hippocampal and amygdala kindling are facilitated, because in naive susceptible rats amygdala kindling is not different from controls. We confirmed the same data in WARs and demonstrated also that this phenomenon is permanent since even 40 days after ASK, amygdala kindling is accelerated (Galvis-Alonso et al., 2004). By contrast, GEPRs naive to AS have already an enhanced response to limbic kindling (Savage et al., 1987) and also brainstem epileptiform responses after forebrain stimulation (Coffey et al., 1996). The advantage of these combined protocols is that we can evaluate the interaction between the genetic background of the strains and the seizure experience imposed by the electrical protocols such as amygdala kindling or MES, or chemical protocols such as PTZ or pilocarpine. In the latter, the induction of SE (Garcia-Cairasco et al., 2004) and SRS (unpublished observations) in genetically developed strains such as WARs are a welcome mix because most of the SE protocols are made with normal rats, and as it is also the case with amygdala electrical kindling, the interaction between features of epilepsy genetic predisposition and seizure experience are infrequently considered or even neglected. An excellent exception has been the studies in the so-called slow and fast kindling strains selected for their behavioral and EEG responses to amygdala kindling (Racine et al., 1999; McIntyre et al., 1999).

In the search for eventual co-morbidities associated to the seizure susceptibility of WARs, several behavioral, neuroendocrinological and electrophysiological protocols have shown that these animals are more anxious than their resistant counterparts, in both the elevated plus maze and the open field (Garcia-Cairasco et al., 1998), have abnormal hydro-electrolytic function challenged by water overloads (Garcia-Cairasco et al., 1994b) and have excitatory-inhibitory (GABA-glutamate) balance altered when hippocampal neonatal neurons in culture are evaluated (Mesquita et al., 2005).

Another example of the combination of these genetic models with pharmacological treatments comes from the work by Del Bel et al. (1997). Briefly, the inhibitor of the NO synthase (L-NOArg) was capable to modify seizure activity depending on the epilepsy model used. First, it increased seizure responses to subconvulsant doses of pilocarpine, second it did not modify AS in WARs and GEPRs and finally it was pro-convulsant with low doses of PTZ and anticonvulsant with high doses of PTZ (Del Bel et al., 1997). The use of the genetic models, in combination with others, because the formers represent better cellular and molecular alterations of the epileptic, endogenously ill brain (gene alterations, channelopathies), have been highlighted as the ideal strategies for future AEDs research (Meldrum, 2002; White et al., 2006).

See in *figures 1 and 2* an overview of integrated neuroethological, EEG and cellular approaches to the study of acute and kindled AS in WARs.

■ Concluding remarks and future perspectives

The questions of relevance to clinical neurology that this chapter has raised, and as precise as possible answered, were: What are the sequels of GTCS repetition? Are the models considering progression? Usually GTCS are developed in acute protocols. Are in the clinical situation numbers on how many patients begin their seizures experience with GTCS? How much PTZ and MES repetition, as well as ASK could model this situation? Are there other neurological or neuro-psychiatric disorders co-morbid with epilepsy? Therefore, that is why is so relevant to distinguish between ictal fear, ictal flight and consequences of seizures such as fear, anxiety and psychosis. How much ASK is a model of limbic seizure recruitment and epilepsy progression? What happened when we combined ASK with amygdala kindling? Did this mimic similar situations in clinical neurology? How many of the changes after ASK are negative? Cell loss, lack of sprouting; how many are positive? Limbic seizures, EEG epileptiform activity in limbic regions and neurogenesis. What happened if we induce SE with pilocarpine in WARs? Is this a good model of genetic background-seizure experience interactions? What if pilocarpine is injected not systemically but intra-hippocampally? How good are these combinations of models for new AEDs development?

Most of the answers to these questions, although sometimes incomplete, were obtained with literature data and with our own experience, mostly with acute and kindled audiogenic seizures. We concluded then that we should combine genetic and acquired models of epilepsy to further understand basic mechanisms, to look for markers of epilepsy and to simulate clinical situations as close as possible. The integrated addition of all these strategies will help to produce relevant data to epileptology, no matter whether is a contribution to epileptogenesis, to the prediction of seizures, to the field of AEDs development or hopefully to finding a cure.

Thus, accepting that we are modeling partial aspects of the human epilepsies and that we are in some way distant from the evolutionary characteristics of the subject to be modeled, we can discuss if the question is more about developing ideal research strategies than of the use of limited models alone. In that direction we presented in this chapter some basic characteristics on the so-called classical models of GTCS (MES and PTZ), more recent views on AS and ASK as models in the genetically selected strain WAR, and the most important point, the multifaceted effects of GTCS repetition and exponential effects of combinations of the AS and ASK with other seizure types (MES, PTZ, amygdala kindling and SE after pilocarpine). The rationale

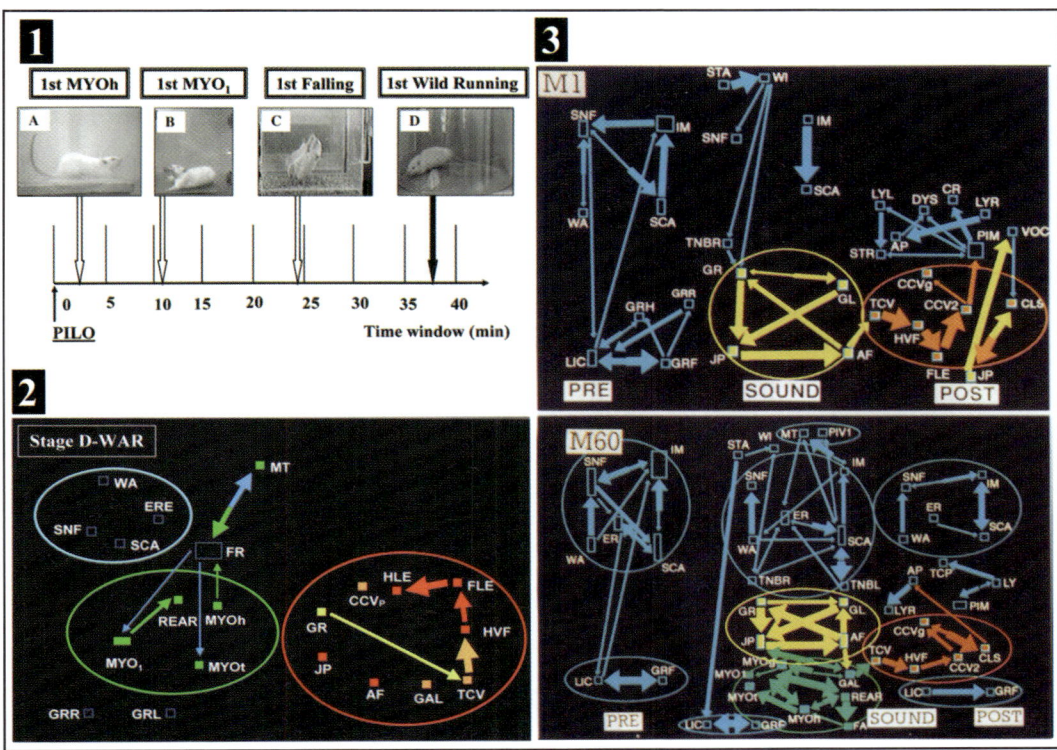

Figure 1. Flowchart representation of behavioral sequences after pilocarpine-induced SE in WARs **(1,2)** and in AS and ASK in WARs **(3)**. **(1)** Main behavioral items during limbic seizures. Behavioral triggers mark the beginning of the observation window after pilocarpine injection: First MYOh= First Head Myoclonus; First MYO_1= First forelimb myoclonus; First Falling; First Wild Running. **(2)** Neuroethological studies with WARs during pilocarpine-induced SE illustrating, in contrast to Wistars (not shown), the expression of a partial limbic seizure (green cluster) followed by a secondary GTCS (orange and red cluster). Exploratory behaviors are part of the so-called background cluster (blue). Behaviors are illustrated as rectangles with height and base proportional to frequency and duration, respectively. See details in the text and additional discussion in Garcia-Cairasco et al. (2004).**(3)** Flowcharts of behavioral sequences of male WARs after acute AS (M1= males at stimulus 1) and ASK.(M60= males at stimulus 60). PRE=before sound stimulation; SOUND=during sound stimulation; POST=after sound stimulation. Observe in M1 and M60, at the PRE-sound phase, the presence of exploration and grooming clusters (blue symbols; behavioral background). At the SOUND phase, in M1 are, besides background behaviors, a clear wild running pattern (gyri, jumping and atonic falling; yellow symbols) that at the POST-sound phase, is followed by GTCS (tonic convulsion, generalized clonic seizures; red symbols). In M60, there is the co-expression of a wild running cluster (yellow symbols) and recruited limbic seizures (green cluster; a clear-cut marker of ASK) very similar to the one shown in **(2)** with pilocarpine. At the POST-sound phase it is clear the presence of a GTCS not as strong as the one in M1 (acute AS). See details in the text and in Garcia-Cairasco et al. (1996a).
Reproduced with permission from Elsevier.

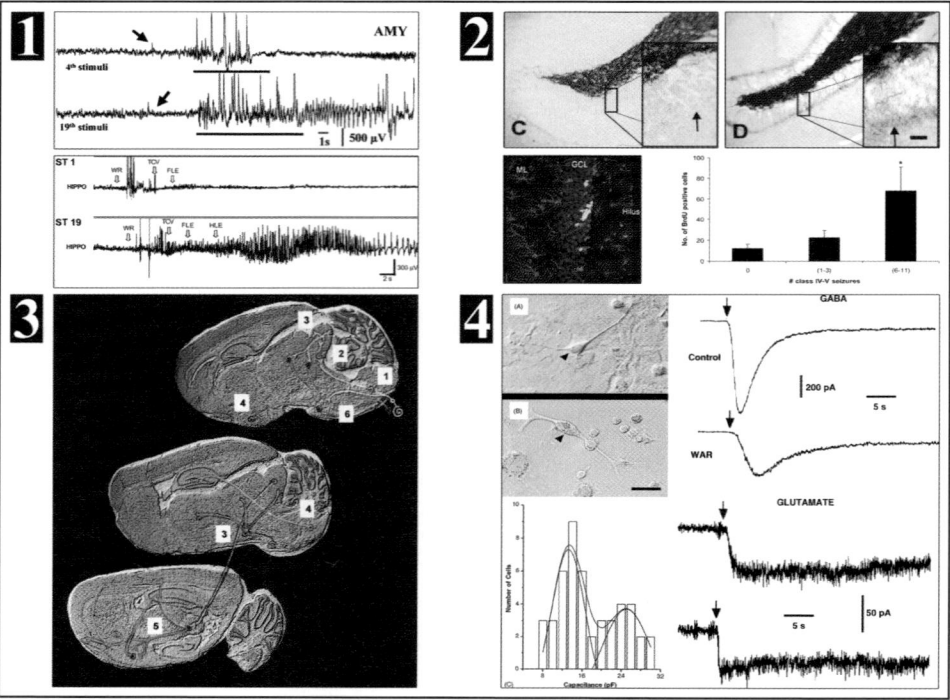

Figure 2. Besides the neuroethological studies shown in *figure 1*, we characterized, by means of Video-EEG coupling and histological studies, the evolution of epileptogenicity after ASK in WARs. **(1)** Progression of epileptiform EEG activity in amygdala (top recordings) and hippocampus (bottom recordings) after repeated ASK in WARs. See details in the text and in Moraes *et al.* (2000) and Romcy-Pereira and Garcia-Cairasco (2003). **(2)** Although behavioral and EEG changes accompany ASK (in this case 80 acoustic stimuli; two per day and additional 16 electrical stimuli of amygdala kindling after ASK), there was no signal of mossy fiber sprouting (MFS) in the inner molecular layer of the dentate gyrus (arrow; left top panel), whereas animals treated with pilocarpine (arrow; top right panel; positive control) developed strong MFS. However, the participation of the hippocampus in ASK is confirmed with the EEG data as shown in **(1)** and by the presence of neurogenesis indicated by BrdU-positive cells (green label), negative for GFAP (red label). The histogram shows that the amount of BrdU cells is proportional to the quantity of limbic seizures after ASK. See details in the text and in Galvis-Alonso *et al.* (2004; top panels) and in Romcy-Pereira and Garcia-Cairasco (bottom panels). **(3)**. It is proposed that there is a dynamic interaction of selective networks, either for the expression of acute AS or ASK. In the case of acute AS, there is a brainstem network with an auditory trigger and inferior colliculus-superior colliculus-substantia nigra-central grey-pontine nuclei network, as the most prominent regions. In the case of ASK the auditory trigger is still needed, but there is an interaction between the brainstem complex network, just described for AS, and the newly recruited, amplified network, composed mainly by amygdala, hippocampus, piriform and perirhinal cortices, among other forebrain structures. See details in the text and in Garcia-Cairasco (2002). **(4)** Identification of endogenous or genetic alterations of specific regions or even cell populations in WARs will be tremendously important for the confirmation of this strain as genetically predisposed to epilepsy. As an example, we recently described a consistent failure of GABAergic and glutamatergic neurotransmission in post-natal day 2 (well distant from the age of functional activation of auditory structures) hippocampal cells maintained in culture. See details in Mesquita *et al.* (2005).
Reproduced with permission from Elsevier.

of these combinations was not only to see whether facilitation occurs or seizures are stronger, but to develop a multidisciplinary strategy to evaluate how known combinations simulate better the clinical conditions.

Acute AS pathways include IC, SC, SNR, reticular formation and other brainstem areas such as PAG. In ASK, however, in addition to those brainstem structures critical for acute AS, amygdala, hippocampus and neocortex appear as some of the more critical substrates of limbic recruitment. Some of these circuits were reviewed elsewhere (Garcia-Cairasco, 2002; Faingold, 2004). We believe that the ASK protocol has opened a new avenue of integrative research, where critical brainstem and forebrain regions cooperate to switch and modulate relevant pro and anti-epileptic information. This activity may be adaptive such as in startle, and flight or maladaptive, such as in limbic seizures recruited after GTCS repetition.

In AS, a model of GTCS triggered by sound, seizures also are expressed in the genetically developed strains (WARs, GEPRs) with a very similar final motor pattern such as the one seen in MES and PTZ, which strengthens the view that common mechanisms (once certain threshold has been reached) make the models interchangeable in terms of information relevant to epileptology. In addition to that, because AS sensitive animals have their seizures triggered by sound, this might make them less attractive for clinical-oriented researchers. Now, because AS have this well controlled sensory trigger, they present advantages over other models where seizure can occur unpredictably.

However, we have highlighted that a combination of AS and ASK genetic models with others such as PTZ, MES, amygdala kindling and SE induced by systemic pilocarpine have given us enormous multidisciplinary data on seizure and epilepsy origin, progression, cellular and circuitry plasticity. We have conducted protocols for characterization of the correlations between behavior, EEG and cellular substrates in acute experiments. Then the questions of relevance for clinical neurology were: What is the sequela of GTCS repetition? Are the models considering progression? How many patients begin their seizures experience with GTCS? How much PTZ and MES repetition, as well as ASK could model this situation? Are there other neurological or neuro-psychiatric disorders co-morbid with epilepsy? How much ASK is a model of limbic seizure recruitment and epilepsy progression? What if we combine ASK with amygdala kindling? Does this mimic similar situations in clinical neurology? How many of the changes after ASK are negative? Cell loss, lack of sprouting; how many are positive? Limbic seizures, EEG epileptiform activity in limbic regions and neurogenesis. What happens if we induce SE with pilocarpine in WARs? Is this a good model of genetic background-seizure experience interactions? What if pilocarpine is injected not systemically but intra-hippocampally? How good are these combinations of models for new AEDs development?

In summary, we should combine genetic and acquired models of epilepsy to further understand basic mechanisms, to look for markers of epilepsy and to simulate clinical situations as close as possible. The integrated addition of all these strategies will help to produce relevant data to epileptology, no matter whether is a contribution to epileptogenesis, to the prediction of seizures, to the field of AEDs development or hopefully to finding a cure.

Acknowledgements

We thank the Graduate and Undergraduate students as well as the Research Technicians of the Neurophysiology and Experimental Neuroethology Laboratory (LNNE) for their continuous creative and competent work. We thank also our former Graduate students, Post-Docs, some of them currently excellent collaborators. Special thanks to Marcelo Rodrigues Cairrão and João Pereira Leite, for critical reading and suggestions on the first draft of this manuscript and to Artur Fernandes for excellent work with the Figures. Thanks also to Brazilian Research Foundations FAPESP, CNPq, PRONEX, CAPES (PROAP-PROEX) and FAEPA for financial support. NGC holds a CNPq-Brazil Research Fellowship.

References

Annegers JF, Hauser WA, Elveback LR. Remission of seizures and relapse in patients with epilepsy. *Epilepsia* 1979; 20: 729-37.

Bagri A, Di Scala G, Sandner G. Wild running elicited by microinjections of bicuculline or morphine into the inferior colliculus of rats: lack of effect of periaqueductal gray lesions. *Pharmacol Biochem Behav* 1992; 41: 727-32.

Bagri A, Sandner G, Di Scala G. Wild running and switch-off behavior elicited by electrical stimulation of the inferior colliculus: effect of anticonvulsant drugs. *Pharmacol Biochem Behav* 1991; 39: 683-8.

Bagri A, Tomaz C, Brandão ML, Carrive P. Increased susceptibility of detelencephalated rats to audiogenic seizures induced by microinjection of bicuculline into the inferior colliculus. *Braz J Med Biol Res* 1989; 22: 1361-70.

Bonhaus DW, Waters JR, McNamara JO. Activation of substantia nigra neurons: role in the propagation of seizures in kindled rats. *J Neurosci* 1986; 6: 3024.

Brandão ML, Cardoso SH, Melo LL, Mota V, Coimbra NC. Neural substrate of defensive behavior in the midbrain tectum. Neurosci. *Biobehav. Rev* 1994; 18: 339-46.

Brandão ML, Tomaz C, Leão Borges PC, Coimbra NC, Bagri A. Defence reaction induced by microinjection of bicuculline into the inferior colliculus. *Physiol Behav* 1988; 44: 361-5.

Browning RA, Wang C, Nelson DK, Jobe PC. Efect of precollicular transection on audiogenic seizures in genetically epilepsy-prone rats. *Exp Neurol* 1999; 155: 295-301.

Browning RA. Anatomy of generalized convulsive seizures. In: Malafosse A, Genton P, Hirsch E, Marescaux C, Broglin D, Bernaconi R. eds. *Idiopathic generalized epilepsies: clinical, experimental and genetic aspects*. London: John Libbey & Company Ltd, 1994: 399-413.

Browning RA, Nelson DK. Modification of electroshock and pentylenetetrazol seizure patterns in rats after precollicular transections. *Exp Neurol* 1986: 93: 546-56.

Caldecott-Hazard S, Engel J Jr. Limbic postictal events: anatomical substrates and opioid receptor involvement. *Prog Neuropsychopharmacol Biol Psychiatry* 1987; 11: 389-418.

Cardoso, SH, Coimbra, NC, Brandão, ML. Defensive reactions evoked by activation of NMDA receptors in distinct sites of the inferior colliculus. *Behav Brain Res* 1994; 63: 17-24.

Cavalheiro EA, Naffah-Mazzacoratti MG, Mello LE, Leite JP. The pilocarpine model of seizures. In: Pitkänen A, Schwartzkroin P and Moshé S, ed. *Models of seizures and epilepsy*. London: Elsevier Academic Press, 2006: 433-48.

Chandler, Karen. Canine epilepsy: What can we learn from human seizure disorders? *The Veterinary Journal*, in press.

Clough RW, Eells JB, Browning RA, Jobe PC. Seizure and proto-oncogene expression of C-fos in the brain of adult genetically epilepsy-prone rats. *Exp Neurol* 1997; 146: 341-53.

Coimbra NC, Brandão ML. GABAergic nigro-collicular pathways modulate the defensive behaviour elicited by midbrain tectum stimulation. *Behav Brain Res* 1993; 59: 131-9.

Coimbra NC, Eichenberg GCD, Gorchinski RT, Maisonnette S. Effects of the blockade of opioid receptor on defensive reactions elicited by electrical stimulation within the deep layers of the superior colliculus and DPAG. *Brain Res* 1996; 736: 348-52.

Dailey JW, Reigel CE, Mishra PK, Jobe PC. Neurobiology of seizure predisposition in the genetically epilepsy-prone rat. *Epilepsy Res* 1989; 3: 3-17.

Danscher G. Histochemical demonstration of heavy metals. *Histochemistry* 1981; 71: 1-16.

Dal-Col ML, Terra-Bustamante VC, Velasco TR, Oliveira JA, Sakamoto AC, Garcia-Cairasco N. "Neuroethology application for the study of human temporal lobe epilepsy: From basic to applied sciences". *Epilepsy Behav* in press.

Dean P, Redgrave P, Westby GW. Event or emergency? Two response systems in the mammalian superior colliculus. *Trends Neurosci* 1989; 12: 137-47.

Del-Bel EA, Oliveira PR, Oliveira JAC, Mishra PK, Jobe PC, Garcia Cairasco N. Anticonvulsant and proconvulsant roles of nitric oxide in experimental epilepsy models. *Braz J Med Biol Res* 1997; 30: 971-9.

Del-Bel EA, Silveira MC, Graeff FG, Garcia-Cairasco N, Guimarães FS. Differential expression of c-fos mRNA and Fos protein in the rat brian aafter rstraint stress or pentylenetetrazol-induced seizures. *Cell Mol Neurobiol* 1998; 18: 339-46.

Depaulis A, Marescaux C, Liu Z, Vergnes M. GABAergic nigro-collicular pathway is not involved in the inhibitory control of audiogenic seizures in the rat. *Neurosci Lett* 1990; 111: 269-74.

Deransart C, Le-Pham BT, Hirsch E, Marescaux C, Depaulis A. Inhibition of the substantia nigra suppresses absences and clonic seizures in audiogenic rats, but not tonic seizures: evidence for seizure specificity of the nigral control. *Neuroscience* 2001; 105: 203-11.

De Vasconcelos AP, Vergnes M, Boyet S, Marescaux C, Nehlig A. Forebrain metabolic activation induced by the repetition of audiogenic seizures in Wistar rats. *Brain Research* 1997; 762: 114-20.

Donan G, Pelligra R. A unifying concept of seizure onset and termination. *Medicla Hypothesis* 2004: 62: 740-5.

Doretto MC, Burger R, Mishra PK, Garcia-Cairasco N, Dailey JW, Jobe PC. A microdialysis study of amino acid concentration in the extracellular £uid of the substantia nigra of freely behaving GEPR-9s: Relationships to seizure predisposition. *Epilepsy Res* 1994; 17: 157-65.

Doretto MC, Garcia-Cairasco N. Diferential audiogenic seizure sensitization by selective unilateral substantia nigra lesions in resistant Wistar rats. *Phys & Behav* 1995; 58: 273-82.

Doretto MC, Fonseca CG, Lobo RB, Terra VC, Oliveira JA, Garcia-Cairasco N. Quantitative study of the response to genetic selection of the Wistar audiogenic rat strain (WAR). *Behav Genet* 2003; 33: 33-42.

Doretto MC, Oliveira-e-Silva M, Ferreira-Alves DL, Pires SG, Garcia-Cairasco N, Reis AM. Effect of lactation on the expression of audiogenic seizures: association with plasma prolactin profiles. *Epilepsy Res* 2003; 54: 109-21.

Eells JB, Clough RW, Miller JW, Jobe PC, Browning RA. Fos expression and 2-deoxyglucose uptake following seizures in developing genetically epilepsy-prone rats. *Brain Res Bull* 2000; 52: 379-89.

Engel JJr. A proposed diagnostic scheme for people with epileptic seizures and with epilepsy: report of the ILAE Task Force on classification and terminology. *Epilepsia* 2001; 42: 796-803.

Engel JJr, Schwartzkroin P. What should be modeled? In: Pitkänen A, Schwartzkroin P and Moshé S, eds. *Models of seizures and epilepsy*. London: Elsevier Academic Press, 2006: 1-14.

Faingold CL, Fromm GH. Actions on neuronal networks involved in seizure disorders. In: Faingold CL, Fromm GH, eds. *Drugs for Control of Epilepsy: Actions on Neuronal Networks Involved in Seizure Disorders*. Boca Raton, CRC Press, 1991: 1-21.

Faingold CL. Neuronal networks in the genetically epilepsy-prone rats. In: Delgado-Escueta AV, Wilson WA, Olsen RW, Porter RJ, eds. Jasper's Basic Mechanisms of the Epilepsies, Third Edition. *Advances in Neurology*, Vol. 79. Philadelphia: Lippincot Williams and Wilkins, 1999. 311-21.

Faingold CL. Emergent properties of CNS neuronal networks as targets for pharmacology: application to anticonvulsant drug action *Progress in Neurobiology*, 2004; 72: 55-85.

Feng HJ, Faingold CL. Synaptic plasticity in the pathway from the medial geniculate body to the lateral amygdala is induced by seizure repetition, *Brain Res* 2002; 946: 198-205.

Fentress JC, Stilwell FP. Grammar of a movement sequence in inbred mice. *Nature* 1973: 52-3.

Ferland RJ, Applegate CD. Decreased brainstem seizure threshold and facilitated seizure propagation in mice exposed to repeated flurothyl-induced generalized forebrain seizures. *Epilepsy Res* 1998; 30: 49-62.

Fisch BJ. Generalized tonic-clonic seizures. In: Willye E, ed. *The treatment of epilepsy. Principles and practice*. Baltimore: Williams and Wilkins, 1997: 502-21.

Fisher RS. Animal models of the epilepsies. *Brain Res Rev* 1989; 14: 245-78.

Franck JE, Schwartzkroin PA. The genetic epilepsy prone rat has altered GABA receptor binding in substantia nigra but not inferior colliculus. *Soc Neurosci Abstr* 1987; 13: 944.

Freitas RL, Ferreira CMR, Ribeiro SJ, Carvalho A, Elias-Filho DH, Garcia-Cairasco N, Coimbra NC. Intrinsic neural circuits between dorsal midbrain neurons that control fear-induced responses and seizure activity and nuclei of the pain inhibitory system elaborating postictal antinociceptive processes: a functional neuroanatomical and neuropharmacological study. *Experimental Neurol* 2005; 191: 225-42.

Frye GD, McCown TJ, Breese GR. Characterization of susceptibility to audiogenic seizures in ethanol-dependent rats after microinjection of gamma-aminobutyric acid (GABA) agonists into the inferior colliculus, substantia nigra and medial septum. *J Pharmacol Exp Ther* 1983; 227: 663-70.

Galvis-Alonso OY, Cortes de Oliveira JA, Garcia-Cairasco N. Limbic epileptogenicity, cell loss and axonal reorganization induced by audiogenic and amygdala kindling in Wistar Audiogenic Rats (WAR strain). *Neuroscience* 2004: 125: 787-802.

Garant DS, Gale K. Intranigral and muscimol attenuates electrographics signs of seizure activity induced by intravenous bicuculline in rats. *Eur J Pharmacol* 1986; 124: 365-9.

Garcia-Cairasco N, Sabbatini RME. Role of the substantia nigra in audiogenic seizures: A neuroethological study in the rat. *Braz J Med Biol Res* 1983; 16: 171-83.

Garcia-Cairasco N, Doretto MC, Lobo R. Genetic selection of a strain of Wistar rats susceptible to audiogenic seizures. A quantitative analysis. *Epilepsia* 1990; 31: 815.

Garcia-Cairasco N, Doretto MC, Prado P, Jorge BPD, Terra VC, Oliveira JAC. New insights into behavioral evaluation of audiogenic seizures. A comparison of two ethological methods. *Behav Brain Res* 1992; 48: 49-56.

Garcia-Cairasco N, Sabbatini RME. Neuroethological evaluation of audiogenic seizures in hemidetelencephalated rats. *Behav Brain Res* 1989; 33: 65-77.

Garcia-Cairasco N, Sabbatini RME. Possible interaction between the inferior colliculus and the substantia nigra in audiogenic seizures in Wistar rats. *Physiol Behav* 1991; 50: 421-7.

Garcia-Cairasco N, Terra VC, Mishra PK, Dailey JW, Jobe PC. Neuroethology of brainstem-induced forebrain seizure kindling in genetically epilepsy-prone rats (GEPRs). *Society for Neuroscience Abstracts* 20[1], 406. 1994a.

Garcia-Cairasco N, Reis LC, Terra VC, Oliveira JAC, Antunes-Rodrigues J. Diuresis and natriuresis in non-seizing and kindled rats from a genetically audiogenic susceptible strain. *NeuroReport* 1994b; 5: 1853-76.

Garcia-Cairasco N, Terra VC, Doretto MC. Midbrain substrates of audiogenic seizures in rats. *Behav. Brain Res.* 1993; 58: 57-67.

Garcia-Cairasco N, Wakamatsu H, Oliveira JAC, Gomes ELT, Del Bel EA, Mello LEAM. Neuroethological and morphological (Neo-Timm staining) correlates of limbic recruitment during the development of audiogenic kindling in seizure susceptible Wistar rats. *Epilepsy Res* 1996a; 26: 77-192.

Garcia-Cairasco N, Doretto MC, Ramalho MJ, Rodrigues JA, Nonaka KO. Audiogenic and audiogenic-like seizures: locus of induction and seizure severity determine post-ictal prolactin patterns. *Pharmacol Biochem Behav* 1996b; 53: 503-10.

Garcia-Cairasco N, Oliveira JAC, Wakamatsu H, Bueno STB, Guimarães FS. Reduced exploratory activity of audiogenic seizures susceptible Wistar rats. *Physiol Behav* 1998; 64: 671-4.

Garcia-Cairasco N. A critical review on the participation of inferior colliculus in acoustic-motor and acoustic-limbic networks involved in the expression of acute and kindled audiogenic seizures. *Hearing Res* 2002; 168: 208-22.

Garcia-Cairasco N, Rossetti F, Oliveira JAC, Furtado MA. Neuroethological study of status epilepticus induced by systemic pilocarpine in Wistar Audiogenic rats (WAR Strain). *Epilepsy & Behavior* 2004; 5: 455-63.

Gonzalez LP, Hettinger MK. Intranigral muscimol suppresses ethanol withdrawal seizures. *Brain Res* 1984; 298: 163-6.

Gotman J. Interhemispheric relations during bilateral spike and wave activity. *Epilepsia* 1981; 22: 453-66.

Hagiharaa H, Haraa M, Tsunekawaa K, Nakagawaa Y, Sawadac M, Nakanoa K. Tonic-clonic seizures induce division of neuronal progenitor cells with concomitant changes in expression of neurotrophic factors in the brain of pilocarpine-treated mice. *Molecular Brain Research* 2005; 139: 258-66.

Herrera M, Sanchez del Campo F, Ruiz A, Smith-Agreda V. Neuronal relationships between the dorsal periaqueductal nucleus and the inferior colliculus (nucleus commissuralis) in the cat. A Golgi study. *J Anat* 1988; 158: 137-45.

Hirsch E, Maton B, Vergnes M, Depaulis A, Marescaux C. Positive transfer of audiogenic kindling to electrical hippocampal kindling in rats. *Epilepsy Res* 1992; 111: 59-166.

Hirsch E, Danober L, Simler S, Pereira de Vasconcelos A, Maton B, Nehlig A, Marescaux C, Vergnes M. The amygdala is critical for seizure propagation from brainstem to forebrain. *Neuroscience* 1997; 4: 975-84.

Hjeresen D, Franck J, Amend D. Ontogeny of seizure incidence, latency and severity in genetically epilepsy-prone rats. *Dev Psychobiol* 1987; 20: 355-63.

Holmes GL, Thompson JL, Marchi TA, Gabriel PS, Hogan MA, Carl FG, Feldman DS. Efects of seizures on learning, memory and behavior in the genetically epilepsy-prone rat. *Ann Neurol* 1990; 27: 24-32.

Iadarola MJ, Gale K. Substantia nigra: site of anticonvulsant activity mediated by gamma-aminobutyric acid. *Science* 1982; 218: 1237-40.

Itoh K, Watanabe M, Yoshikawa K, Kanaho Y, Berlinder J, FujiII H. Magnetic resonance and biochemical studies during pentylenetetrazol-kindling development: the relationship between nitric oxide, neuronal nitric oxide synthase and seizures. *Neuroscience* 2004; 129: 757-66.

Jeha LE, Morris HH, Burgess RC. Coexistence of focal and idiopathic generalized epilepsy in the same patient population. *Seizure*, in press.

Jobe PC, Picchioni AL, Chin L. Role of brain 5-hydroxytryptamine in audiogenic seizure in the rat. *Life Sciences* 1973; 13: 1-13.

Jobe PC, Mishra PK, Adams-Curtis LE. Deoskar VU, Ko KH, Browning RA, Dailey JW. The genetically epilepsy-prone rat (GEPR). *Ital J Neurol Sci* 1995; 16: 91-9.

Jobe PC, Mishra PK, Ludvig N, Dailey JW. Scope and contribution of genetics models to an understanding of the epilepsies. *Crit Rev Neurobiol* 1991; 6: 183-220.

Kajiwara K, Nagawawa H, Shimizu-Nishikawa K, Ookura T, Kimura M, Sugaya E. Molecular Characterization of Seizure-Related Genes Isolated by Differential Screening. *Biochem Biophysical Res Com* 1996; 219: 795-9.

Kesner RP. Subcortical mechanisms of audiogenic seizures. *Exp Neurol* 1966; 15: 192-205.

Kiesmann M, Marescaux C, Vergnes M, Micheletti G, Depaulis A, Warter JM. Audiogenic seizures in Wistar rats before and after repeated auditory stimuli: clinical, pharmacological and electroencephalographic studies. *J Neural Transm* 1988; 72: 235-44.

King PH, Shin C, Mansbach HH, Chen LS, McNamara JO. Microinjection of a benzodiazepine into substantia nigra elevates kindled seizure threshold. *Brain Res* 1987; 423: 261-8.

Klein BD, Fu YH, Ptacek LJ, White HS. C-Fos immunohistochemical mapping of the audiogenic seizure network and tonotopic neuronal hyperexcitability in the inferior colliculus of the Fring mouse. *Epilepsy Res* 2004.

Krushinski LV. L'Étude physiologique des differents types de crises convulsives de l'épilepsie audiogene du rat. In: Colloques Internationaux du Centre National de la Recherche Scienticque, no. 112, *Psychophysiologie, Neuropharmacologie et Biochimie de la Crise Audiogene*. Éditions du Centre National de la Recherche Scientifique, Paris, 1963. pp. 71-92.

Lasley SM. Roles of neurotransmitter amino acids in seizure severity and experience in the genetically epilepsy-prone rat. *Brain Res* 1991; 701: 117-28.

Lee Y, Lopez DE, Meloni EG, Davis M. A primary acoustic startle pathway: obligatory role of cochlear root neurons and the nucleus reticularis pontis caudalis. *J Neurosci* 1996; 16: 3775-89.

Ledoux J, Farb CB, Ruggiero DA. Topographic organization of neurons in the acoustic thalamus that project to the amygdala. *J Neurosci* 1990; 10: 1043-54.

Leite JP, Bortolotto ZA, Cavalheiro EA, Spontaneous recurrent seizures in rats: an experimental model of partial epilepsy. *Neurosci Biobehav Rev* 1990; 14: 511-7.

Leite JP, Garcia-Cairasco N, Cavalheiro EA. New insights from the use of pilocarpine and kainate models. *Epilepsy Res* 2002; 50: 93-103.

López DE, Saldaña E, Nodal FR, Merchán MA, Warr WB. Projections of cochlear root neurons, sentinels of the rat auditory pathway. *J Comp Neurol* 1999; 415: 160-74.

Lopes da Silva FH, Post R. Evaluation and prediction of effects of antiepileptic drugs in a variety of other CNS disorders. *Epilepsy Research* 2002; 50: 191-3.

Löscher W. New visions in the pharmacology of anticonvulsion. *European Journal of Pharmacology* 1998; 342: 1-13.

Löscher W, Schmidt D. Which animal models should be used in the search for new antiepileptic drugs? A proposal based on experimental and clinical considerations. *Epilepsy Res* 1988; 2: 145-81.

Löscher W, Schmidt D. Strategies in antiepileptic drug development: Is rational drug design superior to random screening and structural variation? *Epilepsy Res* 1994; 17: 95-134.

Löscher W. Animal models of intractable epilepsy. *Progress in Neurobiology* 1997; 53: 239-58.

Magalhães LHM, Garcia-Cairasco N, Massenssini AR, Doretto MC, Moraes MFD. Evidence for augmented brainstem activated forebrain seizures in Wistar Audiogenic Rats subjected to transauricular electroshock. *Neuroscience Letters* 2004; 369: 19-23.

Magistris MR, Mouridian MS, Gloor P. Generalized convulsions induced by pentylenetetrazol I the cat: Participation of forebrain, briantem and spinal cord. *Epilepsia* 1988; 29: 379-88.

Marescaux C, Vergnes M, Kiesmann M, Depaulis A, Micheletti G, Warter JM. Kindling of audiogenic seizures in Wistar rats: and EEG study. *Exp Neurol* 1987; 97: 160-8.

McCown TJ, Breese GR. Seizure interactions between the inferior collicular cortex and the deep prepiriform cortex. *Epilepsy Res* 1991; 8: 21-9.

McCown TJ, Duncan GE, Breese GR. Neuroanatomical characterization of inferior collicular seizure genesis: 2-deoxyglucose and stimulation mapping. *Brain Res* 1991; 567: 25-32.

McCown TJ, Grenwood RS, Breese GR. Inferior collicular interactions with limbic seizure activity. *Epilepsia* 1987; 28: 234-41.

McCown TJ, Grenwood RS, Frye GD, Breese GR. Electrically elicited seizures from the inferior colliculus: a potential site for the genesis of epilepsy? *Exp Neurol* 1984; 86: 527-42.

McIntyre DC, Kelly ME, Dufresne C. FAST and SLOW amygdala kindling rat strains: comparison of amygdala, hippocampal, piriform and perirhinal cortex kindling. *Epilepsy Research* 1999; 35: 197-209.

McNally KA, Blumenfeld H. Focal network involvement in generalized seizures: new insights from electroconvulsive therapy. *Epilepsy & Behavior* 2004; 5: 3-12.

Meeren HKM, Jan Pieter MP, Egidius LJM, Van Luijtelaar, Coenen AML and Lopes da Silva FH. Cortical Focus Drives Widespread Corticothalamic Networks during Spontaneous Absence Seizures in Rats. *The Journal of Neuroscience* 2002: 22: 1480-95.

Meeren H, van Luijtelaar G, Lopes da Silva F, Coenen A, Schridde U, van Luijtelaar G. Evolving concepts on the pathophysiology of absence seizures: the cortical focus theory. *Arch Neurol* 2005; 62: 371-6.

Meldrum B. Do preclinical seizure models preselect certain adverse effects of antiepileptic drugs. *Epilepsy Research* 2002; 50: 33-40.

Mello LL, Cardoso SH, Brandão ML. Antiaversive action of benzodiazepines on escape behavior induced by electrical stimulation of the inferior colliculus. *Physiol Behav* 1992; 51: 557-62.

Merlis JK. Proposal for an international classification of the epilepsies. *Epilepsia* 1970; 11: 114-9.

Merritt HH, Putnam TJ. A new series of anticonvulsant drugs tested by experiments on animals. *Arch Neurol Psychiatry* 1938; 39: 1003-15.

Mesquita F Jr, Aguiar JF, Oliveira JAC, Garcia-Cairasco N, Varanda WA. Electrophysiological properties of cultured hippocampal neurons from Wistar Audiogenic Rats. *Brain Re Bull* 2005; 65: 177-83.

Midzyanovskayaa IS, Kuznetsovaa GD, Vinogradovaa LV, Shatskovaa AB, Coenenb AML, van Luijtelaarb G. Mixed forms of epilepsy in a subpopulation of WAG/Rij rats. *Epilepsy & Behavior* 2004; 5: 655-61.

Millan MH, Meldrum BS, Faingold CL. Induction of audiogenic seizure susceptibility by focal infusion of excitant amino acids or bicuculline into the inferior colliculus of normal rats. *Exp Neurol* 1986; 91: 634-9.

Millan MH, Meldrum RS, Boersma CA, Faingold CL. Excitant amino acids and audiogenic seizures in the genetically epilepsy-prone rat. II. Eferent seizure propagating pathway. *Exp Neurol* 1988; 99: 687-98.

Miller JW, Ferrendelli JA. Brainstem and diencephalic structures regulating experimental generalized (pentylenetetrazol) seizures in rodents. In: Meldrum BS, Ferrendelli JA, Wieser HG, eds. *Anatomy of epileptogenesis*. London: Libbey, 1988: 57-69.

Moraes MFD, Galvis-Alonso OY, Garcia-Cairasco N. Wistar audiogenic rat kindling: An epilepsy model for secondary limbic structures recruitment. *Epilepsy Res* 2000; 39: 251-9.

Moraes MF, Mishra PK, Jobe PC, Garcia-Cairasco N. An electrographic analysis of the synchronous discharge patterns of GEPR-9s generalized seizures. *Brain Res* 2005; 1046: 1-9.

Morimoto K, Fahnestock M, Racine RJ. Kindling and status epilepticus models of epilepsy: rewiring the brain. *Progress in Neurobiology* 2004; 73: 1-60.

Naritoku DK, Mecozzi LB, Aiello MT, Faingold CL. Repetition of audiogenic seizures in genetically epilepsy-prone rats induces cortical epileptiform activity and additional seizure behaviors. *Exp Neurol* 1992; 115: 317-24.

Nehlig A, Vergnes M, HIrshc E, Marescaux C. Brain metabolism and blood flow in models of generalized idiopathic epilepsy in rodents. In: Malafosse A, Genton P, Hirsch E, Marescaux C, Broglin D, Bernaconi R. eds. *Idiopathic generalized epilepsies: clinical, experimental and genetic aspects*. London: John Libbey & Company Ltd, 1994: 169-76.

N'Gouemo P, Faingold L. Periaqueductal grey neurons exhibit increased responsiveness associated with audiogenic seizures in the genetically epilepsy-prone rat. *Neuroscience* 1998; 84: 619-25.

N'Gouemo P, Faingold L. Periaqueductal grey is a critical site in the neuronal network for audiogenic seizures: modulation by GABAA, NMDA and opioid receptors. *Epilepsy Res.* 1999; 35: 39-46.

Norden AD, Blumenfeld H. The role of subcortical structures in human epilepsy. *Epilepsy Behav* 2002; 3: 219-31.

Olazabal UE, Moore K. Nigrotectal projection to the inferior colliculus: horseradish peroxidase immunohistochemical studies in rats, cats and bats. *J Comp Neurol* 1989; 282: 98-118.

Pierson MG, Smith KL, Swann JW. A slow NMDA mediated synaptic potential underlies seizures originating from midbrain. *Brain Res* 1989; 486: 381-6.

Pinel JP, Rovner LI. Electrode placement and kindling-induced experimental epilepsy. *Exp Neurol* 1978; 58: 335-46.

Pitkanen, A, Schwartzkroin, PA, Moshé, SL. *Models of Seizures and Epilepsy*. London, Elsevier Academic Press, 2006, 687 p.

Plotnikoff NA. A neuropharmacological study of escape from audiogenic seizures. In: *Psychopharmacologie, neuropharmacology et Biochimie de la crise audiogene*. CNRS, Paris, 1963. VIII.

Post RM. Do the epilepsies, pain syndromes, and affective disorders share common kindling-like mechanisms? *Epilepsy Research* 2002; 50: 203-19.

Racine RJ. Modification of seizure activity by electrical stimulation: II. Motor seizure. *Electroenceph Clin Neurophysiol* 1972; 32: 281-94.

Racine RJ, Steingart M, McIntyre DC. Development of kindling-prone and kindling-resistant rats: selective breeding and electrophysiological studies. *Epilepsy Research* 1999; 35: 183-95.

Raisinghani M, Faingold CL. Evidence for the perirhinal cortex as a requisite component in the seizure network following seizure repetition in an inherited form of generalized clonic seizures. *Brain Res* 2005; 1048: 193-201.

Redgrave P, Marrow LP, Dean P. Anticonvulsant role of nigrotectal projection in the maximal electroshock model of epilepsy. II. Pathways from substantia nigra pars lateralis and adjacent peripeduncular area to the dorsal midbrain. *Neuroscience* 1992a; 46: 391-406.

Redgrave P, Simkins M, Overton P, Dean P. Anticonvulsant role of nigrotectal projection in the maximal electroshock model of epilepsy. I. Mapping of dorsal midbrain with bicuculline. *Neuroscience* 1992b; 46: 379-90.

Ribak CE, Byun MY, Ruiz, GT, Reifenstein RJ. Increased levels of amino acid neurotransmitters in the inferior colliculus of the genetically epilepsy-prone rat. *Epilepsy Res* 1988; 2: 9-13.

Ribak CE, Lauterborn JC, Navetta MS, Gall CM. The inferior colliculus of GEPRs contains a greater number of cells that express glutamate decarboxylase (GAD67) mRNA. *Epilepsy Res* 1993; 14: 105-13.

Ribak CE, Lanterborn JC, Benson DL, Gall CM. Inferior colliculus of genetically epilepsy-prone rats contains increased numbers of cells that express the mRNA from glutamate decarboxylase. *Epilepsia* 1990; 31: 609.

Ribak CE, Khurana V, Lien NT. The effect of midbrain collicular knife cuts on audiogenic seizure severity in the genetically epilepsy-prone rat. *J Brain Res* 1994; 35: 303-11.

Ribak CE, Manio AL, Navetta MS, Gall CM. In situ hybridization for C-fos mRNA reveals the involvement of the superior colliculus in the propagation of seizure activity in genetically epilepsy-prone rats. *Epilepsy Res* 1997; 26: 397-406.

Roberts RC, Ribak CE, Oertel WH. Increased number of GABAergic neurons in the inferior colliculus of an audiogenic model of epilepsy. *Brain Res* 1985; 361: 324-8.

Romcy-Pereira RN, Garcia-Cairasco N. Hippocampal cell proliferation and epileptogenesis after audiogenic kindling are not accompanied by mossy fiber sprouting or fluoro-jade staining. *Neuroscience* 2003; 119: 533-46.

Ross KC, Coleman JR. Developmental and genetic audiogenic seizure models: behavior and biological substrates. *Neurosci Biobehav Rev* 2000; 24: 639-53.

Rossetti F, Rodrigues MCA, Oliveira JAC, Garcia Cairasco N. EEG frequency alterations in substantia nigra pars reticulata and superior colliculus during phenobarbital anticonvulsant effect and during natural recovery from audiogenic seizures in Wistar Audiogenic Rats. Submitted to *Epilepsy Research*.

Sahibzada N, Dean P, Redgrave P. Movements resembling orientation or avoidance elicited by electrical stimulation of the superior colliculus in rats. *J Neurosci* 1986; 6: 723-33.

Scarlatelli-Lima AV, Magalhaes LH, Doretto MC, Moraes MF. Assessment of the seizure susceptibility of Wistar Audiogenic rat to electroshock, pentyleneterazole and pilocarpine. *Brain Res* 2003; 960: 184-9.

Sakurada O, Kennedy C, Jehle J, Brown JD, Carbin GL, Sokoloff L. Measurement of local cerebral blood flow with [^{14}C]iodoantipyrine. *Am J Physiol* 1978: 234: H59-H66.

Sarkisian MR. Overview of the Current Animal Models for Human Seizure and Epileptic Disorders. *Epilepsy & Behavior* 2001; 2: 201-16.

Savage DD, Reigel CE, Jobe PC. Angular bundle kindling is accelerated in rats with a genetic predisposition to acoustic stimulus-induced seizures *Brain Research* 1986; 376: 412-5.

Schwartzkroin P, Engel J Jr. What good are animal models In: Pitkänen A, Schwartzkroin P and Moshé S, eds. *Models of seizures and epilepsy*. London: Elsevier Academic Press, 2006: 659-68.

Lopes da Silva F, Post RM. Evaluation and prediction of effects of antiepileptic drugs in a variety of other CNS disorders. *Epilepsy Research* 2002; 50: 191-93.

Shaw CA, Wilson JMB. Analysis of neurological disease in four dimensions: insight form ALS-PSC epidemiology and animal models. *Neuroscience and Biobehavioral Reviews* 2003; 27: 493-505.

Simler S, Hirsch E, Danober L, Motte J, Vergnes M, Marescaux C. C-fos expression after single and kindled audiogenic seizures in Wistar rats. *Neurosci Lett* 1999; 175: 58-62.

Snyder-Keller AM, Pierson MG. Audiogenic seizures induce c-fos in a model of developmental epilepsy. *Neurosci Lett* 1992; 135: 108-12.

Spencer PS, Nunn PB, Hugon J, Ludolph AC, Ross SM, Roy DN, Robertson RC. Guam amyotrphic lateral sclerosis-parkinsonism-dementia linked to aplant excitant neurotoxin. *Science* 1987: 237: 517-22.

Spiegel EA. Quantitative determination of the convulsive reactivity by electrical stimulation of the brain with the skull intact. *J Lab Clin Med* 1937; 22: 1274-6.

Sutula T, He XX, Cavazos J, Scott G. Synaptic reorganization in the hippocampus induced by abnormal function activity. *Science* 1988; 239: 1147-50.

Sutula T, Lauersdorf S, Lynch M, Jurgella C, Woodard A. Deficits in radial arm maze performance in kindled rats. Evidence for long-lasting memory dysfunction induced by repeated brief seizures. *J Neurosci* 1995; 15: 8295-301.

Sutula TP. Mechanisms of epilepsy progression: current theories and perspectives from neuroplasticity in adulthood and development. *Epilepsy Res* 2004; 60: 161-71.

Swann JW, Pierson MG, Smith KL, Lee CL. Developmental neuroplasticity: role in early life seizures and chronic epilepsy. In: Delgado-Escueta, AV, Wilson WA, Olsen RW, Porter RJ. eds. *Jasper's Mechanisms of the Epilepsies. Third Edition: Advances in Neurology*, Vol. 79. Philadelphia: Lippincott Williams and Wilkins, 1999: 203-16.

Terra VC, Garcia-Cairasco N. Neuroethological evaluation of audiogenic seizures and audiogenic-like seizures induced by microinjection of bicuculline into the inferior colliculus II. Efects of nigral clobazam microinjections. *Behav Brain Res* 1992; 52: 19-28.

Terra VC, Garcia-Cairasco N. NMDA-dependent audiogenic seizures are differentially regulated by inferior colliculus subnuclei. *Behav Brain Res* 1994; 62: 29-39.

Theodore WH, Fisher RS. Brain stimulation for epilepsy. *Lancet Neurol* 2004; 3: 111-18.

Tokunaga A, Sugita S, Otani K. Auditory and non-auditory subcortical ajerents to the inferior colliculus in the rat. *J Hirnforsch* 1984; 25: 461-71.

Tsutsui J, Terra VC, Oliveira JAC, Garcia-Cairasco, N. Neuroethological evaluation of audiogenic seizures and audiogenic-like seizures induced by microinjection of bicuculline into the inferior colliculus. I. Effects of midcollicular knife cuts. *Behav Brain Res* 1992; 52: 7-17.

Tükel K, Jasper H. The electroencephalogram in parasaggital lesions. *Electroencephalography Clin Neurophysiol* 1952; 4: 481-94.

Valente T, Domínguez MI, Bellmann A, Journot L, Ferrer I, Auladell C. Zac1 is up-eguated in neural cells of the limbic system of mouse brain following seizures that provoke strong cell activation. *Neuroscience* 2004; 128: 323-36.

Van Camp N, D'Hooge R, Verhoye M, Peeters RR, De Deyn PP, Van der Linden A. Simultaneous electroencephalographic recording and functional magnetic resonance imaging during pentylenetetrazol-induced seizures in rat. *NeuroImage* 2003; 19: 627-36.

Velísek L, Veliskova J, Moshe SL. Electrical Stimulation of Substantia Nigra Pars Reticulata Is Anticonvulsant in Adult and Young Male Rats. *Experimental Neurology* 2002; 173: 145-52.

Veliskova J, Loscher W, Moshe SL. Regional and age specific effects of zolpidem microinfusions in the substantia nigra on seizures. *Epilepsy Res* 1998; 30: 107-14.

Velizkova J, Miller AM, Nunes ML, Brown LL. Regional neural activity within the substantia nigra during peri-ictal flurothyl generalized seizure stages. *Neurobiology of Disease* 2005; 20: 752-9.

Von Meduna L. Biologic control of outcome of schizophrenia by producing epipetic attacks with injections of camphor and metrazol. *Z Neurol Psychol* 1935; 152: 235-62.

White S, Smith-Yockman M, Srivastava A, Wilcox KS. Therapeutic assays for the identification and characterization of antiepileptic and antiepileptogenic drugs? In: Pitkänen A, Schwartzkroin P and Moshé S, eds. *Models of seizures and epilepsy*. London: Elsevier Academic Press, 2006: 539-49.

Willot JF, Lu SM. Midbrain pathways of audiogenic seizures in DBA/2 mice. *Exp Neurol* 1980; 70: 288-99.

Zhao DY, Wu XR, Pei YQ, Zuo QH. Kindling phenomenon of hyperthermic seizures in the epilepsy-prone *versus* the epilepsy resistant rat. *Brain Res* 1985; 358: 390-3.

The semiology and pathophysiology of the secondary generalized tonic-clonic seizures

Samden Lhatoo, Hans Lüders

The Cleveland Clinic Foundation, Cleveland, USA

Gastaut and Broughton (1972), in their authoritative work, *"Epileptic Seizures: Clinical and Electrographic Features, Diagnosis and Treatment"*, provided a detailed description of generalized tonic-clonic seizures. They correctly commented on the difficulty in distinguishing seizures that were truly generalized at the onset, and those that had short, clinically inobvious partial onsets prior to secondary generalization. Thus, their classical description of the generalized tonic-clonic seizure (GTCS) appears to present a composite of "grand mal" primary as well as secondary generalized tonic-clonic seizures (SGTCS). Modern epilepsy semiology literature is reliant on their observations and there are few contemporary analyses that provide more information.

■ Descriptions of seizure semiology

The few modern descriptions of SGTCS that exist refer to Gastaut and Broughton's work as a benchmark with which to relate their findings, and given the exquisite, all encompassing detail that they provide, it is not difficult to see why. Their analyses included semiology, electroencephalography, electrocardiography, electrodermography, sphygmomanometry, pupillary measurement, intravesical pressure measurements, audiometry and spirometry. Gastaut divided the various phases of the GTCS thus:

1. Pre-ictal manifestations
2. The ictal phase
    a. The tonic phase (including an "intermediate vibratory period")
    b. The clonic phase
    c. (Concurrent) Autonomic changes
3. Immediate postictal features
4. Late postictal features

It is the first two phases – the preictal phase and the ictal phase, that have been of greatest semiological interest, mainly because of the clinical information that they provide which may cast light on seizure localization and lateralization.

The preictal "myoclonic" phase (such as occurs in juvenile myoclonic epilepsy [JME]) was thought to occur in the majority and constituted a "succession of brief, bilateral and massive muscle contractions which usually last a total of several seconds and are frequently accompanied by a spasmodic cry". The tonic phase followed or comprised the initial manifestation in others. It was accompanied by loss of consciousness and was characterized by a brief phase in flexion followed by a longer one in extension, in all lasting ten to twenty seconds. A typical flexion was described as one similar to the response to the command "Put up your hands!" where contraction of the trapezius and levator scapulae led to shoulder elevation, serratus anterior and deltoid contraction caused arm elevation and the elbows were held in semi-flexion. The lower limbs were described as being less involved but often with flexion, abduction and external rotation of the thighs and legs, completing an emprosthotonic posture.

This tonic flexion was followed by tonic extension where the deep paravertebral and sub-occipital muscles produced neck and back extension into an opisthotonic position. Contraction of the thoraco-abdominal musculature produced the "tonic epileptic cry". The arms became semiflexed in front of the chest but also at times became extended, with forearm pronation and either wrist flexion and finger extension or wrist extension and fist clenching. The legs went into forced extension, adduction and external rotation along with extension of the feet and toes into a Babinski-like posture. In contrast to the flexion phase, the body assumed an opisthotonic position. This "tetanic" phase subsequently became less complete and the rigidity was replaced by a fine tremor that grew in amplitude and slowed in frequency from 8/second to 4/second because of recurrent decreases in muscle tone – a so-called "intermediate vibratory period".

The clonic phase lasted about 30 seconds and was said to occur when each of the recurrent muscular contractions responsible for the vibratory phase became sufficiently prolonged to completely interrupt the tonic contraction, the resultant flexor spasms of the entire body appearing to resemble an "an epileptic form of bilateral myoclonus". This myoclonus progressively slowed until seizure cessation. Variations to this entire theme were considered occasional and unusual. Asynchrony between two sides during the tonic or clonic phases was one such deviation. This asynchrony could be clinical or only evident on EMG recordings when clinically unnoticed.

Two important studies have addressed the issue of the importance of two semiological features at the onset of secondary generalization in focal epilepsies that can be an invaluable aid to lateralization. Wyllie *et al.* studied head version in 61 seizures in 27 patients and reported that this occurred contralateral to the hemisphere of seizure onset in all patients (Wyllie E *et al.*, 1986). It is important to emphasize here that the definition of head version is crucial to correct lateralization. Only forced and prolonged head turning, usually in a clonic motion with the chin pointing upwards, with eye version to the same side as head version allows precise lateralization *(Figure 1)*. Very frequently, such a version is also accompanied by pulling of the face towards the contralateral, clonic, twitching side. Kotagal *et al.* reported the "sign of 4"

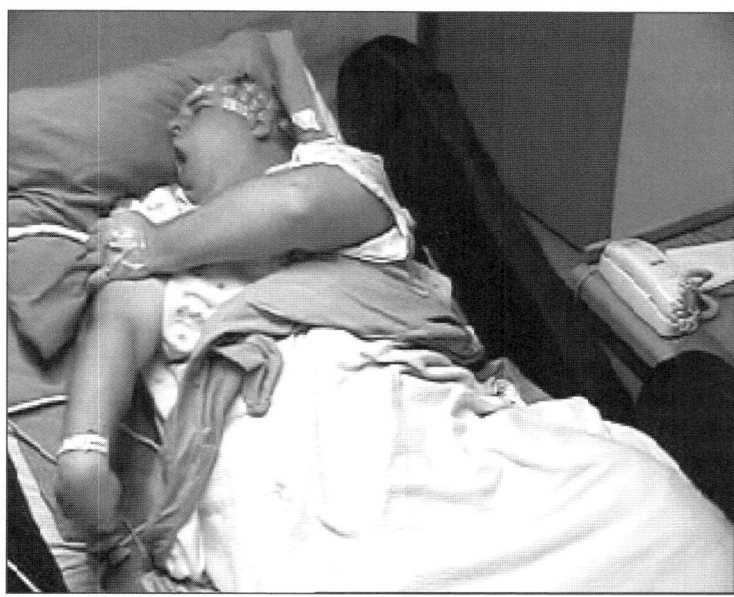

Figure 1. The sign of 4 with right elbow extension indicating left hemisphere seizure onset. Also notice version of the head to the right.

or the "figure 4 sign" where the elbow contralateral to the hemisphere of seizure onset extends and the ipsilateral elbow flexes over the chest to produce an upper limbs posture that resembles a figure 4 (Kotagal P *et al.*, 2000) *(Figure 1)*. In a study that looked at 39 patients with focal epilepsy, correct lateralization with this sign was seen in 90%. However, both head version and the sign of 4 are unreliable semiological features once the seizure is well established and their main value is derived at the onset of generalization.

A few studies have since examined the progression of the SGTCS *(Table I)*. A study from Bethesda, Maryland in 1994 presented a videotape analysis of 120 SGTCS in 47 patients with focal epilepsy with an age range between 11 to 56 years (Theodore WH *et al.*, 1994). Seizure semiology analysis was carried out jointly by three observers and the generalized phase was divided into 5 phases that constituted onset of generalization, pretonic clonic, tonic, tremulousness and clonic phases. 84% of the seizures had the "onset" phase characterized by vocalization, head version or some form of movement. 48% had a pretonic clonic phase where patients had irregular and asymmetric jerking, 95% had a tonic phase and 98% had a clonic phase. Only 27% of these seizures exhibited all 5 phases. The authors noted that generalization was not uniform or symmetric and noted the marked heterogeneity in GTCS phenomenology. Another study that examined SGTCS progression in temporal lobe epilepsy patients in 2001 found the classically described sequence of progression in only half their patients and in a third, a clonic phase preceded the tonic and in a quarter, the progression was one of tonic to clonic to tonic. Asynchrony in the clonic phase was noted in only two patients (Jobst BC *et al.*, 2001).

Table I. Studies of seizure semiology in secondary generalized tonic-clonic seizures.

Study	*No of Seizures	**Seizure progression – % of patients				Asynchrony*** yes/no – %
		T→C	C→T→C	T→C→T	C	
Theodore 1994	120		48			
Niaz 1999	10	80	10		10	yes (80)
Jobst 2001	286	52	31	28		yes
Trinka 2002	39					yes (60)
Leutmezer 2002	74					yes (43)
Kirton 2003	64					yes (38.5)

*Number of seizures specified rather than number of patients because of seizure heterogeneity in the same patient.
**T = Tonic, C = Clonic.
***Asynchrony is used synonymously with asymmetry.

An unblinded videotape analysis from Nashville, Tennessee in 1999 compared 10 GTCS in nine patients with idiopathic generalized epilepsy and 10 GTCS in 10 patients with temporal lobe epilepsy (Niaz FE et al., 1999). Interestingly, and this has been noted by subsequent studies, focal features were seen before generalization in 7 idiopathic generalized seizures, most commonly comprising head turning, in one patient occurring in different directions in two different seizures. The authors noted that the tonic phase was always symmetric but that in the last generalized clonic phase, asymmetry or asynchrony of motor activity was seen transiently in three seizures. In contrast, in the temporal lobe epilepsy patients, focal tonic activity occurred in 4 seizures, with variable lateralization and there was asymmetric or asynchronous activity in the clonic phase in 8 seizures. Seizure progression in these patients was tonic to clonic in 8, clonic to tonic to clonic in one and only clonic in one.

A 2003 study from Calgary attempted to distinguish primary from SGTCS in children aged 18 months to 17 years by examining 64 GTCS in 13 children with medically refractory epilepsy (Kirton A et al., 2004). The study highlighted mouth movements and motor activity following clinical and EEG seizure end as distinctive features of the SGTCS although these conclusions and their value in clinical practice is debatable. However, these authors too, noted the asymmetry in arm movements in 7 out of 12 children and in leg movements in 9 out of 12 children during secondary generalization. In 5 patients, seizure activity continued on one side, with varying lateralization.

Two common themes emerge from these studies. Firstly, that there is considerable heterogeneity in seizure progression during the phase of secondary generalization as compared to Gastaut's classical description and secondly, there is asynchrony (disparity of rhythm between the two sides) and/or asymmetry (disparity in amplitude of limb movement between the two sides) during the seizure in a substantial proportion of patients. Apportioning any great clinical weight to the lateralizing value of these phenomena during the SGTCS may not be justifiable, but studies that have examined seizure termination in the SGTCS of temporal lobe epilepsy have pointed out that in 80-83% of seizures that end in an asynchronous fashion, the final clonic movements occurred on the side ipsilateral to the hemisphere of seizure onset (Leutmezer F et al., 2002b; Trinka E et al., 2002). Contrary to the caution required in interpreting late ictal phenomena, forced head version immediately prior to the onset of secondary generalization and the asymmetric "sign of 4" tonic posturing at the onset of the SGTCS are known to be useful lateralizing features where head version or elbow extension in the sign of 4 occur contralateral to the hemisphere of seizure onset (Kotagal P et al., 2000). However, there is literature to suggest that focal features arise in the GTCS of idiopathic generalized epilepsy too, although definitions of head version for example, may differ in their interpretation (Leutmezer F et al., 2002a).

Methods

We studied 24 SGTCS in 14 patients (12 male, 2 female) aged 9-39 years who underwent video-EEG monitoring as part of their pre-surgical investigation for medically refractory focal epilepsy. All 14 patients had invasive evaluations with subdural grid electrodes and/or depth electrodes. The duration of epilepsy ranged from 1-22 years. Clinical details are provided in *table II*. In each case, the epilepsy diagnosis was made with a combination of seizure semiology, imaging, inter-ictal and ictal EEG findings.

Results and discussion

Seizure semiology was studied from the point of onset of secondary generalization. We employed a practical definition for generalization as that clinical stage where there was clear evidence of bilateral motor arm and/or leg involvement along with complete loss of consciousness. We did not include head or eye version in this definition. Mode of onset, progression of generalization, duration of various motor stages, symmetry of seizures, synchrony of the clonic phase and the presence or absence of paradoxical lateralization were all studied. Asymmetry was defined as a greater than 50% difference in amplitude of movement between the two sides of the body. Asynchrony was defined as a clear difference in the rhythm of movement between the two sides of the body. *Table III* summarizes these findings.

Seizure onset

The sign of 4 was seen in eight (7 patients) of 24 (33%) seizures. In seven of these seizures (87.5%), it predicted the side of seizure onset correctly, with arm extension contralateral to the side of seizure onset. In one patient, two further seizures occurred without a sign of 4, suggesting that this does not consistently occur in all seizures in the same patients. In 6/24 (25%) seizures, there was an asymmetric tonic onset to the seizures that did not amount to a sign of 4. In 6/24 (25%), there was a symmetric tonic onset to the generalization. In 4/24 (17%) there was a clonic onset that was asymmetric in all.

Table II. Clinical Characteristics of Patients with Secondary Generalized Tonic-Clonic Seizures.

Patient	Sex	Age	Duration of Ep.	Diagnosis	Pathology
1.	F	26	12	Left Temporal Lobe Epilepsy	Temporal hamartoma
2.	M	27	15	Right Tempero-Parieto-Occipital Epilepsy	Bihemispheric MCD*
3.	M	18	13	Right Mesial Frontal Lobe Epilepsy	Remote infarct
4.	M	25	21	Left Basal Temporal Lobe Epilepsy	Focal subpial gliosis
5.	M	19	10	Left Lateral Temporal Lobe Epilepsy	Focal subpial gliosis
6	M	14	9	Right Tempero-Parietal Epilepsy	Focal cortical dysplasia
7.	F	35	19	Right Hemispheric Epilepsy	Bi-hemispheric MCD
8	M	25	15	Left Hemispheric Epilepsy	Unknown
9.	M	18	15	Right Mesial Frontal Lobe Epilepsy	Remote infarct/contusion
10.	M	20	9	Right Parieto-Occipital Epilepsy	Focal cortical dysplasia
11.	M	39	22	Right Tempero-Occipital Epilepsy	Bi-hemispheric MCD
12.	M	23	20	Left Lateral Frontal Lobe Epilepsy	Focal subpial gliosis
13.	M	9	7	Right Lateral Temporal Lobe Epilepsy	Unknown
14.	M	13	1	Right Tempero-Occipital Epilepsy	DNET**

MCD* – Malformation of Cortical Development.
DNET** – Dysembryoplastic neuroepithelial tumor.

Seizure progression

Progression of generalization through various phases also varied. In 13/24 (54%) of seizures, there was a tonic phase followed by the vibratory phase, followed by a clonic phase. In 6/24 (25%) seizures, there was no intervening vibratory phase. In 1 patient, there was progression from a tonic to a focal arm clonic phase. The clonic to tonic to clonic progression noted by Gastaut was seen in only 3/24 (13%) of seizures and in one patient, the seizure remained clonic throughout. All seizures had a clonic phase.

Table III. Characteristics of Secondary Generalization in SGTCS.

Pt.	Onset	Tonic Phase	Vibratory Phase	Clonic Phase	Asynchrony	Paradoxical Lat.
1.	ST	S	S	S	No	No
2.	AST	A	S	S	Yes	No
3.	Sign of 4 – Rt arm	S	S	S	No	No
4	Bilat. arm clonic	S	S	A	No	No
5a.	ST	S	S	A	Yes	No
5b.	ST	S	No	S	No	No
5c.	Sign of 4 – Rt arm	S	No	S	Yes	Yes
5d.	ST	A	No	S	Yes	Yes
6.	Bilat. Leg clonic	No	No	A	Yes	Yes
7.	AST	A	No	S	No	No
8.	Sign of 4 – Rt arm	S	No	A	No	No
9a.	AST	S	S	S	No	No
9b	AST	S	A	A	Yes	No
9c.	Sign of 4 – Lt arm	A	S	A	Yes	No
9d.	Sign of 4 – Lt arm	A	A	A	Yes	No
10a.	ST	S	No	S	Yes	No
10b.	ST	S	S	A	Yes	No
10c.	Sign of 4 – Lt arm	S	S	S	Yes	No
10d.	Bilat. Arm clonic	A	S	A	Yes	No
11.	Sign of 4 – Lt arm	A	No	A	Yes	No
12a.	Sign of 4 – Rt arm	S	No	S	No	No
12b.	Bilat. Arm clonic	A	S	S	Yes	Yes
13.	AST	A	No	A	Yes	No
14.	AST	A	No	A	Yes	Yes

AST – Asymmetric tonic.
ST – Symmetric tonic.
S – symmetric.
A – Asymmetric.

The Tonic Phase

During the tonic phase, the dominant posture varied with different patients and with different seizures in the same patients. These postures could be categorized into the following types *(Figure 2)*:

1. **Type 1** (35%) – The upper limbs were held in a position of shoulder adduction, elbow flexion, wrist flexion and finger flexion or extension. The lower limbs were held extended with plantar flexion. The neck was flexed *(Figure 2a)*.

2. **Type 2** (26%) –   The body was held in the same position as in Type 1 but with persistent elbow extension rather than flexion (*Figure 2b*).
3. **Type 3** (9%) –   The body was held in the same position as in Type 1 but with hip and knee flexion rather than extension (*Figure 2c*).
4. **Type 4** (30%) –   The body was held in a position of bilateral asymmetric tonicity with upper and/or lower limb flexion on one side and upper and/or lower limb extension on the other (*Figure 2d*).

The Clonic Phase and Paradoxical Lateralization

During the clonic phase, there were asymmetric movements in 13/24 (54%) seizures and asynchrony of limb movements in 15/24 (62%) of seizures. During both the tonic phase as well as the clonic phase, asymmetry and/or asynchrony had no lateralizing value.

Focal clonic limb movements occurred at the end of the bilateral motor seizure in 8/24 (33%) seizures in 7 patients. These comprised strictly unilateral arm clonic movements in 7 and clonic movements of the face, arm and leg in one patient. In 6 (75%), these lateralizing movements occurred paradoxically ipsilateral to the side of seizure onset, a figure that is keeping with similar observations made by previous studies that have examined seizure termination in temporal lobe epilepsy (Leutmezer F et al., 2002b; Trinka E et al., 2002). This may reflect on earlier seizure cessation in the hemisphere of seizure onset due to factors such as neuronal fatigue, an exhaustion of excitatory processes or a predominance of inhibitory processes. The marked slowing usually seen on scalp EEG during this phase in the hemisphere ipsilateral to the paradoxical movements lends support to this. Paradoxical movements are most likely to be generated in the contralateral cortex and propogated by the pyramidal tract rather than originating in the brainstem, not least because there is a clear relationship between ipsilateral cortical discharges and strictly contralateral clonic signs. There appears to be some lateralizing value to this sign although it is important to emphasize that the seizure should always be viewed in its entirety and the value of lateralizing signs at seizure onset outweigh the importance of phenomena that occur during or towards the end of seizures.

Thus, asymmetry and asynchrony at any stage of the secondary GTCS seems a common phenomenon. This is at variance with the primary GTCS where symmetry and synchrony are more often found (Niaz FE et al., 1999). However, there are an increasing number of studies that report clinical as well as electroencephalographic focality in patients with primary GTCS. Usui et al. reported 26 patients with JME, only two of whom had both JME and a focal epilepsy. 46% of these patients had focal semiological features that included focal myoclonus, sign of 4 tonic posturing, forced head version and left arm clonic movements. EEG seizures in these patients were all generalized at the onset although in two patients with left head version at onset, the EEG lateralized to the right side during the seizure (Usui N et al., 2005). It is likely therefore that primary and secondary GTCS represent a semiological

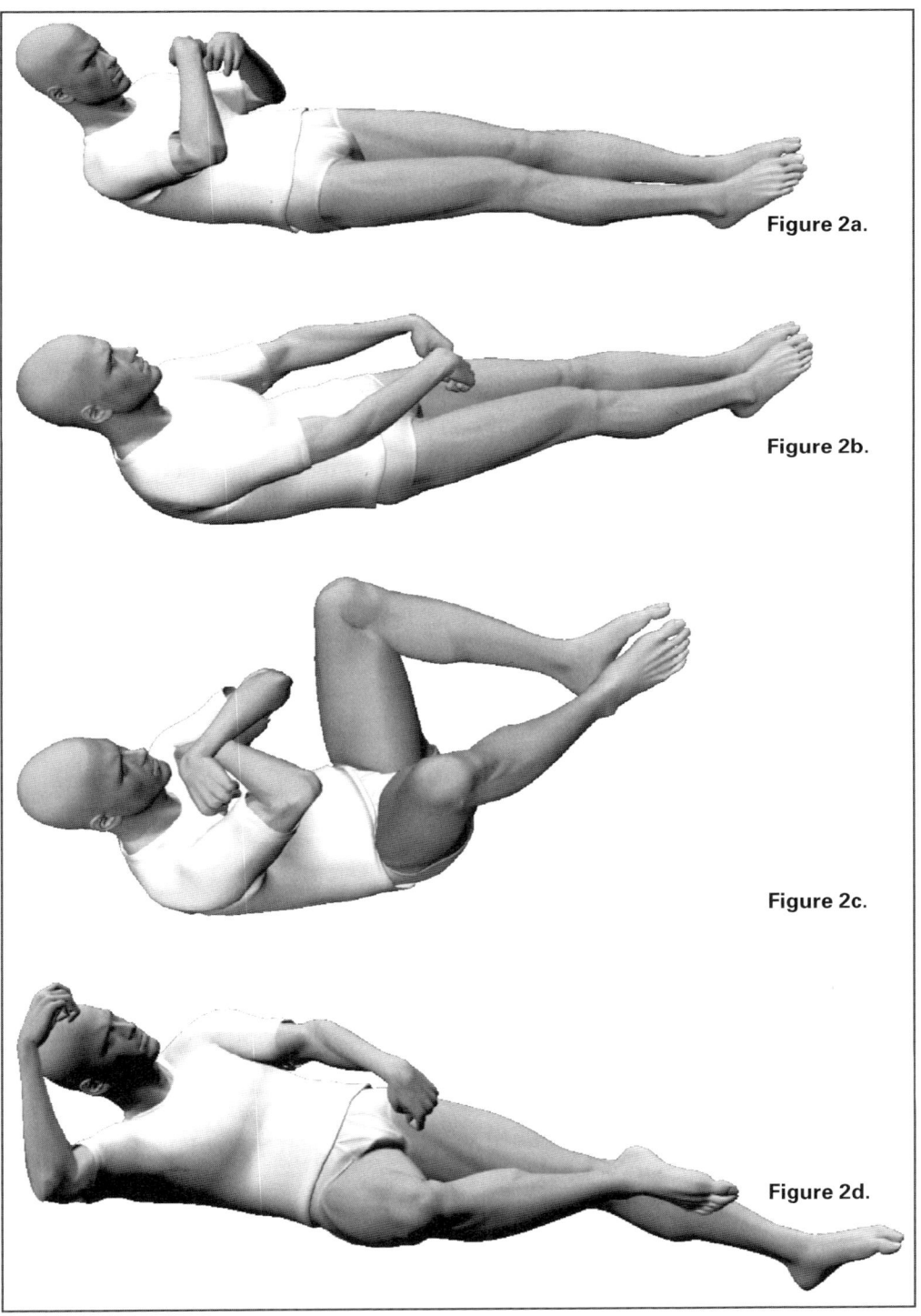

Figure 2a.

Figure 2b.

Figure 2c.

Figure 2d.

spectrum where symmetry and synchrony are seen most often in primary GTCS, with increasing asymmetry and asynchrony across the continuum towards a typical secondary GTCS *(Figure 3)*.

■ From clinical asynchrony to brain asynchrony – pathophysiology of the secondary GTCS

Gastaut, commenting on asynchronous generalized seizures, speculated on the possibility of two independent unilateral seizures occurring, one in each hemisphere. The traditionally held view of ictal cortical activity during a generalized seizure is one of complete synchronization of widespread brain activity. Recently, there has been some debate as to whether this is true. Investigators have attempted to address these questions with human EEG analyses, both scalp as well invasive, and with magnetoencephalography (MEG) (Dominguez LG *et al.*, 2005; Le Van Quyen M *et al.*, 2001; Mormann F *et al.*, 2000; van Putten MJ, 2003).

Synchronization implies the agreement in time of a particular property of two dynamical systems, usually in the time and frequency domains, and biological synchronization (particularly phase synchronization) has been studied in various ways

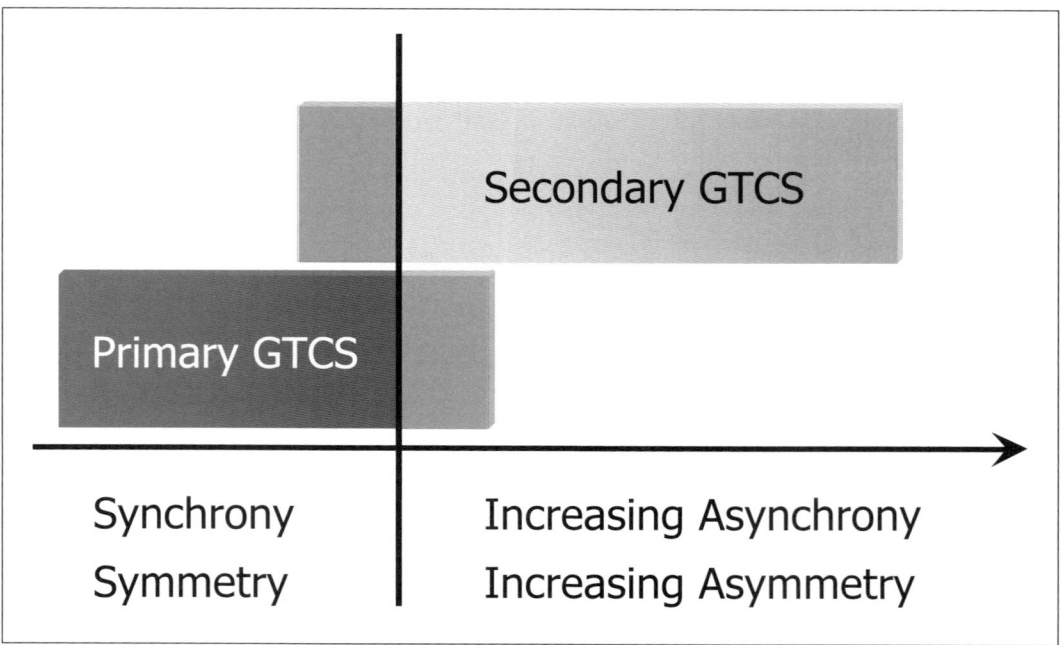

Figure 3. The semiological spectrum of primary and secondary generalized tonic-clonic seizures.

(Brown R and Kocarev L, 2000). In the context of epilepsy, nearest neighbor phase synchronization (NNPS) has been used in scalp EEGs as a means to more sensitive seizure detection (van Putten MJ, 2003). Whilst synchronization of adjacent brain areas is a not a biologically counterintuitive premise and the results are therefore not surprising, this method does not address the issue of distant brain synchronization during seizures. Furthermore, scalp EEG studies are subject to reference contamination and volume conduction artifacts, issues that may be particularly prominent during generalized seizures.

Le Van Quyen used the Hilbert transform method and wavelet methods to analyze neural synchrony in a patient with mesial temporal lobe epilepsy undergoing a depth electrode evaluation (Le Van Quyen M *et al.*, 2001). A contact each in the ipsilateral amygdala and hippocampus was used against an ear (scalp) electrode that was thought to be quiet. The raw data was digitized at 200Hz and passed to a 32 channel amplifier system with band-pass filter settings of 0.5-99Hz. Pre-seizure recordings showed phase relationship of neuronal activity in the 30-80Hz range. At seizure onset, (presumably with a seizure that remained focal) there was a transition to synchrony in the 12-15Hz and 3 Hz range. As the seizure progressed, there was synchrony in the 3Hz range that persisted but there was strong desynchronization in the high frequency range. Following the seizure, there was synchrony again in the 30-80Hz range. Thus, despite the relative proximity of the electrodes studied, there was some evidence of asynchrony. Another patient with orbitofrontal epilepsy was studied with subdural grids. Here, seizure onset was characterized by abrupt synchrony at 8-10Hz followed by synchronies at 25-90Hz. As the seizure progressed, there was a progressive decline in synchronization frequency. However, it is not clear if this patient had secondary generalization to the seizure and what precise electrodes, near or distant, showed asynchrony. Gotman *et al.* in 1987 described interhemispheric interactions in focal seizures after examining the intracranial recordings of 8 patients with epilepsy. They compared, where possible, homologous brain regions in each hemisphere and found that interhemispheric coherence or broadly, phase synchrony, was surprisingly low. However, sampling of brain areas was limited to a few depth electrodes and no data on the clinical semiology was presented. Other observers (Mormann) have made observations on pathological synchrony in epileptogenic brain in focal epilepsy through invasive recordings although again, conclusions are restricted by the limited areas covered by the electrode contacts (Mormann F *et al.*, 2000).

A magneto-encephalographic study with scalp EEG examined local and distant phase synchronization in generalized seizures (Dominguez LG *et al.*, 2005). Interestingly, distant synchronization was observed to be better in primary generalized absence seizures as compared to secondarily generalized motor seizures in focal epilepsy, although in the latter, there was evidence of strong local synchrony in keeping with the scalp EEG data presented by van Putten (van Putten MJ, 2003).

Thus, although it makes intuitive sense that there should be generalized synchrony in extended brain regions during generalized seizures, the true picture is less clear and there is evidence in literature that significant asynchrony may occur in SGTCS. Patient undergoing invasive monitoring with subdural grids and/or depth electrodes provide an opportunity to examine these issues.

Methods

We analyzed the SGTCS of 9 seizures in 9 of the above patients who underwent an invasive presurgical evaluation for medically refractory epilepsy. Electrodes of seizure onset were screened and referenced to an uninvolved/artifact free intracranial electrode. Pre and post-operative 3D MRI reconstruction was used with data from somatosensory evoked potentials and cortical electrical stimulation to determine the position of the central sulcus in order to locate electrodes over the motor strip. These were screened and referenced to an uninvolved/artifact free intracranial electrode. The seizure patterns at onset and during each phase of the secondary GTCS were analyzed with particular emphasis on synchrony of EEG rhythms. Synchrony was not defined quantitatively but in practical terms as the consistent agreement in time and/or frequency between the electrical activities of one brain region with another.

Thus, this definition does not allow an estimation of time relationships at the sub-second time scale.

Results and discussion

Results of the analysis of synchrony are detailed in *Table IV*. Synchrony between the motor strip and the brain region of seizure onset was seen only in three patients (33%), one during the tonic phase only and two during the clonic phase only. Thus, in the majority of patients, there was a clear asynchrony with very different seizure rhythms occurring in the two hemispheres or even within one hemisphere. This appeared to confirm Gastaut's suspicion that there is indeed more than one seizure occurring in the brain during a generalized seizure. In patient 1 for example (*Figures 4, 5 et 6*), where there is coverage of both motor strips as well as of the region of seizure onset. A clear difference in seizure rhythms can be visualized between the frontal lobes on either side and between the frontal lobe and temporal lobe in the hemisphere of seizure onset.

Thus, synchronization of brain regions does not appear to be necessary during SGTCS. Indeed, different seizures appear to occur simultaneously in different brain regions during the same clinical seizure.

Table IV. Brain synchrony between different brain regions in secondary generalized tonic clonic seizures.

Patient	Diagnosis	EEG Synchrony between regions	
		Tonic phase	Clonic Phase
1.	Lt Hemispheric E	–	–
2.	Rt TLE	+	–
3.	Rt TLE		–
4.	Rt Mesial FLE	–	–
5.	Lt Hemispheric E	–	–
6.	Lt TLE	–	–
7.	Rt TOE	–	+
8.	Rt TPE	–	–
9.	Rt POE	–	+

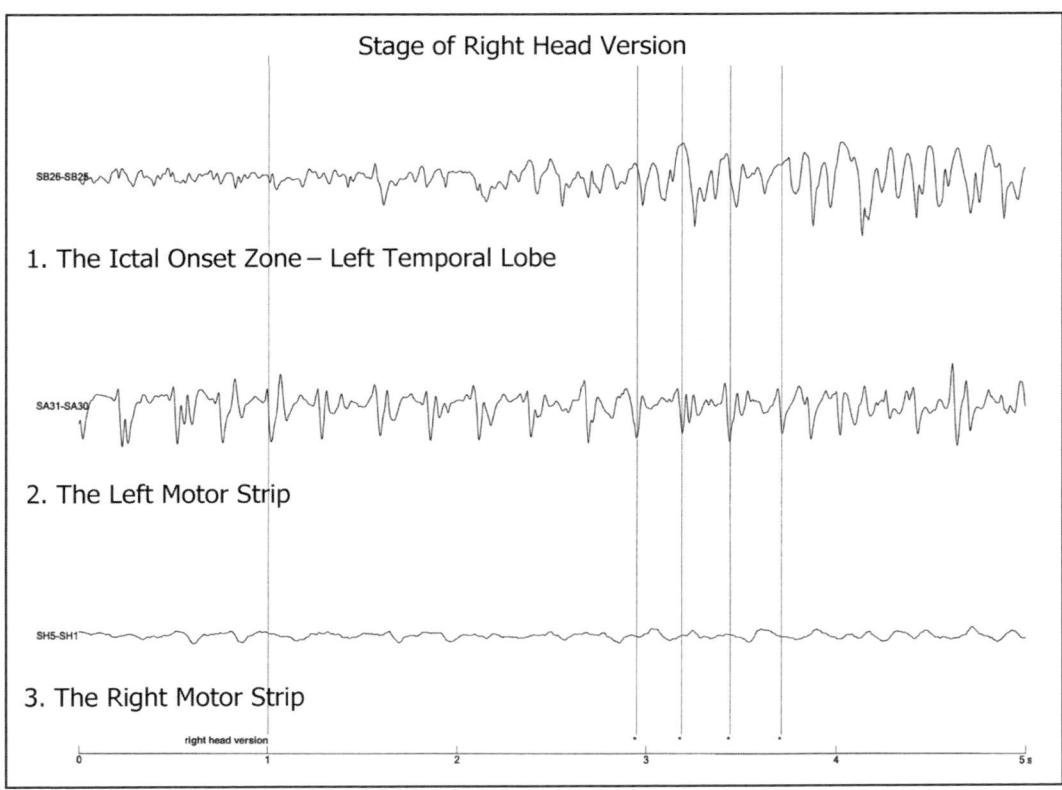

Figure 4. Left hemisphere epilepsy – stage of right head version: asynchrony between left temporal lobe and left motor strip. No activity in the right motor strip (Patient 1).

■ Brainstem or cortex?

As is evident from discussions elsewhere in this book, there is some animal evidence of brainstem seizure generation. However, it is far from clear that the same is true in humans. It appears likely however, that involvement of the cortex is critical to seizure generation. In all our patients, clinical seizure end always preceded EEG seizure end, suggesting that for the production of clinical seizure symptoms, a cortical discharge is always necessary, unlike the situation with brainstem seizure generation for example, where clinical symptoms could be expected to occur in the absence of cortical discharge. However, it is extremely likely that the brainstem plays an important part in the modulation of the secondary GTCS. Whilst it is easy to visualize the corticospinal tract as the main pathway for the clinical motor expression of the cortical seizure discharge, there are several other pathways that originate in the frontal cortex that relay in the human brainstem. These include projections to the brainstem reticular nuclei, the vestibular nuclei, the superior colliculus, the red nucleus and the olivary nuclei amongst others. There are interneuronal connections between these structures in the brainstem that probably form networks as part of central pattern generators. From here, the vestibulospinal and reticulospinal tracts project downwards

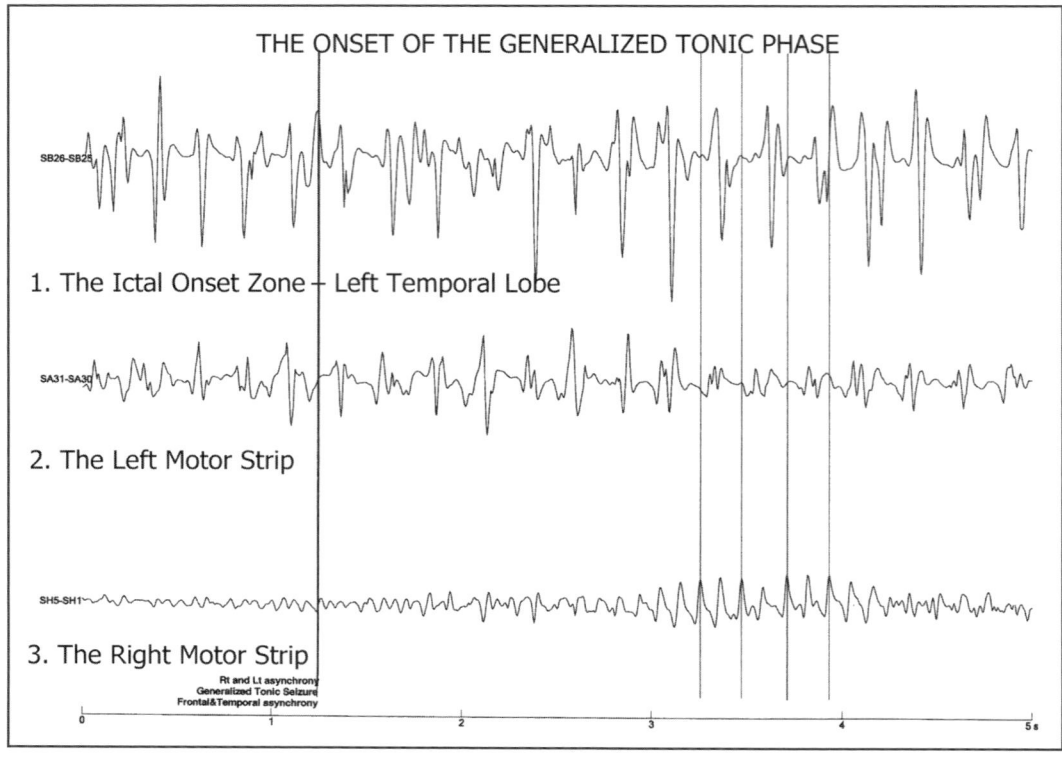

Figure 5. Onset of the generalized tonic phase. EEG asynchrony between motor strips and between left temporal lobe and left motor strip in the presence of clinical synchrony (Patient 1).

into the spinal cord and are likely candidates for the structures that subserve the variability in tonic posturing that is seen with the secondary GTCS. The vestibulospinal tract for example, produces upper limb flexion and lower limb extension whereas the reticulospinal tract produces the converse.

Patients who have undergone anatomical hemispherectomies may provide the best human evidence of brainstem seizure modulation. The video 2 demonstrates a generalized tonic-clonic seizure in a 3 1/2 year old post-hemispherectomy patient who has no residual cortex on the right side. The patient first presented with infantile spasms from birth due to an extensive right hemispheric malformation of cortical development. A right functional hemispherectomy was carried out with removal of the pericentral and temporal cortices. Following this, the patient continued to have medically refractory seizures although these were now left arm tonic seizures evolving into bilateral asymmetric tonic seizures and generalized clonic seizures, indicating a right frontal lobe onset. An anatomical hemispherectomy was then carried out with complete removal of all cortical structures. Following this surgery, the patient continued to have seizures that now originated from the left frontal region as shown in *figure 7*.

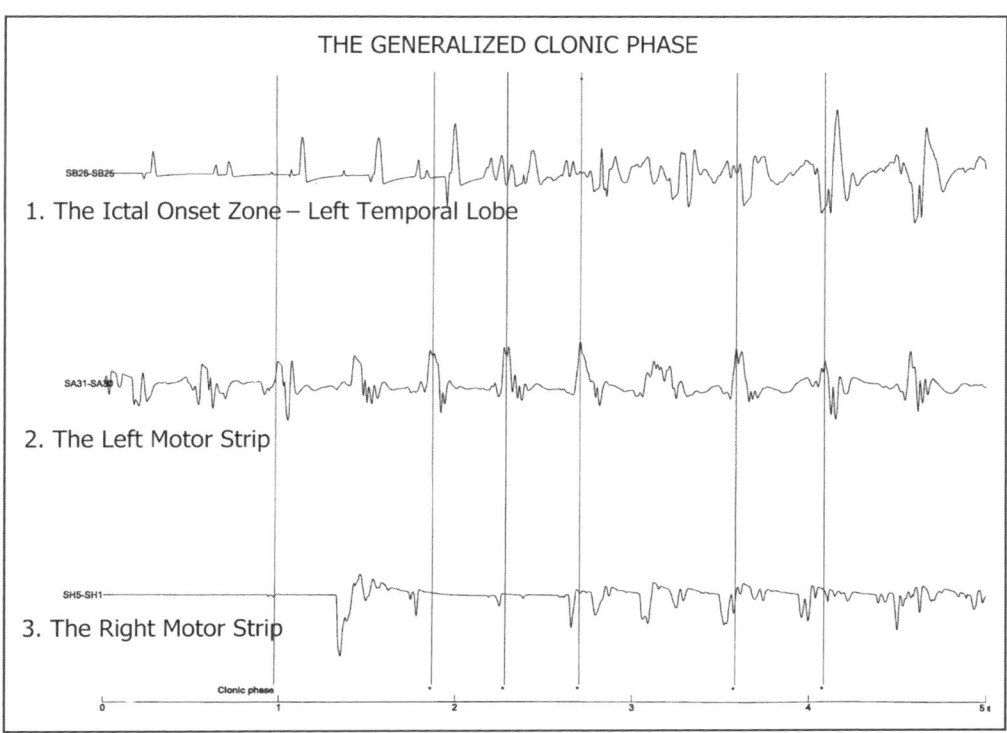

Figure 6. The generalized clonic phase with. Persistent EEG asynchrony between motor strips, between the left temporal lobe and the left motor strip during apparent clinical synchrony (Patient 1).

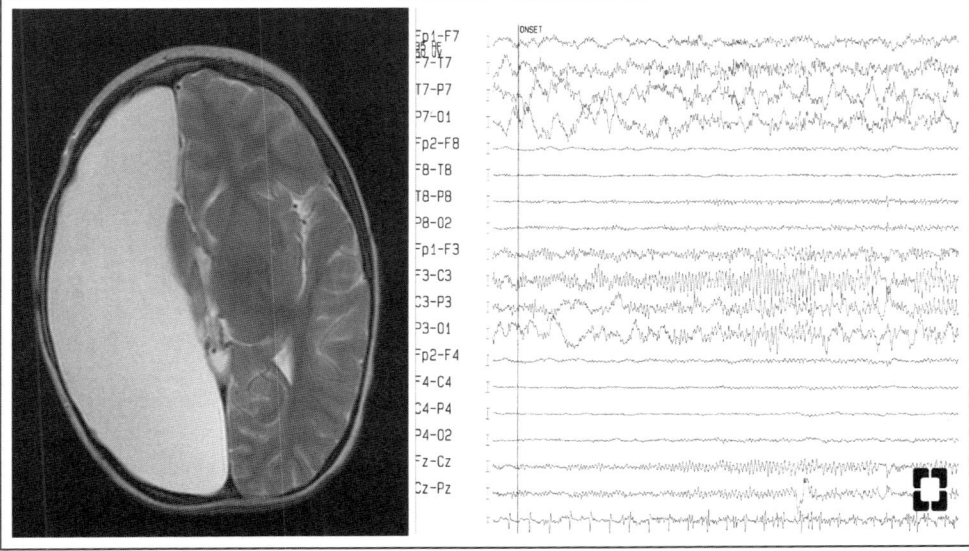

Figure 7. MRI image of patient with right anatomical hemispherectomy. EEG showing seizure onset in the left frontal region (Patient 1).

The tonic and clonic manifestations of the seizure are very symmetric in their expression, rendering it unlikely that the uncrossed ipsilateral corticospinal tract or the ipsilateral supplementary motor cortex have a role in their generation. Both these pathways have a clear predominance of contralateral projections and therefore tend to produce either strictly or predominantly contralateral motor seizures. Therefore, it is more probable that the ipsilateral cortical seizure discharge is being modulated in the brainstem to produce bilateral motor phenomena expressed through the vestibulospinal and/or reticulospinal tracts.

■ Conclusions

In summary, the semiology of the secondary GTCS is phenomenologically heterogeneous, with asynchrony and asymmetry displayed prominently in a substantial proportion of seizures, unlike the GTCS of primary generalized epilepsy where seizures are mostly synchronous and symmetric. Clinical asynchrony and asymmetry are accompanied by electrical asynchrony in the majority of patients as evidenced by the study of seizure rhythms in patients with secondary GTCS undergoing invasive evaluations. Electrical synchronization of brain activity does not appear necessary in secondary GTCS and indeed, there may be more than one seizure occurring in different brain regions at the same time. In humans, seizure generation is most likely to occur only in the cortex although evidence from patients who have undergone anatomical hemispherectomies strongly suggests that significant seizure modulation takes place in the brainstem. Thus, both areas of the brain (cortex ands brainstem) are important in the shaping of the semiology of the secondary GTCS.

References

Brown R, Kocarev L. A unifying definition of synchronization for dynamical systems. *Chaos* 2000; 10: 344-9.

Dominguez LG, Wennberg RA, Gaetz W, Cheyne D, Carter Snead III O, Velazquez JL. Enhanced synchrony in epileptiform activity? Local *versus* distant phase synchronization in generalized seizures. *J Neurosc* 2005; 25: 8077-84.

Gastaut H, Broughton R. *Epileptic seizures: clinical and electrographic features, diagnosis and treatment.* Springfield IL: Charles C Thomas, 1972: 25-90.

Jobst BC, Williamson PD, Neuschwander TB, Darcey TM, Thadani VM, Roberts DW. Secondarily generalized seizures in mesial temporal epilepsy: clinical characteristics, lateralizing signs, and association with sleep-wake cycle. *Epilepsia* 2001; 42: 1279-87.

Kirton A, Darwish H, Wirrell E. Unique clinical phenomenology can help distinguish primary from secondary generalized seizures in children. *J Child Neurol* 2004; 19: 265-70.

Kotagal P, Bleasel A, Geller E, Kankirawatana P, Moorjani B, Rybicki L. Lateralizing value of asymmetric tonic limb posturing observed in secondarily generalized tonic-clonic seizures. *Epilepsia* 2000; 41: 457-62.

Le Van Quyen M, Foucher J, Lachaux JP, Rodriguez E, Lutz A, Martinerie J, Varela F. Comparison of Hilbert transform and wavelet methods for the analysis of neuronal synchrony. *J Neurosc Meth* 2001; 111: 83-98.

Leutmezer F, Lurger S, Baumgartner C. Focal features in patients with idiopathic generalized epilepsy. *Epilepsy Res* 2002a; 50: 293-300.

Leutmezer F, Woginger S, Antoni E, Seidl B, Baumgartner C. Asymmetric ending in secondarily generalized seizures – a lateralizing sign in TLE. *Neurology* 2002b; 59: 1252-4.

Mormann F, Lehnertz K, David P, Elger CE. Mean phase coherence as a measure for phase synchronization and its application to the EEG of epilepsy patients. *Physica D* 2000; 144: 358-69.

Niaz FE, Abou-Khalil B, Fakhoury T. The generalized tonic-clonic seizure in partial *versus* generalized epilepsy: semiologic differences. *Epilepsia* 1999; 40: 1664-6.

Theodore WH, Porter RJ, Albert P, Kelley K, Bromfield E, Devinsky O, Sato S. The secondarily generalized tonic-clonic seizure. *Neurology* 1994; 44: 1403-7.

Trinka E, Walser G, Unterberger I, Luef G, Benke T, Bartha L, Eibl G, Ortler M, Bauer G. Asymmetric termination of secondarily generalized tonic-clonic seizures in temporal lobe epilepsy. *Neurology* 2002; 59: 1254-6.

Usui N, Kotagal P, Matsumoto R, Kellinghaus C, Luders HO. Focal semiologic and electroencephalographic features in pateints with juvenile myoclonic epilepsy. *Epilepsia* 2005; 46: 1668-76.

van Putten MJ. Nearest neighbour phase synchronization as a measure to detect seizure activity from scalp EEG recordings. *J Clin Neurophysiol* 2003; 20: 320-5.

Wyllie E, Luders HO, Morris HH, Lesser R, Dinner DS. The lateralizing significance of versive head and eye movements during epileptic seizures. *Neurology* 1986; 36: 606-11.

Tonic-clonic and clonic-tonic-clonic seizures in human primary generalized epilepsies

[*†‡]Reyna M. Durón, [**‡]Julia N. Bailey, [†‡*]Marco T. Medina,
[§*‡]Iris E. Martínez-Juárez, [*‡]Miyabi Tanaka, [§‡]María Elisa Alonso,
[¶‡]Ramón H. Castro Ortega, [*‡]Katerina Tanya Perez-Gosiengfiao,
[#‡]Ignacio Pascual-Castroviejo, [§‡]Adriana Ochoa,
[§‡]Aurelio Jara-Prado, [*‡]Jesús Machado-Salas, [***‡]Lizardo Mija,
[*‡]Antonio V. Delgado-Escueta

[*]California Comprehensive Epilepsy Program, David Geffen School of Medicine at UCLA and Department of Veterans Affairs, Greater Los Angeles Healthcare System, Los Angeles, California, USA;
[†]National Autonomous University, Tegucigalpa, Honduras;
[‡]GENetic EpilepsieS Studies (GENESS) International Consortium;
[**]Semel Institute of Neurosciences, and Neuropsychiatry Institute, David Geffen School of Medicine at UCLA;
[§]National Institute of Neurology and Neurosurgery, Mexico City, Mexico;
[¶]Autonomous University of Sonora, Hermosillo, Mexico;
[#]Pediatric Neurology, University Hospital La Paz, Madrid, Spain;
[***]National Institute of Neurological Sciences, Lima, Peru

"At the onset of the severe fit the spasms is tonic in character, -rigid, violent, muscular contraction, fixing the limbs in some strained position... When the cyanosis has become intense, the fixed tetanic contractions of the muscles can be felt to be vibratory, and the vibrations gradually increase until there are slight visible remissions. As these become deeper, the muscular contractions become more shock-like in character..." "Such attacks may commence with tonic spasm, or they may commence by, and sometimes consist only of clonic spasm... Precursory symptoms occasionally precede a fit, sudden jerks of the body or limbs."

Sir W.R. Gowers' description of "major fits" or "grand mal",
Gulstonian Lectures,
Royal College of Physicians of London, February 1880.

The "grand mal" seizure phenotypes

In 1981 the Commission on Classification and Terminology of the International League Against the Epilepsy (ILAE) proposed several generalized forms of seizures amongst whom where tonic-clonic ("the most frequently encountered often known as grand mal"), myoclonic, clonic, tonic, and atonic seizures. To assess the usefulness of this classification, we assessed the frequency of these "grand mal" seizure phenotypes in the GENESS Consortium Database (Martinez-Juarez et al., 2006; Alonso et al., 2005; Medina et al., 2005; Durón et al., 2006). *Figures 1-3* illustrate the various "grand mal" seizure phenotypes in probands and family members of JME subsyndromes and other IGE syndromes. Most common were clonic-tonic-clonic (CTC) convulsions (42%) and tonic-clonic (TC) convulsions (37%). Less frequent was absence immediately evolving into TC (18%) and astatic immediately evolving into tonic-clonic (3%). We encountered generalized clonic seizures in 27% of early childhood myoclonic epilepsy syndrome. Generalized clonic seizures were often associated with myoclonic, CTC and absence seizures in this syndrome. All these varieties of "grand mal" seizure phenotypes are documented on closed circuit television videotape and EEG telemetry when such patients required an inpatient workup.

Figure 2 caricatures the common seizures that associate with the grand mal phenotypes to compose the various idiopathic generalized epilepsy (IGE) syndromes. The most common grand mal phenotypes of CTC and TC comprise 93% of the seizures in probands of classic JME, 95% of CAE evolving to JME, 49% of the absence syndromes and 77% of early childhood myoclonic epilepsy syndrome.

Another way to assess what had been considered the most common phenotype of grand mal is to review published cohort(s) prospectively ascertained through an index case with idiopathic generalized TC seizures and EEG diffuse spike-wave complexes intended for pharmacologic studies. A careful history will easily reveal that one third of patients also have absence seizures, one third of patients obtained also have myoclonic seizures, one fourth will have grand mal only and less than 5% will have rare tonic seizures or rare astatic seizures associated with the tonic-clonic seizures. This agrees with our GENESS Database prospectively ascertained for genetic studies. Similar divisions of patients who have tonic-clonic grand mal seizures turn out to have: 1) clonic-tonic-clonic grand mal convulsions in the syndromes of juvenile myoclonic epilepsy and various forms of progressive myoclonus epilepsies, 2) absence immediately preceding tonic-clonic seizures in the syndrome of childhood absence epilepsy persisting with grand mal tonic-clonic seizures and in childhood absence epilepsy evolving to JME, 3) clonic convulsions in early childhood myoclonic epilepsy, 4) TC-convulsions plus astatic seizures and 5) TC convulsions plus tonic seizures. TC seizures only are less frequent in this prospectively ascertained database (GENESS, 2006). A similar experience is reported by the Centre Saint Paul between 1986 and 2002; where epilepsy with "grand mal on awakening (41 cases) only" is less frequent than the myoclonic and clonic tonic clonic seizures of JME (140 cases) (Genton et al., 2005).

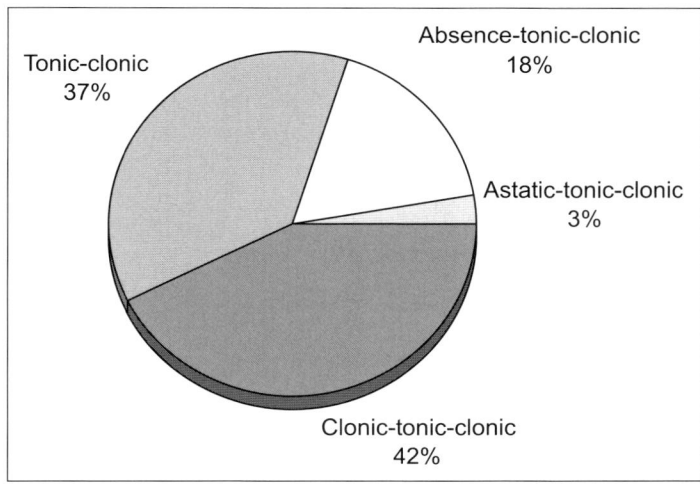

Figure 1. The grand mal seizure phenotypes in probands with JME syndromes (n = 288) according to GENESS database (Martínez-Juárez *et al.*, 2006; Durón *et al.*, 2006).

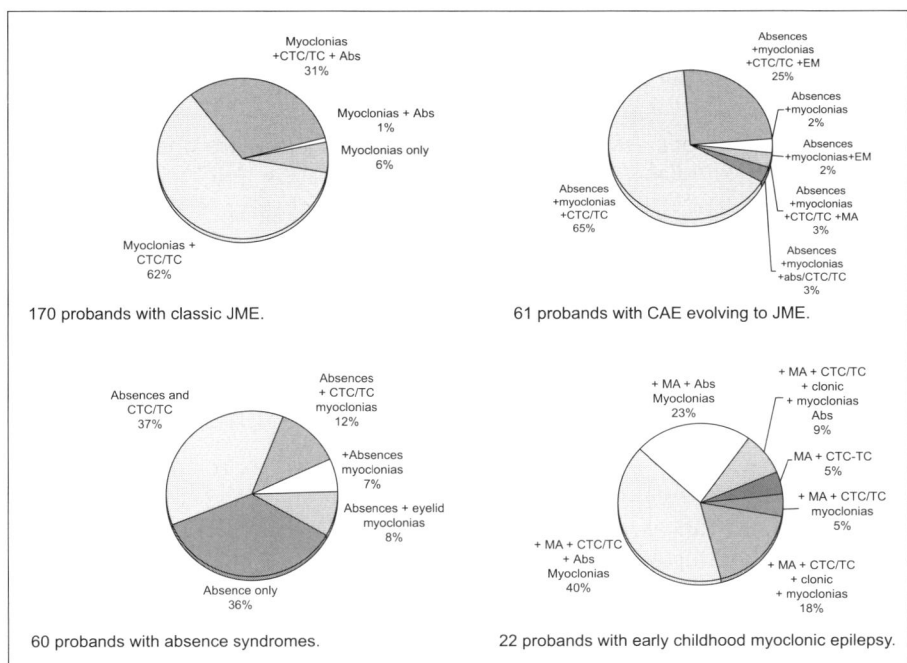

Figure 2. Seizure phenotypes associated with the grand mal seizure phenotypes in probands with IGEs according to GENESS database (Martínez-Juárez *et al.*, 2006; Durón *et al.*, 2006). Abs: absence; EM: eyelid myoclonia; MA: myoclonic astatic; MS: myoclonic seizures.

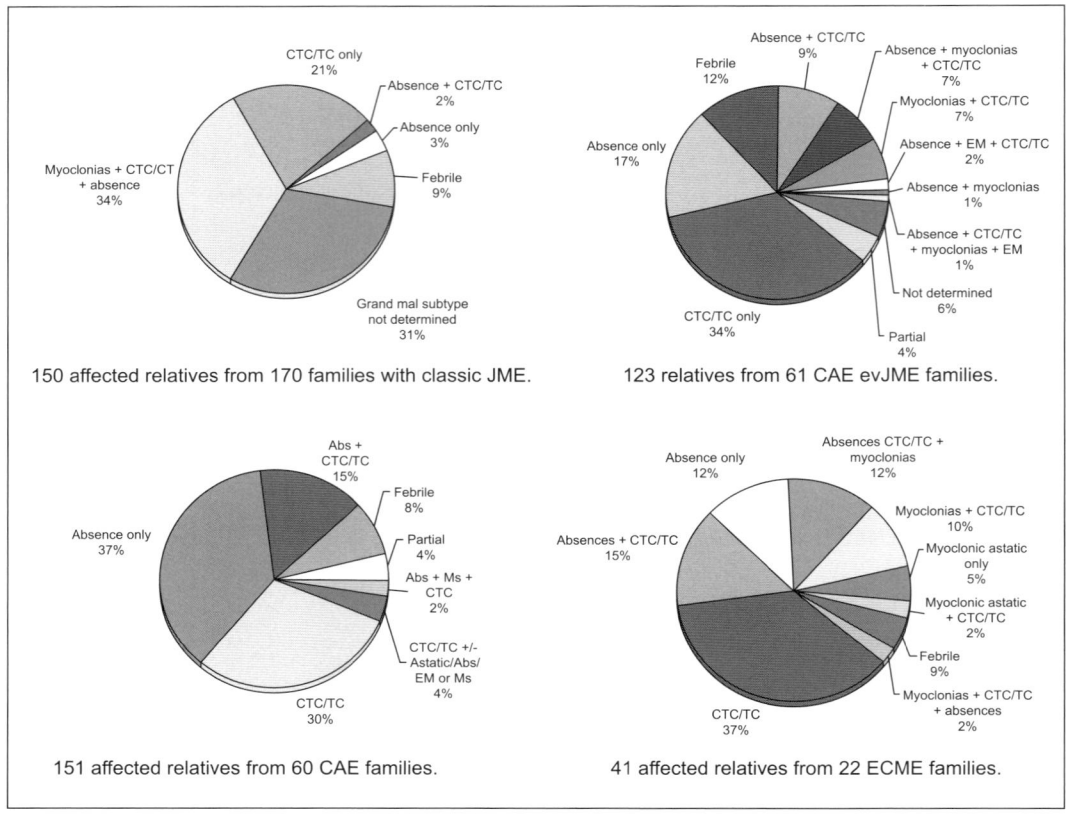

Figure 3. Seizure phenotypes associated with the grand mal seizure phenotypes in affected relatives of probands with IGEs according to GENESS database (Martínez-Juárez et al. 2006; Durón et al., 2006).
Abs: absence; EM: eyelid myoclonia; MA: myoclonic astatic; MS: myoclonic seizures.

Epidemiological studies of the "grand mal" seizure phenotypes differ from prospectively ascertained pharmacological and genetic cohorts

Thus, if clonic-tonic-clonic seizures are as common, if not more common, than tonic-clonic seizures, why do epidemiologic studies conclude that TC grand mal seizures affect more patients than any other type of idiopathic generalized seizures? In epidemiologic studies of epilepsies, generalized TC seizures only or patients experiencing TC seizures exclusively comprised 20.6% (Hauser, 1990). In Denmark, tonic-clonic grand mal seizures accounted for 24.6% of all seizure types in a population of 244,800 (Juul-Jenssen and Foldspan, 1983). In Tokyo, 87% of idiopathic generalized epilepsies were described to have TC seizures exclusively amongst 17,044 children three years and older. Indeed, epidemiologic studies repeatedly emphasize that the majority of patients with IGE have tonic-clonic grand mal seizures.

In epidemiological studies, the segment of patients with "grand mal only" does not usually have their phenotypes described in detail as in prospectively ascertained cohorts for pharmacologic or genetic studies. Moreover, epidemiologic studies usually do not document seizure phenotypes on CCTV-EEG. In patients with "idiopathic TC convulsive seizures" enrolled into prospective cohorts or admitted to CCTV-EEG telemetry units for diagnosis or treatment, absence seizures are recorded preceding the tonic-clonic seizures or myoclonic seizures precede and evolve with TC seizures. Absence at various moments of the days or myoclonic seizures between 4 AM and 9 AM are also observed or videotaped outside the "grand mal" seizure. It is an infrequent patient who has TC seizures as their sole phenotype. Other closed-circuit television-electroencephalogram (CCTV-EEG) studies and polygraphic studies of drug resistant patients with "pure grand mal epilepsy only" show that tonic-clonic seizures are almost always preceded by bilateral myoclonic jerks or absences (Delgado-Escueta, 1996, 2002).

In this chapter, we will review how the more common TC and CTC grand mal phenotypes as well as the less common generalized clonic, absence-tonic-clonic and astatic-tonic-clonic seizure phenotypes exist across the IGE syndromes (Tables I-II), suggesting common neuroanatomical systems (Table III). We discuss how the same "grand mal" seizure phenotypes in various IGEs, respond differently to the same treatment, suggesting different molecular lesions. We will review how advances in molecular epileptology provide a physiopathology for some of these syndromes and bring hopes to curative treatments.

■ Seizure phenotypes commonly associated with "grand mal" in human generalized epilepsies according to published literature

Tonic-Clonic (TC), Clonic-Tonic-Clonic (CTC) and generalized clonic seizures occur in variable frequencies and patterns in the different IGEs, suggesting common neurochemical or anatomical systems. Table I shows the frequency of "grand mal" seizures and other seizure phenotypes in generalized epilepsy syndromes, and Table II shows the temporal profile of seizures in most of these syndromes.

JME is probably the most common form of IGE and the most common cause of primary grand mal seizures. Most hospital and clinical-based reports calculate that JME accounts for at least 12% of all epilepsies (Genton et al., 2005; Janz, 1969), while a house-to-house population survey estimated that 3% were myoclonic epilepsies (Nicoletti et al., 1999).

Epilepsies with typical absence seizures are certainly common forms of IGEs, as exemplified by CAE, juvenile absence epilepsy (JAE), and eyelid myoclonia with absence. CAE accounts for 2% to 10% of children with epilepsies, while JAE constitutes 10% of all IGEs (Delgado-Escueta et al., 1999, 2005; Wolf and Inoue, 2002). Livingston (1975) and Lennox (1945) estimate the prevalence of absence seizures to be 2.3% to 37.7% of all epilepsies. Eyelid myoclonia with absence contributes 2% to all epilepsies and 11% to all IGEs (Giannakodimos and Panayiotopoulos, 1996).

Table I. Frequency of TC or CTC grand mal seizures and other seizure types in some patients with idiopathic generalized epilepsy syndromes.

Epilepsy syndromes (Ref)	Tonic-clonic or clonic-tonic-clonic	Absence	Myoclonic	Febrile seizures	Myoclonic absence	Myoclonic astatic	Eyelid myoclonia	Perioral myoclonias	Atonic Astatic	Tonic	Focal[a]
Benign myoclonic epilepsy of infancy (Dravet, Bureau, 2005)	Rare	–	100%	Rare	–	–	Rare	–	–	–	–
Severe myoclonic epilepsy of infancy (Dravet syndrome) (Dravet et al., 2005)	14%	40-95%[b]	100%	28-48%	–	–	Yes	–	–	14%	53%
Familial myoclonic epilepsy with onset in infancy (Zara et al., 2005)	100%	–	100%	63%	–	–	–	–	–	–	–
Myoclonic astatic epilepsy (Doose syndrome) (Doose et al., 2005)	75%-95%	62-79%	100%	11-28%	–	100%	–	–	–	30%-95%	–
Early childhood myoclonic epilepsy (Delgado-Escueta et al., 1990)	TC – 72% CTC – 27%	68%	100%	14%	–	–	–	–	91%	–	–
Myoclonic absences (Bureau, Tassinari, 2002; Tassinari et al., 1992)	45%	4%	–	Rare	100%	–	4%	–	–	–	–
Eyelid myoclonia with absence (Jeavons syndrome) (Giannakodimos, Panayiotopoulos et al., 1996; Panayiotopoulos et al., 1996)	50%	Rare	34-55%	Rare	100%	–	–	–	–	–	–

(modified from Durón et al., 2005; with permission)

Table I (cont.). Frequency of TC or CTC grand mal seizures and other seizure types in patients with idiopathic generalized epilepsy syndromes.

Epilepsy syndromes	Tonic-clonic or clonic-tonic-clonic	Absence	Myoclonic	Febrile seizures	Myoclonic absence	Myoclonic astatic	Eyelid myoclonia	Perioral myoclonias	Atonic Astatic	Tonic	Focal[a]
GEFS+ and absence with GABRg2 mutation (Baulac et al., 2005)	34%	29%	7%	86%	–	4%	–	–	4%	–	4%
GEFS+ with SCN1A mutation (Charlton, Yahr, 1967)	64%	21%	9%	83%	–	9%	–	–	12%	–	9%
Typical CAE (Wirrel, 2003)	30-60%	100%	–	20-22%	–	–	–	–	–	–	–
CAE evolving to JME (Martinez-Juárez et al., 2006; Alonso et al., 2005)	98%	100%	100%	3%	–	–	30%	–	–	–	–
Typical JME (Delgado-Escueta, Bacsal, 1984; Martinez-Juárez et al., 2006)	80%-95%	7%-38%	100%	13%	–	4%	–	23%	–	–	–
JME with adolescent pyknoleptic absences (Delgado-Escueta, Bacsal, 1984; Martinez-Juárez et al., 2006)	95%	100%	100%	–	–	–	–	–	–	–	–
JME with astatic seizures (Delgado-Escueta, Bacsal, 1984; Martinez-Juárez et al., 2006)	100%	9%	100%	–	–	–	–	–	100%	–	–
JAE (Wolf, Inoue, 2002)	–	100%	15%-20%	–	37-80%	–	–	–	–	–	–
Grand mal on awakening (Janz, 1969; Wolf, 2002)	100%	13-63%	6%-29%	–	–	–	–	–	–	–	4-22%

GEFS+, generalized epilepsy with febrile seizures plus; GABR2, GABA receptor subunit 2; SCN1, sodium channel alfa 1 subunit; CAE, childhood absence epilepsy; JME, juvenile myoclonic epilepsy; JAE, juvenile absence epilepsy.
[a] Consider that focal seizures and segmental myoclonias are often confused with each other.
[b] Refers to family members, not probands.

It is difficult to estimate the contributions of rare to infrequent epilepsy syndromes to all epilepsies in general. Severe myoclonic epilepsy of Dravet, benign myoclonic epilepsy, myoclonic absence, photogenic epilepsies, idiopathic myoclonic astatic epilepsy (MAE) or Doose syndrome, and early childhood myoclonic epilepsies could conservatively add another 2% to 3% to the IGEs (Genton et al., 2005) In all these syndromes, tonic-clonic, clonic-tonic-clonic, generalized clonic, absence preceding tonic-clonic and astatic evolving to TC seizures can be found.

Clonic-tonic-clonic and tonic-clonic "grand mal" seizures

Grand mal CTC or TC seizures are common to almost all epilepsy syndromes. Clonic-tonic-clonic seizures are almost always genetic or biochemical in origin, while tonic-clonic seizures can have a genetic or lesional etiology. As mentioned above, the percentage of TC grand mal as the sole phenotype is low if seizures are studied with videotape and EEG telemetry or polygraphy (Delgado-Escueta et al., 1990). Most of the time, grand mal seizures are preceded or accompanied by absences or myoclonic seizures that are not reported or noticed by patients and clinicians (Roger et al., 2005; Jain et al., 1997). Myoclonic seizures are often mistaken as tics and nervousness (Delgado-Escueta et al., 1996). Additionally, grand mal seizures can be the first seizure type in up to 30% of patients with JME, with myoclonias reported later (Alonso et al., 2005). Epidemiological studies undercount absences with grand mal and JME, listing them instead under generalized tonic-clonic seizures.

Absences immediately preceding TC and CTC "grand mal" seizures

The International Classification of Epilepsies and Epileptic Syndromes includes three types of IGEs with typical absences associated with grand mal seizures: CAE, JAE, JME (Commission on Classification and Terminology 1981 and 1989). More absence syndromes exist in addition to the three listed above. Several varieties of absence syndromes are differentiated from the pyknoleptic CAE that occurs between 4 and 10 years of age and that remits in adolescence. These absence syndromes are (1) absence epilepsy of early childhood starting before 5 years of age (Chaix et al., 2003; Cavazzuti et al. 1989); (2) MAE, in which myoclonias occur simultaneously with absence seizures (Bureau et al., 1992; Tassinari et al., 1992); (3) eyelid myoclonia with absences (Panayiotopoulos, 1996); (4) CAE that persists with grand mal into adulthood (Wirrel et al., 1996; Charlton 1967); and (5) CAE that evolves into JME (Medina et al., 2005). Pyknoleptic CAEs persisting into adolescence and adulthood with grand mal seizures are reported to occur in 12% to 32% of all absence cases (Charlton and Yahr, 1967, Olsson and Hagberg 1991; Bouma and Tassinari 1996; Sato et al., 1983). Many emphasize how absence seizures are frequently misdiagnosed as complex partial seizures, but what is more commonly missed are absences immediately preceding TC convulsions. Electroencephalography, particularly video-electroencephalography, is invaluable in identifying absence-TC seizures.

Myoclonias and the "grand mal" seizure phenotypes

While myoclonias are the sine qua non of JME, grand mal TC or CTC seizures are present in 95% of JME, often during awakening hours between 5 and 9am and sometimes during the first hours of the awake period. As described in the 1981 and 1989

Table II. Temporal profile of TC and CTC grand mal seizures with absences and myoclonias showing their age dependency.

Syndrome	First year of life (months)	Infancy and childhood (years)	Adolescence (years)	Adulthood (years)	Remission and prognosis
	1 2 3 4 5 6 7 8 9 10 11 12	2 3 4 5 6 7 8 9	10 11 12 13 14 15-19	20 25 30 35 40 50+	
Severe myoclonic epilepsy in infancy					High mortality in childhood, stops progressing at 3-4 y
Angelman syndrome					Seizures can remit by 10 y; if persistent, they attenuate; there is psychomotor delay
Generalized epilepsy with febrile seizures plus					Benign, more studies on prognosis needed
Benign myoclonic epilepsy in infancy					Some remit by 1 y; 45/63 cases last more than 5 y
Epilepsy with myoclonic absences					Only 47% remit; more studies needed
Myoclonic astatic epilepsy					Variable, psychomotor delay; persisting seizures; remission in childhood can occur
Early childhood myoclonic epilepsy					Seizures tend to remit in childhood but TC and CTC can recur in adolescence
Remitting childhood absence epilepsy					Benign, 33-78% may remit from 12 y to late adolescence
Juvenile absence epilepsy					60-76% may remit in the third decade of life
Childhood absence epilepsy evolving to juvenile myoclonic epilepsy					Few patients remit; Difficult to treat with AED; Responsive to AEDs
Epilepsy with grand mal on awakening					17% may remit; Responsive to AEDs
Reading epilepsy					Benign course but rarely remits
Juvenile myoclonic epilepsy					Benign course but rarely remits
JME with adolescent pyknoleptic absences					Benign course but rarely remits
JME with astatic seizures					Benign course but rarely remits

Note: Gray boxes indicate the range age at onset; Black boxes indicate the period seizures persist.
Prepared by Dr. Reyna Durón et al. for the Epilepsy Foundation of Greater Los Angeles, adapted and used with permission (Published in Durón et al., Epilepsia, 2005).

Table III. "Grand mal" seizure phenotypes: hypothesized systems.

	Gen. clonic	Clonic-tonic-clonic	Tonic-clonic	Absence evol. tonic-clonic	Astatic evol. tonic-clonic
Some IGE syndromes	SMEI; MAE of Doose; early childhood myoclonic epilepsy (ECME); uncontrolled convulsive status	SMEI; MAE of Doose; early childhood myoclonic epilepsy (ECME); uncontrolled convulsive status	MAE of Doose; early childhood myoclonic epilepsy; JME; eyelid myoclonic with absence, grand mal on awakening (GMA); JAE	Remitting CAE; CAE persisting with grand mal; CAE evolving to JME	MAE of Doose JME with astatic sz.
Systems based on animal models of epilepsy	Caudal pontine reticular formation (RF) *(Raisinghani and Faingold, 2005; Nersesyan et al., 2004; Korinthenberg et al., 2004)*	Caudal pontine RF, pons oralis and caudalis *(Raisinghani and Faingold, 2005; Nersesyan et al., 2004; Korinthenberg et al., 2004)* Midbrain RF, deep layers of sup. Colicullus, inf. Colicullus, periaqueductal gray and pontine RF *(Ishimoto et al., 2004; Zvanovic et al., 2004; Moraes et al., 2005; Rodin, 2005; Merrill et al., 2005; Chen et al. 2005; Merrill et al., 2003)*	Midbrain reticular formation *(Ishimoto et al., 2004; Zvanovic et al., 2004; Moraes et al., 2005; Rodin, 2005; Merrill et al., 2005, Chen et al., 2005)* Caudal pontine RF, pons oralis and caudalis *(Raisinghani and Faingold, 2005; Nersesyan et al., 2004; Korinthenberg et al., 2004)*	T type calcium channels in thalamus *(Coulter et al. 1989a, 1989b, 1990, 1991)* Noebel's hypothesis: balanced HVACC & LVACC prevent thalamic T type LVDCC from generating thalamocortical oscillations & cortical spike waves *(Noebels 1990; Zhang et al. 2002)* GAERs – functional imbalance between cortico-striatal-nigral (---) and cortico-subthalamic nigral (+++) pathways during EEG spikewaves GAERs – ↓ density of GABAA receptors in **cortex; thalamic NR** lesion abolish EEG spikewave discharges WAG/Ri/rats – **cortical focus** in somatosensory cortex is dominant in initiating spike wave discharges thalamic networks as "resonant devise" Penicillin microinjection **Rostral midbrain RF** → Myoclonic **Caudal midbrain RF** → Tonic **Pons RF pons oralis** → **Giganto cellularis** – Hypotonia	Caudal pontine reticular formation pons oralis and gigantocellularis (hypotonia) *(Velasco and Velasco, 1990)*

Table III (continued). "Grand mal" seizure phenotypes: hypothesized systems.

	Gen. clonic	Clonic-tonic-clonic	Tonic-clonic	Absence evol. tonic-clonic	Astatic evol. tonic-clonic
Molecules based on transgenic models of human epilepsy	• Gabrb3 KO • Laforin/epm2a KO • Cystatin/epm1 KO	• Gabrb3 KO	• Scn1a KO (Dravet) • Scn1b KO (GEFS+) • Kcna1 KO and Ki	• Gabrb3 KO • Cacna1a KO	
Systems based on human studies		• (18FDG) PET scan and functional quantitative MRI scans of JME *"increase cortical gray matter in mesial frontal lobes"* *"reduced prefrontal concentrations of NAA and increased levels of glutamate plus glutamine"* (see chapter of M. Koepp, this book)			

ILAE Classification of Seizures and Syndromes, myoclonias consist of bilateral, single or repetitive, arrhythmic, irregular myoclonic jerks, predominantly in the arms. Jerks may cause some patients to fall suddenly. No disturbance of consciousness is noticeable. Depending on the syndrome, the jerks are accompanied by generalized tonic-clonic seizures, absences or astatic seizures. The interictal EEG has 4-6 Hz spike or polyspike and slow-wave complexes, while high voltage 12 to 30 polyspikes accompanied myoclonic seizures.

Myoclonias may also mark the various syndromes of early childhood myoclonic epilepsies, which represent a broad group of heterogeneous clinical and electroencephalographic entities. Between infancy and 5 years of age, myoclonias can appear together with generalized clonic, tonic-clonic, atonic-drop or astatic, and absence seizures. Although seizures appear in various combinations, the predominant type of epileptic attacks has often determined the name given to the syndromes. For instance, several authors recognized cryptogenic myoclonic epilepsies based on the predominance of myoclonic seizures (Aicardi 1971, 1980, 1986).

Primary generalized seizures with EEG generalized irregular spikes and waves was separated from symptomatic West's infantile spasms and hypsarrhythmia, and from symptomatic Lennox-Gastaut syndrome by Doose et al. (1970), Doose (1992), and Doose and Baier (1987). Initially, they designated this syndrome as myoclonic petit mal of early childhood. Doose and colleagues have recently used the term primarily generalized myoclonic astatic petit mal of early childhood to encompass an epilepsy syndrome characterized by myoclonic, astatic, myoclonic astatic, and mostly tonic-clonic seizures with EEG generalized spikes and waves, photosensitivity, and 4-7 Hz bi-parietal theta rhythms. With a high incidence of seizures and genetic EEG patterns in relatives, these children have mostly normal development and no neurological deficits before the onset of seizures. However, a variable course ranging from spontaneous remission to persistence with neurological deterioration can occur.

Because primary generalized myoclonic seizures in childhood are under-recognized and underdiagnosed, their true prevalence is unknown. Pazzaglia et al. (1979) calculated that 1.4% of all epilepsies have myoclonic astatic seizures, while Doose and Sitepu in an epidemiologic study in Germany (1993) reported that 1% to 2% of all childhood epilepsies up to 9 years of age have myoclonic astatic seizures. In the population-based epilepsy study performed by Medina et al. in Salamá, Honduras, only 1% of epilepsies belonged to this syndrome (Medina et al., 2005).

■ Our GENES database: seizures associated with "grand mal" in specific IGES

Early childhood myoclonic epilepsy (Figures 2 and 3)

Seizures in probands and relatives

The full spectrum of the "grand mal" seizure phenotypes are present in 22 probands with early childhood myoclonic epilepsy (ECME). Also known as idiopathic myoclonic astatic seizures (MAS), this epilepsy syndrome starts during late infancy or early childhood. We prefer the term ECME because myoclonic astatic seizures decrease in frequency and eventually remit in childhood, but in 47% of patients, myoclonic or clonic-tonic-clonic seizures persist into adolescence. In contrast to "myoclonic petit mal of early childhood" described by Doose and colleagues, ECME is usually responsive to antiepileptic drugs like valproate and has a good prognosis.

All probands had myoclonias (100%), while a majority had astatic drops (91%), and absences (68%). Generalized tonic-clonic seizures (72%) and less frequently clonic-tonic-clonic and generalized clonic (27%) seizures were present. Bilateral 2-6 Hz spike or polyspike waves appeared in all probands, and classic 3 Hz spike wave was present in three (14%), and 2-3 Hz spike wave complexes were also present in five probands (23%). There was a slight male preponderance (nine female; 12 male) among probands, but affected nonproband family members were often female (31 female, nine male), with a ratio of 3.4:1. Valproate is effective in seizure control in most cases.

Familial history of epilepsy was present in 50% of probands. Maternal transmission was more common than paternal transmission (67% vs 33%), but in both cases, clinically or EEG-affected nonproband members were more often female (75% and 82%, respectively). In nonproband family members, grand mal (72.5%), absences (42.5%), and myoclonic seizures (22.5%) were common, and astatic seizures were infrequently reported (10%).

Juvenile myoclonic epilepsy subsyndromes

We subdivided 258 JME families into four groups according to the combination of seizure types afflicting the proband; the age of probands at onset of seizures; the results of physical, neurological, and brain imaging examinations; and the long-term outcome after treatment with valproate and/or the new generation of antiepileptic drugs (AEDs) (Medina *et al.*, 2005; Alonso *et al.*, 2004; Martínez-Juárez *et al.*, 2006).

Classic juvenile myoclonic epilepsy *(Figures 2 and 3)*

Seizures in probands

This subsyndrome accounts for 73% (n = 186) of all our cases, starting in adolescence as isolated awakening myoclonic seizures or CTC or TC seizures. In 30% of probands (52 of 170) grand mal seizures preceded myoclonias. Almost all (95%) had tonic-clonic or clonic-tonic-clonic grand mal seizures (see *Figure 2*). Myoclonias were most often the first seizure type to appear (117 of 170 cases; 68%). Sometimes rare isolated absence seizures (spanioleptic or sporadic absences) or rare episodes of absences appeared in clusters. In nine cases, the type of seizure at onset was not ascertained. The interictal EEG had 4-6 Hz spike or polyspike and slow-wave complexes, while high voltage 12 to 30 polyspikes accompanied myoclonic seizures. Although females were numerically more common than males among probands (103 females, 83 males; 1.25:1 ratio), the difference was not statistically significant (p = 1.078).

Seizures in relatives

Seizures were present in family members in 92 of 186 cases of classic JME (49%). Epileptic seizures affected 188 of 1764 (11%) of nonproband family members (see *Figure 3*). Specific seizure types could be determined in only 136 of the affected relatives; 11.5% of first-degree relatives had seizures. The most common (46%) were myoclonias with or without CTC or TC grand mal. Rarely were absence seizures present in relatives. Only 4% of second-degree relatives had seizures. Most common were CTC or TC grand mal seizures (41.4%), followed by myoclonic seizures (28%). Abnormal EEGs were found in 24 asymptomatic relatives. Of these 24 relatives, 15 (63%) had 4-6 Hz polyspike waves, four (17%) had bursts of focal or diffuse slowing, three (12%) had 3-5 Hz spike and wave complexes, and two (8%) had bursts of focal or diffuse sharp waves. Most asymptomatic family members with EEG polyspike wave were female (10 females, five males).

Childhood absence epilepsy evolving to juvenile myoclonic epilepsy
(Figures 2 and 3)

This group accounts for 17% of all the idiopathic myoclonic epilepsies in our series and consisted of 45 patients who had absence epilepsy that started in childhood and persisted with myoclonic and CTC or TC grand mal seizures into adulthood *(Figure 2)*.

Seizures in probands

Females were numerically preponderant among probands (29 females, 16 males; 1.8:1 ratio), but this was not statistically significant (χ^2 = 1.91, p = 0.166) because of the small number of cases. Childhood absence seizures were documented as the first seizure in all probands. Absences started at an average age of 6.9 years (1 to 11 years) in 41 probands. Among those with persisting seizures, absences continued to be the chief complaint in 44.4%, and absences mixed or preceding with tonic-clonic or myoclonic seizures were the chief complaint in 16%. Absences occurred at least once a day (range, one to 200 per day), namely pyknoleptic. Myoclonias started at a mean age of 14 years (range 8 to 47 years). Myoclonic seizures preceded grand mal convulsions in 18%, but more often they started in adolescence simultaneously with tonic-clonic seizures (40% of patients). Tonic-clonic seizures appeared for the first time on average at age 12 years (range, 2 to 37 years) (see *Figure 3*).

All probands had the classic 3 Hz single-spike and slow-wave complexes. In addition, 29 probands also had 2-5 Hz single-spike and slow-wave complexes, and 20 probands also had 4-6 Hz polyspike-wave complexes. Thirty-four percent of all cases had both single-spike wave and polyspike waves. We also found diffuse, fast low-amplitude 15-25 Hz rhythms in 22% of cases.

Seizures in relatives

Absence seizures most often affected non-proband family members. Myoclonias only or myoclonias plus TC or CTC grand mal affected only five persons (6%). CAE evolving to JME was documented in 13 (16%) of nonproband affected members (eight females, five males) (see *Figure 3*). When checking for parental affectedness in multiplex/multigenerational pedigrees, nine of 32 mothers had seizures more often (28%) than fathers (two of 32, or 6%).

Juvenile myoclonic epilepsy with adolescent-onset pyknoleptic absences

This group accounted for 7% of all JME cases (18 families). There was a female preponderance in probands (2.6:1 female:male ratio, $\chi^2 = 1.87$, p = 0.171). Pyknoleptic absences started commonly at age 16 years, usually between the ages of 11 and 32 years, and were combined with myoclonia and CTC and TC grand mal seizures. Myoclonic seizures were the first seizure type in 61% (see *Figure 2*). Myoclonic seizures were the main seizure type in 72% of the probands, but in eight cases with persistent seizures, absences with or without myoclonic seizures were predominant (five of eight cases). Interictal EEGs of 14 probands were available for analysis. Seven of 14 had normal 4-5 Hz spike-wave or polyspike waves. Two showed 4-6 Hz polyspike-wave complexes mixed with 3 Hz spike-wave complexes. One had generalized bursts of slow waves, and one had 3 Hz spike-wave complexes. Photoparoxysmal response was found in two of 14 probands. Of 18 probands, 61% (11 of 18) had a family history of epilepsy.

Juvenile myoclonic epilepsy with astatic seizures

This group accounted for 3% of all JME cases (nine families). Aside from the adolescent-onset myoclonia and TC or CTC grand mal seizures, nine patients exhibited astatic seizures between the ages of 8 and 17 years, with a mean age of onset of 14.3 years. No gender predominance was found (five females, four males). Only one of our patients has spanioleptic absences with ons*et al.*so in adolescence. EEGs of four patients showed 4-6 Hz spike-wave or polyspike and slow-wave complexes. One patient had the same pattern, but polyspike-waves were combined with 3 Hz spike-wave complexes. Four probands (44%) had family history of epilepsy.

■ The same TC or CTC "grand mal" seizure phenotypes respond differently to the same treatment in IGEs

Primary generalized seizures share a particular pharmacological sensitivity not found in seizure types produced by lesions. They respond well to valproate and the new generation AEDs levetiracetam, topiramate, and zonisamide. They can also respond well to lamotrigine but lamotrigine can exacerbate myoclonic seizures. They can be exacerbated by phenytoin, carbamezapine, oxcarbazapine, gabapentin, and primidone (Genton *et al.*, 1998; Medina *et al.*, 2005; Alonso *et al.*, 2005). Yet, the same absences and myoclonic, tonic-clonic, and astatic seizures that respond well to valproate in one syndrome, *e.g.*, CAE, classic JME, or ECME, do not respond in another syndrome, *e.g.*, Dravet syndrome, CAE evolving to JME, or MAE of Doose. This is why there is general agreement that selection of the best treatment options should be based not only on the correct determination of seizure types but also on the correct diagnosis of epilepsy syndrome (Camfield and Camfield, 2003). According to the experience of most epileptologists, the more combinations of seizure types a patient has, the harder it is to control seizures with AEDs, especially if absences persist from childhood (Wirrel, 2001 and 2003; Doose and Sitepu, 1983).

Another important observation, only recently emphasized, has been the aggravation of IGEs by the older-generation AEDs, *e.g.*, phenytoin and carbamazepine, as discussed by Dieter Schmidt in a separate chapter in this book. Others have reported that vigabatrin, tiagabine, and gabapentin aggravate myoclonic and absences epilepsies (Genton and McMenaim, 1998) and even induce myoclonic and absence status (Knake *et al.*, 1999; Pedersen *et al.*, 1985). In infrequent cases, lamotrigine has aggravated seizure frequency in myoclonic epilepsies (Biraben *et al.*, 2000).

Clearly, the response of the various grand mal seizure phenotypes, absences, myoclonias, or grand mal seizures to a particular AED must depend on the molecular defect(s) that underlie the specific epilepsy syndrome. This is the force that drives the search for molecular lesions in IGEs. Many posit that solving the molecular mysteries of IGEs will lead to novel remedies. If so, understanding how AEDs work in IGEs could point to the biochemical pathways used in epileptogenesis by epilepsy genes. The mechanisms of seizure-suppressing AEDs such as valproate, levetiracetam, topiramate, zonisamide, and lamotrigine in JME remain unexplained. Similarly, the reasons why ethosuximide has no effect, and phenytoin and carbamazepine can worsen seizures in JME, remain unexplained.

■ Molecular pathophysiology of "grand mal seizures" in IGEs

In addition to electroclinical-anatomical state, modern brain imaging, long-term outcome, and response to treatment, discoveries in the molecular pathophysiology of the epilepsies have helped improve nosology and has brought hope for a curative treatment. Perhaps none has been more dramatic than the unraveling of the myoclonic epilepsies of infancy and early childhood by discoveries of de novo mutations in SCN1A in sporadic severe myoclonic epilepsy of infancy (Dravet syndrome) and germline mutations in SCN1B, SCN2A, and SCN1A in generalized epilepsies with febrile seizures plus (GEFS+). In GEFS+, genetic pleiotropism played out as febrile seizures, myoclonic, atonic, grand mal, and absence seizures were observed in members of the same family ascertained through a proband with myoclonic astatic seizures. These discoveries have led to the separation of Dravet syndrome and GEFS+ from idiopathic MAE of Doose and ECME, which do not have mutations in SCN1A (Claes *et al.*, 2001), SCN1B, and SCN2A (Wallace *et al.*, 1998). Mutations in CLCN2 and myoclonin/EFHC1 substantiate the entity of JME, the latter no longer recognized as a single entity by the 2001 ILAE classification of epilepsy syndromes.

Similarly, mutations in GABRA1, GABRG2, and GABRB3 are associated with syndromes that have in common the presence of absence seizures. Finding separate chromosomal loci in specific IGEs can also help nosology. Three subvarieties of absence syndromes previously suggested by clinical epileptologists have different chromosome loci indicating different molecular lesions, namely: remitting CAE in chromosome 15q11-12 (Delgado-Escueta *et al.*, 2000); CAE that persists into adulthood with tonic-clonic convulsions in chromosome 8q24 (Fong, *et al.*, 1998); and CAE evolving to JME, nonallelic to all presently known epilepsy loci (Medina *et al.*, 2005). Future molecular genetic studies should tell us if the other subsyndromes of absence epilepsies such as absence epilepsy of early childhood starting before 5 years of age, myoclonic absence epilepsy in which myoclonias occur simultaneously with absence seizures, eyelid myoclonia with absences, and juvenile absence epilepsy truly exist as separate entities.

Similar advances in JME have occurred, providing us a glimpse of its complex genetics. *Table IV* shows the loci and genes currently associated with JME. Three mutation-harboring genes for JME have been identified to date. One is the GABA-receptor gene, which is unique to two large French-Canadian families with JME and one index case with absence epilepsy (Cossette *et al.*, 2002). The second gene is CLNC2, which was found in a large German family (Haug *et al.*, 2003). These two genes appear to be unique to these families and have not been found in other samples. The third gene found for JME was recently discovered in our laboratories (Suzuki *et al.*, 2004). Missense mutations in Myoclonin/EFHC1 in 6p12 co-segregated with 21 affected members from six of 24 unrelated families of native American-European ancestry with Hispanic culture from California and Mexico.

In 2004, we hypothesized that JME mutations, by compromising EFHC1's apoptotic activity through $Ca_v2.3$, prevent pruning and elimination of unwanted neurons/synapses during CNS development, lead to increased density of dystopic neurons (and synaptic trees) with dysregulated calcium homeostasis, produce thick cerebral cortex and scattered dystopic neurons predisposing to myoclonias and tonic clonic convulsions *(Figure 4)*. Noebels and colleagues suggest that dysregulated $Ca_v2.3$ tilts the balance to more low voltage activated T type calcium currents in thalamus, leading to cortical spike waves and absences.

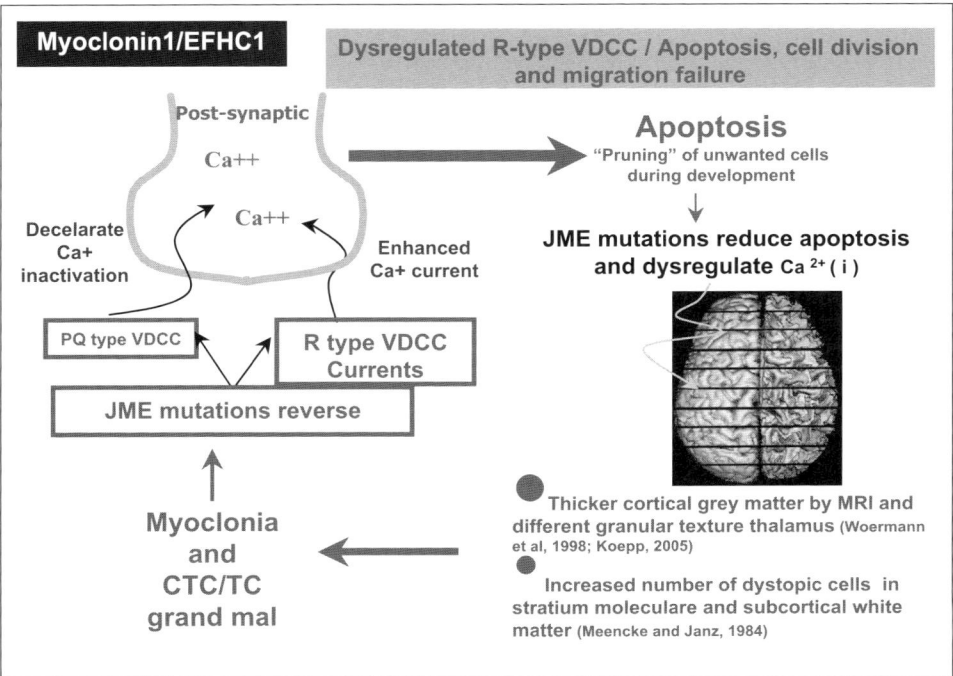

Figure 4. Pathogenesis of seizures in JME: Dysregulated $Ca_v2.3$ and apoptosis failure.

Table IV. Genes identified for grand mal, myoclonic and absence seizures in JME to date.

Locus		Country/Ethnic group	No. of families	Mode of inheritance	Phenotype	Author, year
6p12-11	EFHC1[a]	Los Angeles, California	22	AD	Classic JME and pCAE evolving to JME	Liu et al., 1996
		Belize	1	AD	Classic JME	Serratosa et al., 1996
		Mexico[b]	31	AD	Classic JME	Bai et al., 2002; Suzuki et al., 2004
6p12-11		Netherlands	18	AD	JME	Pinto et al., 2005
6p21.3	BRD2[a]	Los Angeles, California	24	AD	Classic JME	Greenberg et al., 1988
		New York[c]	85	AD	Classic JME mixed with CAE evolving to JME	Greenberg et al., 2000; Pal et al., 2003
6p21.3		Germany	29	AD	JME	Sander et al., 1997
15q14	CX36[d]	United Kingdom, Denmark, France, Greece, Portugal, Sweden	25	AR	JME	Elmslie et al., 1997; Mas et al., 2004
6q24		Saudi Arabia	34	AR	JME, some nonproband members with mild gait ataxia and tremors	Bate et al., 2000
2q22-2q23	CACNB4[a]	Germany	1	?	Classic JME with absences	Escayg et al., 2000
5q34GABR1	GABRA1[a]	French Canadian	1	AD	4/8 affected family members had pCAE. One with epilepsy onset at 5 y	Cossette et al., 2002
3q26	CLCN2[a]	Germany	1	AD	Classic JME	Haug et al., 2001, 2003
18	ME2[d]	European American	–	?	Classic JME	Greenberg et al., 2005

[a]Mutations; [b]European Amerind (Hispanics); [c]European American; [d]SNP associated variants; AD, autosomal dominant; AR, autosomal recessive; JME, juvenile myoclonic epilepsy; CAE, childhood absence epilepsy. See Durón et al., 2005 for further references.

Most recently, novel missense, nonsense, deletion and deletion/frameshift mutations have been found in Mexican, Honduran, and Japanese families. Myoclonin/EFHC1 mutations have now been found in 3 separate cohorts from our database accounting for 10% of JME at large. However, mutations and polymorphisms in Myoclonin/EFHC1 do not account for all our JME families in the Americas. There are obviously additional loci to be found that work alone or in conjunction with other loci to produce the JME phenotype and related syndromes presenting with tonic-clonic, clonic-tonic-clonic or clonic seizures.

References

Aicardi J. Myoclonic epilepsies of infancy and childhood. *Adv Neurol* 1986; 43: 11-31.

Aicardi J, Chevrie J. Myoclonic epilepsies of childhood. *Neuropädiatrie* 1971; 3: 177-90.

Aicardi J. Course and prognosis of certain childhood epilepsies with predominantly myoclonic seizures. In: Wada JA, Penry JK, eds. *Advances in epileptology: XIIth Epilepsy International Symposium*. New York: Raven Press, 1980: 159-63.

Alonso ME, Medina MT, Martínez-Juárez IE, *et al*. Familial juvenile myoclonic epilepsy. In: Delgado-Escueta AV, Guerrini R, Medina MT, Genton P, Bureau M, Dravet C, eds. *Myoclonic Epilepsies. Adv Neurol* 2005; 95: 227-44.

Baulac M, Gourfinkel-An I, Baulac S, Leguern E. Myoclonic seizures in the context of generalized epilepsy with febrile seizures plus (GEFS+). In: *Myoclonic Epilepsies*, Ed. A.V. Delgado-Escueta, R. Guerrini, M.T. Medina, P. Genton, M. Bureau, C. Dravet. *Adv Neurol* 2005; 95: 119-26.

Biraben A, Allain H, Scarbin JM, Schuck S, Edan G. Exacerbation of juvenile myoclonic epilepsy with lamotrigine. *Neurology* 2000; 55: 1758.

Bouma PA, Westendorp RG, van Dijk JG, Peters AC, Brouwer OF. The outcome of absence epilepsy: a meta-analysis. *Neurology* 1996; 47: 802-8.

Bureau M, Tassinari C. Myoclonic absences: the seizure and the syndrome. In: Roger J, Bureau M, Dravet C, Dreifuss FE, Perret A, Wolf P, eds. *Epileptic syndromes in infancy, childhood and adolescence*. 2ed. London: John Libbey, 2002: 175-83.

Camfield P, Camfield C. Childhood epilepsy: what is the evidence for what we think and what we do? *J Child Neurol* 2003; 18: 272-87.

Commission on Classification and Terminology of the International League against Epilepsy. Proposal for revised classification of epilepsies and epileptic syndromes. *Epilepsia* 1989; 30: 389-99.

Commission on Classification and Terminology of the International League Against Epilepsy. Proposal for revised clinical and electrographic classification of epileptic seizures. *Epilepsia* 1981 22: 489-501.

Cossette P, Loi L, Brisebois K, *et al*. Mutation of GABRA1 in an autosomal dominant form of juvenile myoclonic epilepsy. *Nat Genet* 2002; 31: 184-9.

Chaix Y, Daquin G, Monteiro F, Villeneuve N, Laguitton V, Genton P. Absence epilepsy with onset before age three years: a heterogeneous and often severe condition. *Epilepsia* 2003; 44 (7): 944-9.

Cavazzuti GB, Ferrari F, Galli B, Benatti A. Epilepsy with typical absence seizures with onset during the first year of life. *Epilepsia* 1989; 30: 802-6.

Charlton M, Yahr M. Long-term follow-up of patients with petit mal. *Arch Neurol* 1967; 16: 595-8.

Claes L, Del-Favero J, Ceulemans B, *et al*. De novo mutations in the sodium channels gene SCN1A cause severe myoclonic epilepsy of infancy. *Am J Hum Genet* 2001; 68: 1327-32.

Coulter DA, Huguenard JR, Prince DA. Characterization of ethosuximide reduction of low-threshold calcium current in thalamic neurons. *Ann Neurol* 1989; 25: 582-93.

Coulter DA, Huguenard JR, Prince DA. Differential effects of petit mal anticonvulsants and convulsants on thalamic neurones: calcium current reduction. *Br J Pharmacol* 1990; 100 (4): 800-6.

Delgado-Escueta AV, Serratosa JM and Medina MT. Juvenile Myoclonic Epilepsy. In: Elaine Wyllie, ed. *The Treatment of Epilepsy: Principles and Practice*. 2nd Ed. Baltimore: Williams and Wilkins, 1996; 33: 484-501.

Delgado-Escueta AV, Enrile BF. Juvenile myoclonic epilepsy of Janz. *Neurology* 1984; 34: 285-95.

Delgado-Escueta AV, Alonso M, Medina MT, Gee M, Fong CY. The search for epilepsy genes in juvenile myoclonic epilepsy: discoveries along the way. In: Schmitz B, Sander T, eds. *Juvenile myoclonic epilepsy: the Janz syndrome*. Petersfield: Wrightson Biomedical Publishing, 2000: 145-70.

Delgado-Escueta AV, Greenberg D, Weissbecker K, *et al*. Gene mapping in the idiopathic generalized epilepsies. Juvenile myoclonic epilepsy, childhood absence epilepsy, epilepsy with grand mal seizures and early childhood myoclonic epilepsy. *Epilepsia* 1990; 31 (Suppl 3): S19-29.

Delgado-Escueta AV, Medina MT, Bai D, *et al*. Genetics of Idiopathic myoclonic Epilepsies: An Overview. In: Myoclonus and Paroxysmal Dyskinesias. Fahn S, Frucht S, Hallett M, Truoung D. *Adv Neurol* 2002; 89: 161-84.

Doose H, Gerken H, Leonhardt R, *et al*. Centrencephalic myoclonic-astatic petit mal. Clinical and genetic investigations. *Neuropädiatrie* 1970; 2: 59-78.

Doose H. Myoclonic-astatic epilepsy. *Epilepsy Res* 1992; 6 (Suppl): 163-8.

Doose H, Baier WK. Epilepsy with primarily generalized myoclonic-astatic seizures: a genetically determined disease. *Eur J Pediatr* 1987; 146: 550-4.

Doose H, Sitepu B. Childhood epilepsy in a German city. *Neuropediatrics* 1983; 14: 220-4.

Durón RM, Medina MT, Martinez-Juarez IE, Bailey JN, Perez-Gosiengfiao KT, Ramos-Ramirez R, *et al*. Seizures of idiopathic generalized epilepsies. *Epilepsia* 2005; 46 (Suppl 9): 34-47.

Durón RM, Bailey JN, Maertinez-Juarez IE, Medina MT, Alonso ME, *et al*. The grand mal seizure phenotypes: Semiology, frequency and long-term follow-up in idiopathic generalized epilepsies. Submitted for publication, 2006.

Dravet C, Bureau M. Benign myoclonic epilepsy in infancy. In: *Epileptic Syndromes in Infancy, Childhood and Adolescence*, Ed. J. Roger, M. Bureau, C. Dravet, P. Genton, CA Tassinari, P. Wolf, 2005 : 77-88.

Dravet C, Bureau M, Oguni H, Fukuyama Y, Cokar O. Severe myoclonic epilepsy in infancy: Dravet syndrome. *Adv Neurol* 2005; 95: 71-102.

Fong C, Shan P, Huang Y, *et al*. Childhood absence epilepsy in and Indian (Bombay) family maps to chromosome 8q24. *Neurology* 1998; 50: A357.

Genton P, Gonzales-Sanchez MdS, Thomas P. Epilepsy with grand mal on awakening. In: Roger P, Bureau M, Dravet Ch, Genton P, Tassinari CA, Wolf P, eds. *Epileptic syndromes in infancy, childhood and adolescence*. 4ed. Montrouge: John Libbey Eurotext, 2005: 389-94.

Genton P, Roger J, Guerrini R, *et al*. History and classification of "myoclonic" epilepsies: from seizures to syndromes to diseases. *Adv Neurol* 2005; 95: 1-14.

Genton P, McMenamin J. Aggravation of seizures by antiepileptic drugs: what to do in clinical practice. *Epilepsia* 1998; 38: 26-9.

Giannakodimos S, Panayiotopoulos CP. Eyelid myoclonia with absences in adults: a clinical and video-EEG study. *Epilepsia* 1996; 37: 36-44.

Gowers WR. *A Manual of diseases of the nervous system*. 2ed. Philadelphia: P. Blakiston's Son & Co, 1901: vol. II, 735-6.

Haug K, Warnstedt M, Alekov AK, *et al*. Mutations in CLCN2 encoding a voltage-gated chloride channel are associated with idiopathic generalized epilepsies. *Nat Genet* 2003; 33: 527-32.

Hauser WA, Hesdorffer DC. *Epilepsy-frequency, causes and consequences*. New York: Demos Medical Publishing, 1990: 1-51.

Ishimoto T, Chiba S, Omori N. Convulsive seizures induced by alpha-amino-3-hydroxy-5-methyl-4-isoxazolepropionic acid microinjection into the mesencephalic reticular formation in rats. *Brain Res* 2004; 1021 (1): 69-75.

Jain S, Padma M, Maheshwari MC. Occurrence of only myoclonic jerks in juvenile myoclonic epilepsy. *Acta Neurol Scand* 1997; 95: 263-7.

Janz D. *Die Epilepsien*. Stuttgart: George Thieme Verlag, 1969.

Jallon P. Epilepsy in developing countries. *Epilepsia* 1997; 38: 1143-51.

Juul-Jenssen P, Foldspang A. Natural history of epileptic seizures. *Epilepsia* 1983: 24; 297-312.

Medina MT, Duron RM, Alonso ME, Dravet C, Leon L, Lopez-Ruiz M, Ramos-Ramirez R, et al. *Adv Neurol* 2005; 95: 197-215.

Livingston S, Torres I, Pauli LL, Rider RV. Petit mal epilepsy. Results of a prolonged follow-up study of 117 patients. *JAMA* 1965; 194: 227-32.

Knake S, Hamer HM, Schomburg U, Oertel WH, Rosenow F. Tiagabine-induced absence status in idiopathic generalized epilepsy. *Seizure* 1999; 8: 314-7.

Kelly KM, Gross RA, MacDonald RL. Valproic acid selectively reduces the low-threshold (T) calcium current in rat nodose neurons. *Neurosci Lett* 1990; 116: 233-8.

Koepp MJ. Juvenile myoclonic epilepsy – a generalized epilepsy syndrome? *Acta Neurol Scand* 2005; 181 (Suppl): 57-62.

Korinthenberg R, Bauer-Scheid C, Burkart P, Martens-Le Bouar H, Kassubek J, Juengling FD. 18FDG-PET in epilepsies of infantile onset with pharmacoresistant generalized tonic-clonic seizures. *Epilepsy Res* 2004; 60 (1): 53-61.

Kuzmiski JB, Barr W, Zamponi GW, MacVicar BA. Topiramate inhibits the initiation of plateau potentials in CA1 neurons by depressing R-type calcium channels. *Epilepsia* 2005; 46: 481-9.

Lennox W. The petit mal epilepsies. *JAMA* 1945; 129: 1069-73.

Martínez-Juárez IE, Alonso ME, Medina MT, Durón RD, Bailey JN, López-Ruiz M, et al. Juvenile myoclonic epilepsy subsyndromes: family studies and long term follow-up. *Brain* 2006; 129: 1269-80.

Medina, MT, Durón RM, Martínez, Osorio JR, Estrada AL, Zúñiga C, Cartagena D, Collins JS, Holden KR. Prevalence, incidence and causes of epilepsy in rural Honduras: the Salamá study. *Epilepsia* 2005; 46 (5): 1-8. Nicoletti A, Reggio A, Bartoloni A, et al. Prevalence of epilepsy in rural Bolivia: a door-to-door survey. *Neurology* 1999; 53: 2064-9.

Medina MT, Durón RM, Alonso ME, et al. Childhood absence evolving to juvenile myoclonic epilepsy: electroclinical and genetic features. *Adv Neurol* 2005; 95: 197-216.

Moraes MF, Mishra PK, Jobe PC, Garcia-Cairasco N. An electrographic analysis of the synchronous discharge patterns of GEPR-9s generalized seizures. *Brain Res* 2005; 1046 (1-2): 1-9.

Nail-Boucherie K, Le-Pham BT, Gobaille S, Maitre M, Aunis D, Depaulis A. Evidence for a role of the parafascicular nucleus of the thalamus in the control of epileptic seizures by the superior colliculus. *Epilepsia* 2005; 46 (1): 141-5.

Nersesyan H, Herman P, Erdogan E, Hyder F, Blumenfeld H. Relative changes in cerebral blood flow and neuronal activity in local microdomains during generalized seizures. *J Cereb Blood Flow Metab* 2004; 24 (9): 1057-68.

Niespodziany I, Klitgaard H, Margineanu DG. Levetiracetam: modulation of high-voltage-activated Ca+ currents in CA1 pyramidal neurons of rat hyppocampal slices. *Epilepsia* 2000; 31: 347.

Noebels JL. Modeling human epilepsies in mice. *Epilepsia* 2001; 42 (Suppl 5): 11-5.

Noebels JL. Exploring new gene discoveries in idiopathic generalized epilepsy. *Epilepsia* 2003; 44 (Suppl 2): 16-21.

Oguni H, Tanaka T, Hayashi K, et al. Treatment and long-term prognosis of myoclonic -astatic epilepsy of early childhood. *Neuropediatrics* 2002; 33: 122-32.

Olsson I, Hagberg G. Epidemiology of absence epilepsy. III. Clinical aspects. *Acta Paediatr Scand* 1991; 80: 1066-2.

Panayiotopoulus CP, Agathonikou A, Koutroumanidis M, Giannakodios S, Rowlinson S, Carr CP. Eyelid myoclonia with absences: the symptoms. In: Duncan J, Panayiotopoulos CP, eds. *Eyelid myoclonia with absences*. London: John Libbey, 1996: 17-26.

Pazzaglia P, Giovanardi R, Cirignotta F, et al. Nosografia delle epilessie miocloniche. *Rivista Italiana di EEG e Neurofisiología Clinica* 1978; 2: 245-52.

Pedersen SA, Klosterskow P, Gram L, Dam M. Long-term study of gamma-vinyl GABA in the treatment of epilepsy. *Acta Neurol Scand* 1985; 72: 295-8.

Raisinghani M, Faingold CL. Pontine reticular formation neurons are implicated in the neuronal network for generalized clonic seizures which is intensified by audiogenic kindling. *Brain Res* 2005 ; 1064 (1-2): 90-7.

Rodin E. Paper recordings of ultrafast frequencies in experimental epilepsy. *Clin EEG Neurosci* 2005; 36 (4): 263-70.

Sato S, Dreifuss FE, Penry JK, Kirby DD, Palesch Y. Long-term follow-up of absence seizures. *Neurology* 1983; 33: 1590-5.

Suzuki S Kawahami K, Nishimura S, et al. Zonisamide blocks T-type calcium channel in cultured neurons of rat cerebral cortex. *Epilepsy Res* 1992; 12: 21-7.

Suzuki T, Delgado-Escueta A, Aguan K, et al. Mutations in EFHC1 cause juvenile myoclonic epilepsy. *Nat Genet* 2004; 36: 842-9.

Tassinari CA, Bureau M, Thomas P. Epilepsy with myoclonic absences. In: Roger J, Bureau M, Dravet C, Dreifuss FE, Perret A, Wolf P, eds. *Epileptic syndromes in infancy, childhood and adolescence*. 2ed. London: John Libbey, 1992: 151-60.

Velasco M, Velasco F, Alcala H, Diaz de Leon AE. Wakefulness-sleep modulation of EEG-EMG epileptiform activities: a quantitative study on a child with intractable epilepsia partialis continua. *Int J Neurosci* 1990; 54 (3-4): 325-37.

Wallace RH, Wang D, Singh R, et al. Febrile seizures and generalized epilepsy associated with a mutation in the Na+ -channel beta 1 subunit gene SCN1B. *Nature Genet* 1998; 19: 366-70.

Wirrel EC, Camfield CS, Camfield PR, et al. Long-term prognosis of typical childhood absence epilepsy: remission of progression to juvenile myoclonic epilepsy. *Neurology* 1996; 47: 912-8.

Wirrell E. Natural history of absence epilepsy in children. *Can J Neurol Sci* 2003; 30: 184-8.

Wirrel E, Camfield C, Camfield D, et al. Prognostic significance of failure of the initial antiepileptic drugs in children with absence epilepsy. *Epilepsia* 2001; 42: 760-3.

Woermann FG, Sisodiya SM, Free SL, Duncan JS. Quantitative MRI in patients with idiopathic generalized epilepsy. Evidence of widespread cerebral structural changes. *Brain* 1998; 121 (Pt 9): 1661-7.

Wolf P, Inoue Y. Juvenile absence epilepsy. In: Roger J, Bureau M, Dravet C, Genton P, Tassinari CA, Wolf P, eds. *Epileptic syndromes in infancy, childhood and adolescence*. 3ed. London: John Libbey, 2002: 331-4.

Zara F, De Falco FA. Autosomal recessive benign myoclonic epilepsy of infancy. In: *Myoclonic Epilepsies*, Ed. A.V. Delgado-Escueta, R. Guerrini, M.T. Medina, P. Genton, M. Bureau, C. Dravet. *Adv Neurol* 2005; 95: 139-46.

Zhang X, Velumian AA, Jones OT, et al. Modulation of high voltage-activated calcium channels in dentate granule cells by topiramate. *Epilepsia* 2000; 41 (Suppl): S52-60.

Zhang Y, Vilaythong AP, Yoshor D, Noebels J. Elevated thalamic low-voltage-activated currents precede the onset of absence epilepsy in the SNAP25-deficient mouse mutant coloboma. *J Neurosci* 2004; 24 (22): 5239-48.

Zhang YF, Gibbs III JW, Coulter DA. Anticonvulsant drug effects on spontaneous thalamocortical rhythms *in vitro*: ethosuximide, trimethadione, and dimethadione. *Epilepsy Res* 1996; 23: 15-36.

Zivanovic D, Stanojlovic O, Stojanovic J, Susic V. Induction of audiogenic seizures in imipenem/cilastatin-treated rats. *Epilepsy Behav* 2004; 5 (2): 151-8.

Section VI:
The "cortical" and "centrencephalic" theories revisited

Cortical trigger in generalized seizures

Fernando Lopes da Silva

Center of Neurosciences, Swammerdam Institute for Life Sciences, Faculty of Science, University of Amsterdam, The Netherlands.

■ Absence-type seizures: generalized or not? Experimental evidence for a focal nature

Classically absence seizures or "petit mal" seizures are considered par excellence the paradigm of primary generalized epilepsies (PGE). They are characterized by a sudden arrest of ongoing behaviour and conscious awareness, while the electroencephalogram (EEG) displays the abrupt onset and cessation of bilaterally synchronous 3/second spike-and-wave discharges (SWDs) over wide cortical areas (Niedermeyer and Lopes da Silva 2005). The generalized nature of the discharges led to the hypothesis of a common central (midline subcortical) pacemaker (Jasper & Kershman, 1941). However, the relative contributions of thalamus and cortex to the pathophysiology of this kind of disorder are still a matter of debate among clinicians and experimental researchers.

Extensive investigation of the feline penicillin generalized epilepsy (FPGE) model revealed that the generation of SWDs is closely linked to the mechanisms that mediate spindles (Gloor et al., 1990). The cellular mechanisms that underlie the generation of *spindle oscillations* in the thalamic *microcircuits* have been elucidated to a great extent (*e.g.* reviewed in Steriade & Llinás, 1988; McCormick & Bal, 1997, Steriade et al., 1997). The prevalent common assumption is that the same neuronal mechanisms also apply for the generation of generalized SWDs. It has been assumed also that the generalization process requires the synchronization of widely distributed thalamocortical networks. As mechanism responsible for this massive synchronization the recurrent oscillatory activity in the network between cells of the reticular thalamic nucleus (RTN) and thalamocortical relay (TCR) cells (*e.g.* Buzsáki, 1991, McCormick & Bal, 1997; Avanzini et al., 2000) has been proposed, but no experimental proof for this interpretation has, as yet, been advanced. We approached this issue using a genetic model of absence epilepsy, the WAG/Rij rat (Coenen et al.,

1992). The basic question that we formulated was the following: *In the intact brain of WAG/Rij rats is it possible to find out whether SWDs are initiated in the cortex or in the thalamus, and to estimate how these discharges evolve in the brain?*

This question was approached by a quantified analysis of the interrelations of local EEG signals recorded simultaneously from multiple cortical and thalamic sites, during SWDs in the freely moving WAG/Rij rat. The dynamics of the evolution of SWDs, both on the cortical surface and in the thalamus, was quantified using signal analysis methods based on the estimation of nonlinear signal associations (Pijn et al., 1989).

A cortical "focus" was found within the peri-oral sub-region of the somatosensory cortex *(Figure 1)*. This leading focus was found consistently in the first 500 ms of a SWD. This timing was essential, since as the SWDs evolve in the course of time the relationships become more complex. Thalamic and other cortical sites were consistently found to lag behind this focal site, with time delays that increased with electrode distance, resulting in a "whole seizure" propagation velocity over the cortex of 1.4 m/s averaged over animals. These results show that the large-scale synchronization during the initial stage of generalized SWDs primarily arises from intracortical processes. After the initial period of 500 ms the time relations between cortex and thalamus could switch directions in an unpredictable way, indicating that during the whole SWDs cortex and thalamus forms one complex oscillatory network, where a leading area cannot be identified. The leading role for the cortex is corroborated by our observation that cortical spike-and-waves could sometimes occur without concomitant thalamic spike-and-waves, whereas the reverse was never observed.

These results challenge two common assumptions. First, instead of being non-focal, Absence-type seizures are of focal origin. The generalized and apparent "synchronous" character of the SWDs from the outset is caused by an extremely fast cortical spread of seizure activity. Second, the primary driving source for the rhythmic discharges is, in the WAG/Rij experimental model, not the thalamus but the cortex. However, after the oscillation has started cortex and thalamus form one complex oscillatory network, in which oscillations in both structures are interlocked. The role of the thalamus probably lies in providing a resonant circuit to amplify and sustain the SWDs. The latter can be considered an emerging property of this neuronal circuit.

■ Routes to Absence-type seizures. Lessons from computational modeling

SWDs are complex phenomena that depend on the activity of neuronal networks interconnected by a diversity of synaptic connections and neurons with a variety of ionic channels and receptor mediated processes. This complexity makes a comprehensive analysis of the underlying cellular and network phenomena rather cumbersome. We thought that computational modelling could help understanding the complex behaviour of these networks leading to the generation of SWDs. It is currently believed that the mechanisms underlying SWDs may be related to the thalamocortical mechanisms of sleep spindle generation (Steriade 2005; Avoli et al., 2001; McCormick and Contreras, 2001). With respect to understanding the pathophysiology of Absence-type seizures, however, it is necessary to understand how *spontaneous*

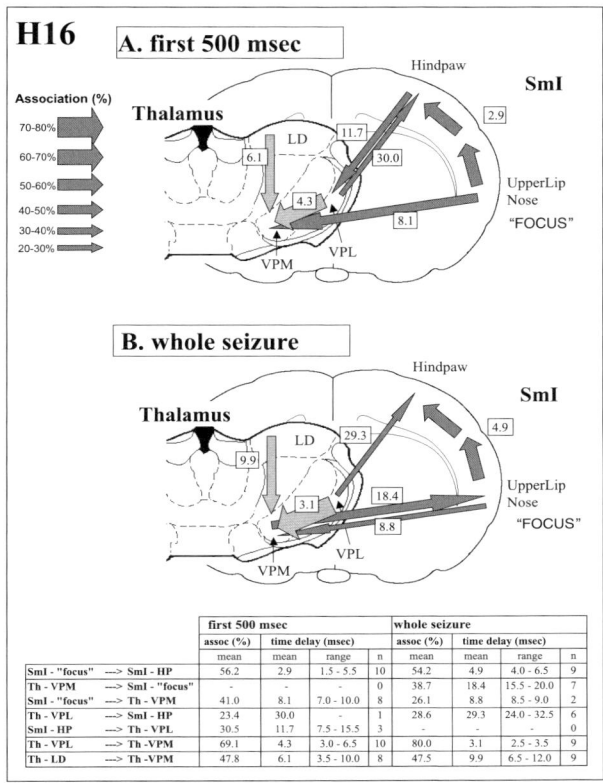

Figure 1. Summary of the cortico-cortical (represented by the black arrows), intra-thalamic (light gray arrows), and cortico-thalamic (dark gray arrows) interdependencies during spontaneous absence seizures in the WAG/Rij rat as established by the nonlinear association analysis. The thickness of the arrow represents the average strength of the association, and the direction of the arrowhead points to the direction of the lagging site. The values represent the corresponding average time delays in milliseconds. For this rat, 10 seizures were analyzed.
A, The relationships as found for the first 500 msec of the generalized seizure. A consistent cortical focus was found in the upper lip and nose area of the somatosensory cortex (SmI), because this site consistently led the other cortical recording sites. The hindpaw area, for instance, was found to lag by 2.9 msec on average with respect to this focal site. Within the thalamus, the laterodorsal (LD) nucleus was found to consistently lead other thalamic sites. The ventroposterior medial (VPM) nucleus was found to lag behind the ventroposterior lateral (VPL) nucleus, with an average time delay of 4.3 msec. Concerning corticothalamic interrelationships, the cortical focus site consistently led the thalamus (VPM), with an average time delay of 8.1 msec. Within the somatosensory system of the hindpaw, the (nonfocal) cortical site led the thalamic site (VPL) during 3 of 10 seizures; the thalamus led the cortex during 1 seizure, whereas for the other 6 seizures no direction of the delay could be established.
B, The relationships as found when the whole seizure is analyzed as one epoch. The same cortical focus as during the first 500 msec was found consistently. Compared with the first 500 msec, the time delay from the cortical focus with respect to the nonfocal cortical sites has increased. Furthermore, the strength of association between VPL and VPM has increased. The direction of the cortico-thalamic couplings has changed. For the nonfocal cortical sites, the thalamus was found to lead during all seizures. For the focal cortical site, the cortex was found to lead during two seizures, whereas the thalamus was found to lead during seven seizures. (Adapted from Meeren et al., 2002).

transitions between normal on-going oscillations and paroxysmal SWDs occur. Of course, a patient is not seizing all the time. Thus a realistic model network has to account for *both the normal oscillatory activity and the SWDs, as well as for the transition between these two kinds of activities*. The main point is that a general hypothesis that may account for these dynamical phenomena has not been forthcoming. Therefore we constructed such a general model that may account for the generation of SWDs out of a background of on-going normal EEG oscillations. We assumed that a computational model that takes into account the most relevant (patho)physiological experimental findings (reviewed in McCormick, 2002; Destexhe and Sejnowski, 2003) would be an appropriate tool that could contribute to reach such a comprehensive view. A number of detailed, distributed models of thalamic and thalamocortical networks were developed (*e.g.*, Wang at al., 1995, Lytton *et al.*, 1997, Destexhe 1998, 1999). These models have given insight into some basic neuronal mechanisms of SW discharges, but do not address specifically the most essential issue of this type of epileptic activity: *that a given thalamocortical loop can display both kinds of activity, normal oscillations and SWDs, without specific adjustments of parameters being expressly made*. Indeed the essence of epilepsy is that a patient displays (long) periods of normal EEG activity (*i.e.* non-epileptiform) intermingled with epileptiform paroxysmal activity only occasionally. Thus, the main aim of the present study was to find out the mechanisms responsible for *transitions* from normal activity to paroxysmal SW discharges.

We developed the model (model scheme in *figure 2*) at the intermediate level between the distributed neuronal network and lumped circuit levels and focussed on EEG activities that are commonly recorded from genetic animal models of absence epilepsy, namely the WAG/Rij rat (van Luijtelaar and Coenen, 1986; Coenen and van Luijtelaar, 2003) and the GAERS (Marescaux *et al.*, 1992), as published in detail by Suffczynski *et al.* (2004). Without entering here into a detailed description, it is sufficient to note that the model can exhibit two qualitatively different types of behavior, such as seen in the experimental animals (WAG/Rij and GAERS) and in patients with Absences. The output signal may display a waxing and waning "spindle-like" oscillation having a spectrum with a peak at approximately 11 Hz or a high amplitude "seizure-like" oscillation or SWDs. We refer to the former behavior as "normal on-going" activity while to the latter as paroxysmal activity. The model output in this regime is shown in *figure 3*, upper panel. The lower panel depicts the corresponding power spectra.

The *bifurcation* behavior of the model depends essentially on the non-linear properties of a number of cellular components. In short, during normal activity the thresholds for the activation of GABA-B receptors in the Thalamo-Cortical (TC) and Pyramidal cells (PY) are not reached. When one of these thresholds is surpassed, GABA-B receptor mediated IPSPs may be triggered, which results in the sudden transition of the model's behavior from "normal on-going" activity to SWDs large amplitude oscillations. The frequency and amplitude of paroxysmal oscillations depend on the relative contribution of GABA-A and GABA-B components.

A dynamical analysis of the model showed that *bifurcations* cannot take place when input signals are constant. This implies that random fluctuations that are introduced into the system by noise in cortical and sensory inputs are necessary for the transitions

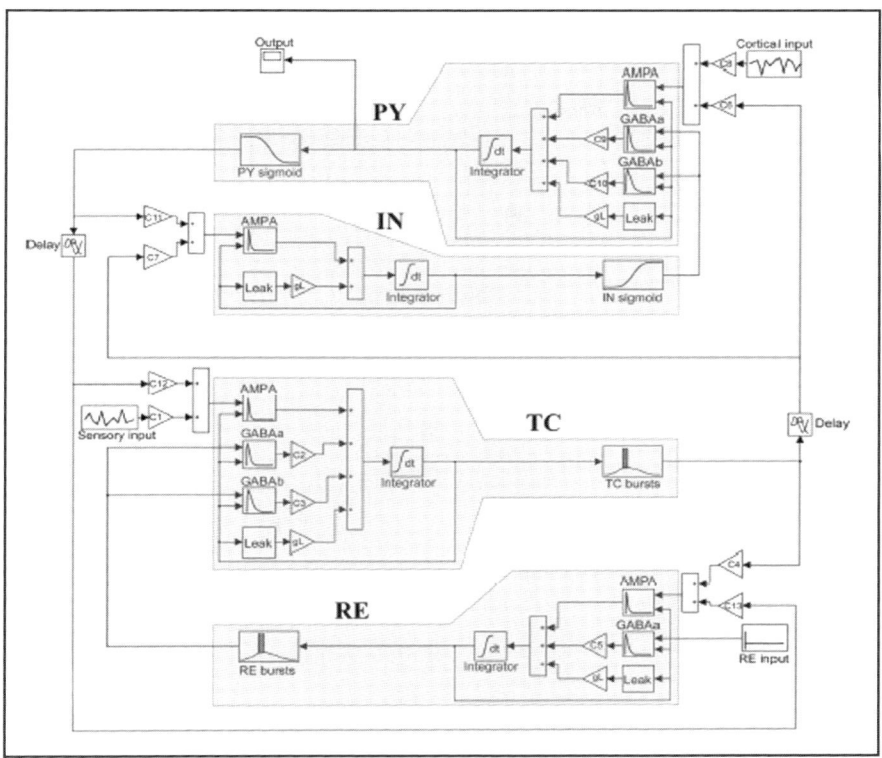

Figure 2. Model diagram: Thalamocortical network model consisting of interconnected cortical and thalamic modules. The cortical module consists of two interconnected populations of pyramidal (PY) cells and cortical interneurons (IN). In both populations membrane leakage and postsynaptic AMPA, and GABA-A, and GABA-B (both in the PY population only) currents are assumed to contribute to the mean membrane potential. Changes of mean membrane potential are transformed into firing densities. In both cortical populations the transformations between mean membrane potential and firing density are described by sigmoidal functions. The PY population receives external excitatory input. The model output is the mean membrane potential of the PY population. The thalamic module consists of two interconnected populations of thalamocortical (TC) and reticular nucleus (RE) neurons. In the TC and RE populations, membrane leakage and postsynaptic AMPA, GABA-A and GABA-B (slow GABA-B is present in the TC population only) currents contribute to mean membrane potential. The latter is transformed into firing density using transformation functions. The TC population receives sensory input whereas the RE population receives external inhibitory input. Coupling constants c1-c13 represent the average numbers of connections between different cell types. (Adapted from Suffczynski *et al.*, 2005).

to occur. A set of simulations revealed that the transition between the "normal on-going" and the SWDs modes occurs when the cortical input increases beyond a given bifurcation point. As the cortical input is subsequently decreased there is a jump from large amplitude limit cycle oscillations (SWDs) back to equilibrium state but this takes place at a lower value of the cortical input. This is manifestation of *hysteresis*. Thus such a network has two dynamical states that are locally stable in the sense that under small perturbations of finite-time duration the system returns to its original state. Therefore we can call such system a *bistable system*.

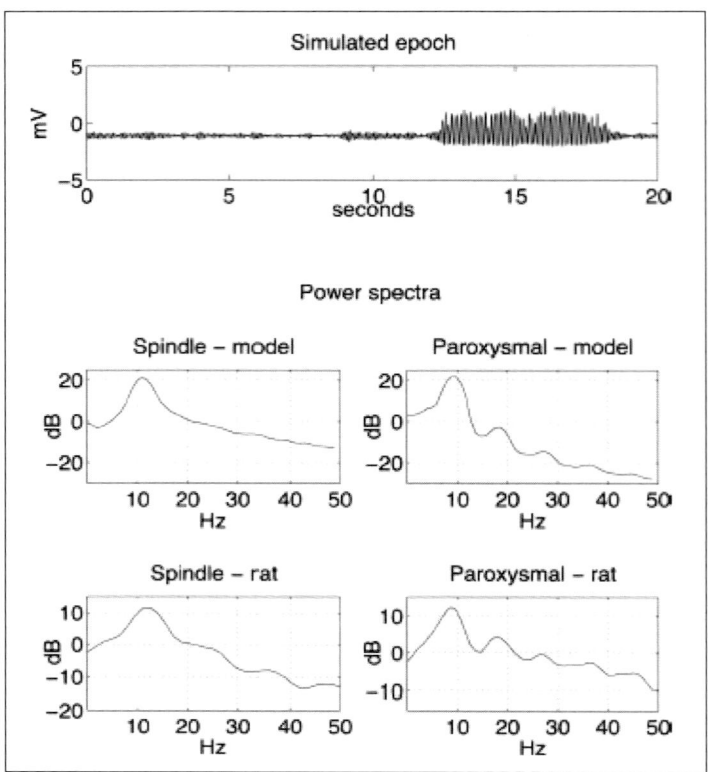

Figure 3. Example of model output.
Upper panel: Twenty seconds of simulation with the occurrence of a spontaneous paroxysmal (SWD) episode. Lower panels: Power spectra of simulated normal and SWD, paroxysmal activity, in the model in the WAG/Rij epileptic rat. Dominant frequency of normal activity is around 11 Hz whereas that of paroxysmal activity is around 9 Hz.
(Adapted from Suffczynski et al., 2005).

A mathematical model acquires added value if it may lead to *predictions* that may be tested experimentally. The present model allowed predicting that the onset and cessation of SWDs should occur randomly over time with certain probabilities. Accordingly, the distribution of the duration of paroxysmal and normal epochs can be predicted to be exponential, or gamma functions. Therefore the construction of histograms of the durations of paroxysmal and normal epochs from simulated and experimental time series offers a way to verify these theoretical predictions regarding the dynamics of the process leading to spontaneous paroxysmal discharges as described in more detail in Suffczynski et al. (2005) and illustrated in *figure 4*. A first observation is that in a number of ictal and interictal data the parameter α (see caption of *figure 4*) is close to one, which is consistent with the model predictions and suggests that epileptic transitions are random in time with fixed probability of occurrence, *i.e.* they represent a Poisson process. The second observation is that the dynamical processes obtaining during ictal epochs are, in general, different with respect to those obtaining during the interictal state. A majority of ictal epochs have the α parameter larger

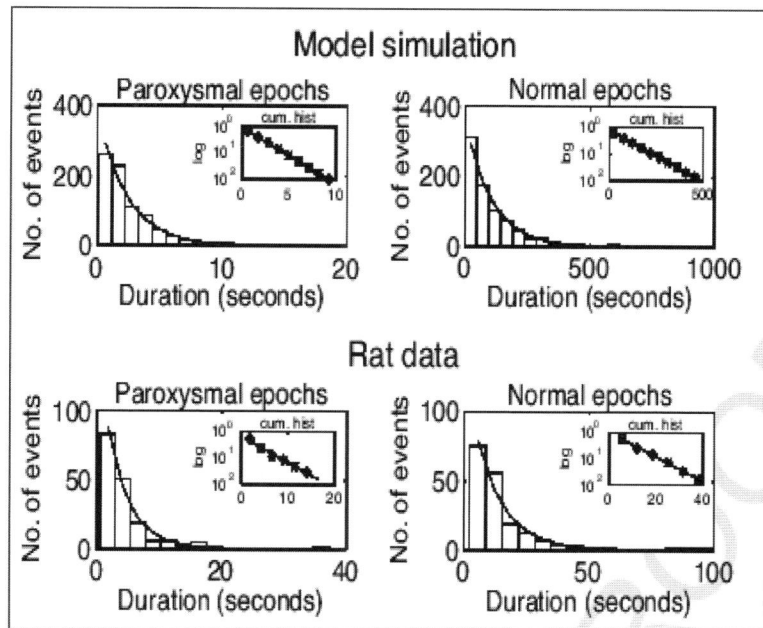

Figure 4. Distributions of lengths of normal and paroxysmal epochs of the simulated signal (upper panel) and of real EEG signal recorded from the rat (lower panel). On each plot an exponential function fitted to the histogram is shown. Model histograms were obtained by simulating 24 h of activity using the reference parameters set. Histograms of rat data were obtained from 30 min recording of EEGs of WAG/Rij rat after administration of high dose of vigabatrin. In all four distributions shown, the divergence between the observed histogram and fitted function is small and we were not able to reject the null hypothesis that the observed histogram scores came from the fitted exponential distribution even when tested at high significance level. Insets in each window depict cumulative histograms shown on logarithmic scale and straight lines fitted to histogram points. In all four plots the lines fit well the histograms' points further confirming exponential distributions. More in general both ictal and interictal durations distributions can be fitted with a gamma distribution:
$y = Cx^\alpha e^{-x/\beta}$ where α and β are distribution parameters and C is a normalization constant. Gamma distributions are flexible in terms of their overall shape. The shape is determined by the shape parameter, α. For $\alpha < 1$ the distribution has the maximum at the origin and is monotonically decreasing, for $\alpha = 1$ the distribution has an exponential shape, and for $\alpha > 1$ the distribution has zero at the origin and maximum at a nonzero value.
(Adapted from Suffczynski *et al.*, 2004, 2005).

than one, which suggests that one or more system parameters are changing gradually after seizure initiation. In such case seizures duration is reproducible to some extent. On the contrary, interictal epochs are described predominantly with α parameter smaller than one; this reveals that the transition probability is not constant and decreases over time measured from the moment of the previous transition. This kind of dynamics results in the occurrence of clusters of seizures, separated by long interictal periods.

Discussion and Conclusions

The experimental and modeling findings presented above allow us to draw a number of conclusions: The experimental results demonstrate that Absence-type seizures are of *focal cortical origin*. These findings have already led to fruitful new investigations in order to determine whether the focal cortical area of the somato-sensory cortex has particular properties that may differentiate it from other cortical areas and make it more prone for the initiation of SWDs. Interestingly bilateral injection of the anti-absence drug Ethosuximide at multiple cortical and thalamic loci in GAERS, leads to a decrease of the incidence of SWDs only in case the drug is injected in the somato-motor cortex and not in other cortical or thalamic areas. Therefore, Ethosuximide to be most effective should affect the focal cortical zone (Manning *et al.*, 2004). Furthermore Sitnikova and Luijtelaar (2004) made unilateral microinjections (1 microl) of 2% lidocaine into the somato-sensory cortex (SmI) in 13 WAG/Rij rats and found that this reduced the incidence of SWDs on the entire cortex in both hemispheres. The number of SWDs gradually reached control level at the end of the second hour after injections of lidocaine, indicating that proper functioning of SmI is important for the occurrence of SWDs. In addition, this focal cortical area appears to have a number of other peculiarities that make it more epilepsy-prone, namely the following, (see also van Luijtelaar *et al.* this Volume); – increase of NMDA-receptor mediated excitatory synaptic activity was found in pyramidal cells of deep layers of the same cortical focal area (D'Antuono *et al.* 2006); – alterations in the expression of voltage sensitive sodium channels mRNA (quantitative PCR) and the corresponding protein (immunocytochemistry) in cortical neurons in the WAG/Rij absence epileptic rat were found (Klein *et al.* 2004); mRNA levels for sodium channels Nav1.1 and Nav1.6, but not Nav1.2, were found to be up-regulated selectively within the facial somatosensory cortex; Protein levels for Nav1.1 and Nav1.6 were up-regulated in layer II-IV cortical neurons in this region of cortex. No significant changes were seen in adjacent regions or other brain areas, including the pre-frontal and occipital cortex. Indeed this region of cortex approximately matches the electrophysiologically determined region of seizure onset.

Furthermore Blumenfeld and collaborators (Nersesyan *et al.* 2004) investigated whether during SWDs the cortical activation had a focal or a generalized character, using blood oxygen level-dependent (BOLD) functional magnetic resonance imaging (fMRI) measurements at 7T with simultaneous EEG recordings. During spontaneous SWDs in WAG/Rij rats they found increased fMRI signals in focal regions including the perioral somato-sensory cortex, whereas the occipital cortex was spared. For comparison this was not the case for bicuculline-induced generalized tonic-clonic seizures under the same conditions, where the fMRI increases were larger and more widespread than during SWDs. These findings support the conclusion that SWDs have a focal cortical origin.

The modelling studies and the subsequent statistical observations regarding the durations of ictal and inter-ictal epochs led to novel insights into physiological mechanisms of ictal transitions. The model assumed, in first instance, that transitions between normal oscillations and SWDs would occur randomly due to fluctuations of cortical input. Although this is the case for a number of experimental observations both in human and in the rat experimental models, some interesting exceptions were noted. In these cases we should assume that there are other physiological mechanisms involved in seizure initiation and termination that have not been implemented in the model. The current analysis offers some clues regarding the additional physiological mechanisms responsible for seizure generation. For instance, in all patients with absence seizures, ictal durations during daytime yield higher values of α than those during night time. Such a variation suggests that at least in these patients deterministic mechanisms of seizure termination are predominantly operating during wakefulness. This may be related to a possible hormonally regulation related to the sleep-waking cycle in patients with IGE (Andermann and Berkovic, 2001, Lin *et al.*, 2002). In addition, in WAG/Rij rats the α parameter is larger than one in all saline rats, while α is equal to one in all vigabatrin treated animals. Since vigabatrin is a GABA transaminase inhibitor and thus increases GABA concentration, such change of the value of α suggests that seizure termination mechanisms depend on endogenous GABA levels in the brain.

In many cases an alpha parameter larger than one was obtained for most of the interictal durations, what corresponds to a tendency for seizures to occur in clusters. Indeed in human day and night recordings, seizure clustering could be *e.g.*, attributed to the fact that seizure incidence depends on the state of vigilance and sleep stage (Nagao *et al.*, 1990; Horita 2001; Amzica, 2002). However this cannot be the only explanation for the seizures clustering phenomenon since it is also present in some relatively short recordings, *e.g.*, lasting 30 minutes in WAG/Rij rats under vigabatrin. One cannot exclude that in these cases changes of extra- or intracellular ion concentrations during SWDs might modulate neuronal excitability, as has been shown experimentally (Moody *et al.*, 1974; McNamara, 1994).

The modelling study permits also to approach the question whether absence seizures may be predicted in a general way. Indeed the prediction of the exact timing of Absence seizure occurrence is not possible and it can be only approached in the probabilistic way.

Acknowledgements: This overview would not be possible without the collaboration of a number of colleagues, namely Hanneke Meeren, Gilles Luijtelaar, Stiliyan Kalitzin, Piotr Suffczynski, Jaime Parra, Dimitri Velis, whose contributions are gratefully acknowledged.

References

Amzica F. Physiology of sleep and wakefulness as it relates to the physiology of epilepsy. *J Clin Neurophysiol* 2002; 19: 488-503.

Andermann F, Berkovic SF. Idiopathic generalized epilepsy with generalized and other seizures in adolescence. *Epilepsia* 2001; 42: 317-20.

Avanzini G, Panzica F, De Curtis M. The role of the thalamus in vigilance and epileptogenic mechanisms. *Clin Neurophysiol* 2000; 111 (Suppl 2): S19-S26.

Avoli M, Rogawski A, Avanzini G. Generalized epileptic disorders: An update. *Epilepsia* 2001; 42: 445-57.

Buzsáki G. The thalamic clock: emergent network properties. *Neurosci* 1991; 41 (2/3): 351-64.

Coenen AML, Drinkenburg WHIM, Inoue M, Van Luijtelaar ELJM. Genetic models of absence epilepsy, with emphasis on the WAG/Rij strain of rats. *Epilepsy Res* 1992; 12: 75-86.

Coenen AML, van Luijtelaar ELJM. Genetic animal models for absence epilepsy: a review of the WAG/Rij strain of rats. *Behav Genet* 2003; 33 (6): 635-55.

D'Antuono M, Inaba Y, Biagini G, D'Argancelo V, Avoli M. Synaptic hyperexcitability of deep layer neocortical cells in a genetic model of absence seizures. *Genes, Brain and Behavior*, 2006 (in press).

Destexhe A. Spike-and-wave oscillations based on the properties of GABAB receptors. *J Neurosci* 1998; 18: 9099-111.

Destexhe A. Can GABAA conductances explain the fast oscillation frequency of absence seizures in rodents? *Eur J Neurosci* 1999; 11: 2175-81.

Destexhe A, Sejnowski TJ. Interactions between membrane conductances underlying thalamocortical slow-wave oscillations. *Physiol Rev* 2003t; 83 (4): 1401-53.

Gloor P, Avoli M, Kostopoulos G. Thalamocortical relationships in generalized epilepsy with bilaterally synchronous spike-and-wave discharge. In: Avoli M, Gloor P, Kostopoulos G, Naquet R, Eds. *Generalized Epilepsy: Neurobiological Approaches*. Boston: Birkhäuser, 1990: 190-212.

Horita H. Epileptic seizures and sleep-wake rhythm. *Psychiatry Clin Neurosci* 2001; 55: 171-2.

Jasper HH, Kershman J. Electroencephalographic classification of the epilepsies. *Arch Neurol Psychiat (Chicago)* 1941; 45: 903-43.

Klein JP, Khera DS, Nersesyan H, Kimchi EY, Waxman SG, Blumenfeld H. Dysregulation of sodium channel expression in cortical neurons in a rodent model of absence epilepsy. *Brain Res* 2004; 1000 (1-2): 102-9.

Lin SH, Arai AC, Espana RA, Berridge CW, Leslie FM, Huguenard JR,Vergnes M, Civelli O. Prolactin-releasing peptide (PrRP) promotes awakening and suppresses absence seizures. *Neuroscience* 2002; 114: 229-38.

Lytton WW, Contreras D, Destexhe A, Steriade M. Dynamic interactions determine partial thalamic quiescence in a computer network model of spike-and-wave seizures. *J Neurophysiol* 1997; 77: 1676-96.

Manning JP, Richards DA, Leresche N, Crunelli V, Bowery NG. Cortical-area specific block of genetically determined absence seizures by ethosuximide. *Neuroscience* 2004; 123 (1): 5-9.

Marescaux C, Vergnes M, Depaulis A. Genetic absence epilepsy in rats from Strasbourg – a review. *J Neural Transm Suppl* 1992; 35: 37-69.

McCormick DA, Bal T. Sleep and arousal: thalamocortical mechanisms. *Annu Rev Neurosci* 1997; 20: 185-215.

McCormick DA, Contreras D. On the cellular and network bases of epileptic seizures. *Annu Rev Physiol* 2001; 63: 815-46.

McNamara JO. Cellular and molecular basis of epilepsy. *J Neurosci* 1994; 14: 3413-25.

Meeren HK, Pijn JP, Van Luijtelaar EL, Coenen AM, Lopes da Silva FH. Cortical focus drives widespread corticothalamic networks during spontaneous absence seizures in rats. *J Neurosci* 2002; 22 (4): 1480-95.

Meeren H, van Luijtelaar G, Lopes da Silva F, Coenen A. Evolving concepts on the pathophysiology of absence seizures: the cortical focus theory. *Arch Neurol* 2005; 62 (3): 371-6.

Moody WJ, Futamachi KJ, Prince DA. Extracellular potassium activity during epileptogenesis. *Exp Neurol* 1974; 42: 248-63.

Nagao H, Morimoto T, Takahashi M, Habara S, Nagai H, Matsuda H. The circadian rhythm of typical absence seizures – the frequency and duration of paroxysmal discharges. *Neuropediatrics* 1990; 21: 79-82.

Nersesyan H, Hyder F, Rothman DL, Blumenfeld H. Dynamic fMRI and EEG recordings during spike-wave seizures and generalized tonic-clonic seizures in WAG/Rij rats. *J Cereb Blood Flow Metab* 2004; 24 (6): 589-99.

Niedermeyer E, Lopes da Silva FH. Electroencephalography: Basic principles, Clinical Applications and Related Fields. Lippincott, Williams and Wilkins, Philadelphia, Fifth edition, 2005.

Pijn JPM, Vijn PCM, Lopes da Silva FH, Van Emde Boas W, Blanes W. The use of signal-analysis for the localization of an epileptogenic focus: a new approach. *Advances in Epileptology* 1989; 17: 272-6.

Sitnikova E, van Luijtelaar G. Cortical control of generalized absence seizures: effect of lidocaine applied to the somatosensory cortex in WAG/Rij rats. *Brain Res* 2004; 1012 (1-2): 127-37.

Steriade M, Jones EG, McCormick DA. Thalamus, Volume I: Organisation and Function. Elsevier; Amsterdam, 1997, etc.

Steriade M, Llinás RR. The functional states of the thalamus and the associated neuronal interplay. *Physiol Rev* 1988; 68 (3): 649-742.

Steriade M. Sleep, epilepsy and thalamic reticular inhibitory neurons. *Trends Neurosci* 2005; 28 (6): 317-24.

Suffczynski P, Kalitzin S, Lopes Da Silva FH. Dynamics of non-convulsive epileptic phenomena modeled by a bistable neuronal network. *Neuroscience* 2004; 126 (2): 467-84.

Suffczynski P, Lopes da Silva FH, Parra J, Velis D, Kalitzin S. Epileptic Transitions: Model Predictions and Experimental Validation. *J Clin Neurophysiol* 2005; 22 (5): 288-99.

Van Luijtelaar ELJM, Coenen AML. Two types of electrocortical paroxysms in an inbred strain of rats. *Neurosci Lett* 1986; 70: 393-7.

Wang XJ, Golomb D, Rinzel J. Emergent spindle oscillations and intermittent burst firing in a thalamic model: Specific neuronal parameters. *Proc Natl Acad Sci USA* 1995; 92: 5577-81.

Section VII:
Phenomenology *versus* networks: clinical consequences

Why can some antiepileptic drugs control certain types of seizures and aggravate others?

Dieter Schmidt

Free University of Berlin, Epilepsy Research Group, Berlin, Germany

■ Clinical evidence for aggravation of partial epilepsies

Partial seizures are usually easy to treat in patients with idiopathic partial epilepsies, particularly those beginning in childhood, where 80-90% of patients become seizure-free and, except in some children with rolandic epilepsy, aggravation is uncommon (Genton and McMenamin, 1998). In adult-onset partial epilepsy only about 50-70% of cases become seizure free, an increase in seizure frequency due to aggravation has been reported in one large series of adult patients with partial seizures (Elger *et al.*, 1998). However, such an increase of the habitual type of seizure is difficult to attribute to aggravation for several reasons. One, a major confounding factor is a spontaneous increase in frequency of partial seizures that has been observed in the placebo arm of add-on trials (Somerville, 2002). Two, an increase of seizures may simply present lack of protection because drug treatment was not efficacious and drug resistant epilepsy has developed (Sillanpää and Schmidt, 2006). It seems that aggravation of partial seizures is either uncommon or is difficult to distinguish because of confounding factors (Sazgar and Bourgois, 2005). In contrast, aggravation has been described much more often in generalized epilepsies as will be discussed in the next paragraph.

■ Clinical evidence for aggravation of generalized epilepsies

Although seizures are fully controlled in 80-90% of patients with AEDs, patients with generalized epilepsies may be vulnerable to seizure aggravation as outlined in several reviews (Lerman, 1986; Perucca *et al.*, 1998; Guerrini *et al.*, 1998; Genton and McMenamin, 1998; Genton, 2000; Bourgeois, 2002; Chaves and Sander, 2005; Sazger and Bourgeois, 2005). Disease-related factors may play a role. The mechanism by which a drug is effective for a seizure type may lower seizure threshold for other seizure types (rapid compensatory correction for disrupted equilibrium). This process may account for more susceptibility of children with multiple types of seizures such as the ones with Lennox-Gastaut syndrome or severe myoclonic epilepsy to AED-induced seizure aggravation (Sazger and Bourgeois, 2005). *Table I* summarizes the aggravating effects of individual AEDs on different types of seizures and syndromes (*Table I*).

Table I. AED-induced seizure aggravation of existing seizures or onset of new seizure types (modified from Chaves and Sander, 2005, Sazger and Bourgeois, 2005).

Seizure type or syndrome	May be controlled by*	May be aggravated by, or more rarely, new onset of
Absences	VPA, ETX, LTG, BZP, (LEV), (ZNS), (TPM), (FBM)	CBZ, PHT, ETX, VPA, OXC, VGB, TGB, LTG
Atypical absences	See absences	CBZ, OXC, PB, LTG
Myoclonic, juvenile myoclonic epilepsy	VPA, BZP, (ZNS), (TPM)	CBZ, PHT, VPA, OXC, VGB, TGB, LTG, LEV, GBP, PGB, BZP
Negative myoclonus	VPA	CBZ, PB, VPA, LTG, ZNS
Severe myoclonic epilepsy of infancy	VPA	CBZ, LTG
Lennox-Gastaut, myoclonic-astatic	VPA, LTG, FBM, TPM, (BZP)	BZ
Generalized	VPA	CBZ, PB, ETX, OXC, VGB, TPM
Landau-Kleffner	VPA	CBZ, PHT
Unverricht-Lundborg	PIR	PHT
Benign rolandic epilepsy	CBZ, STL	CBZ, LTG, VPA

Aggravation seems to be much more common in generalized seizure and epilepsy syndromes compared to few reports of aggravation in benign rolandic epilepsy. As will be discussed in more detail below, most AEDs that aggravate epilepsy are either enhancing GABA-ergic transmission (GBP, PGB, TGB, VGB) or voltage-gated blockers of Na^+ or CA^{++} currents (CBZ, LTG, OXC, PHT). However, our understanding of the mechanism of aggravation (and of therapeutic action) is still very limited. For comparison, commonly used AEDs for treatment of individual seizure types and syndromes are included (French *et al.*, 2004a, 2004b; Rogawski and Löscher, 2004).

Abbreviations: * = incomplete list, + = controlled clinical trials, or, mostly, several open trials and general acceptance of utility, parentheses indicate less extensive base of evidence, AED = Antiepileptic drug, BZP = Benzodiazepine, CBZ = Carbamazepine, ETX = Ethosuximide, FBM = Felbamate, GBP = Gabapentin, LEV = Levetiracetam, LTG = Lamotrigine, OXC = Oxcarbazepine, PHT = Phenytoin, PIR = Piracetam, PGB = Pregabalin, STL = Sulthiame, TGB = Tiagabine, TPM = Topiramate, VPA = Valproic acid, VGB = Vigabatrin, ZNS = Zonisamide.

As a caveat it is important to note that most of the published evidence for AED-induced seizure exacerbation is anecdotal, based on small numbers of patients, qualitative and not placebo-controlled. Because spontaneous increase in seizure frequency and the occurrence of new seizure types may represent a part of the natural course of a patient with epilepsy, anecdotal reports for seizure aggravation by AEDs need to be considered with caution. Increase in seizure frequency could represent the natural history of epilepsy or simply indicate that the drug is not efficacious. In order to attribute worsening of seizure frequency or a new seizure type to a true drug effect, the documentation of drug-induced seizure aggravation must establish a consistent temporal relationship between administration of an individual drug and a specific epilepsy type or syndrome. Other potential criteria include demonstrating that the exacerbation is observed soon after introduction of the AED, that increase in seizures parallels the stepwise increase in the dosage of the drug, and that seizure exacerbation is reversible when the dosage of the drug is reduced (Sazger and Bourgeois, 2005). Although rechallenge with the AED provoking the same effect is one criterion for seizure aggravation, ethical issues need to be considered before a rechallenge. Furthermore, aggravation often occurs in specific clinical situations, which will be discussed in the next section.

■ Clinical circumstances of AED-induced seizure aggravation

AED-induced seizure aggravation may have a number of causes (*Table II*). It is useful to distinguish between these clinical circumstances for two reasons, one, the underlying mechanism(s) of aggravation may differ, which will be discussed in a separate section below, and two, the different circumstances determine management (*Table II*).

Paradoxical Reaction

Paradoxical reaction usually occurs shortly after the introduction of AEDs at nontoxic serum concentrations. This condition is considered when an AED appears to exacerbate or cause new seizures in patients who have a type of seizure against which the drug is usually effective. Snead and Hosey (1985) reported 15 children with complex partial seizures in whom carbamazepine was associated with seizure exacerbation. Eleven patients experienced generalized atypical absences, and four had generalized convulsive seizures (Snead and Hosey, 1985). A generalized paroxysmal spike and-wave discharge of 2.5 to 3 cycles per second was observed in all patients who developed severe atypical absence seizures while receiving carbamazepine. Snead (2005) showed that carbamazepine can produce secondary generalized tonic-clonic seizures in frontal lobe epilepsy and continuous spike wave during sleep in atypical benign rolandic epilepsy. He suggested further that carbamazepine and phenobarbital can evoke epileptic negative myoclonus in benign rolandic epilepsy (Snead, 2005). Lerman-Sagie and coworkers discussed eight patients who experienced an increase in the frequency of absence seizures within days of the introduction of valproic acid (Lerman-Sagie *et al.*, 2001). No case was attributed to valproic acid- induced encephalopathy, and dose increments worsened the condition. All improved after

Table II. Seizure aggravation by AEDs: Causes.

Overdosage
Inappropriate AED choice
Paradoxical effect of AEDs
AED-induced encephalopathy
"Unmasking of seizures"
Indirect effects

(Modified from Chaves and Sander, 2005; Cramer, 2005; Sazger and Bourgeois; 2005, Schmidt and Löscher; 2005, Snead, 2005).
Withdrawal seizures- planned and unplanned *i.e.* poor compliance

discontinuation of valproic acid therapy. In five children, valproic acid was reintroduced, resulting again in seizure aggravation. This effect may have been the result of a pharmacodynamic paradoxical reaction (Hirsch and Genton, 2003). Intravenous administration of benzodiazepines is correlated with precipitation of tonic status epilepticus in patients with Lennox-Gastaut syndrome. Tassinari et al. (1971, 1972) suggest this to be a paradoxical reaction to benzodiazepines (diazepam and nitrazepam) specific to children with Lennox-Gastaut syndrome. Similar experiences have been made by Prior et al. (1971), DiMario and Clancy (1988), and Bittencourt and Richens (1991). Severe underlying pathology in these patients may contribute to the risk of paradoxical seizure responses to benzodiazepines. Alternately, some investigators have argued that somnolence following the use of benzodiazepines may be the cause of increased seizure activity in patients with Lennox-Gastaut syndrome (Tassinari et al., 1971), although this view is controversial (Papini et al., 1984). Finally, valproate has been implicated to produce increased absence seizures in rare cases (Snead, 2005).

Paradoxical Intoxication

Increase in seizure frequency or appearance of new seizure types may occur as a manifestation of overdosage or intoxication. The symptoms are usually reversible by dosage reduction or elimination of overtreatment, i.e. unnecessary polypharmacy or unnecessary high dosage that exposes the patient to a poor risk-benefit balance (Deckers et al., 2003; Schmidt et al., 2003). As the seizure increase may be the only overt sign of toxicity, a vicious cycle may come into play where the dosage is increased further when instead a reduction is required. This mechanism of seizure worsening was first demonstrated with phenytoin intoxication in children with Lennox-Gastaut syndrome or with severe focal epilepsies (Vallarta et al., 1974; Troupin and Ojemann, 1975; Osorio et al., 1989). The nonlinear kinetic properties of phenytoin increase the probability of reaching toxic levels with this medication. Phenytoin at high concentrations can exacerbate seizures or precipitate generalized status. Guerrini et al. (1999) discussed the occurrence of myoclonic status epilepticus after administration of high dose lamotrigine therapy in an 8-year-old with Lennox-Gastaut syndrome. There was rapid disappearance of clinical and electroencephalographic signs of myoclonic status epilepticus after discontinuation of lamotrigine with no recurrence after 2 years of follow-up. Similarly, Janszky et al. (2000) reported their observations in two boys with intractable cryptogenic generalized epilepsy who developed disabling myoclonic jerks at high serum concentrations of lamotrigine. Phenobarbital may aggravate absence seizures particularly at high and sedative serum concentrations. Increases in generalized seizures have also been shown with carbamazepine, tiagabin, vigabatrin, lamotrigine, and gabapentin (Chaves and Sander, 2005). Gabapentin or pregabalin can produce myoclonic jerks, usually in overdose (Snead, 2005).

AED-Induced Encephalopathy

Valproic acid monotherapy or valproate polytherapy with benzodiazepines or phenobarbital can produce encephalopathy with seizure aggravation (Sackellares et al., 1979; Marescaux et al., 1982; Bauer, 1996). This effect of valproic acid is not accompanied by valproic acid overdose or altered hepatic function and was first observed and reported by Völzke and Doose, 1973. Valproic acid encephalopathy usually develops within a week of introduction of the antiepileptic drug, or may be delayed for several months. It is a reversible encephalopathy characterized by somnolence, nausea/vomiting, apathy, slowing of background electroencephalographic activity, irritability, and increase in seizure frequency (Sazger and Bourgeois, 2005). The pathophysiology of valproic acid-induced encephalopathy is unknown, a toxic or metabolic origin or a direct intrinsic central nervous system depressant effect have been suggested (Sazger and Bourgeois, 2005). Although valproic acid encephalopathy is not linked to any particular single epilepsy syndrome, a review of the literature suggests that it occurs most commonly in patients with idiopathic or symptomatic generalized epilepsy (Sazger and Bourgeois, 2005). Phenobarbital (and less frequently phenytoin and carbamazepine) may exacerbate valproic acid-induced hyperammonaemic encephalopathy (Sackellares et al., 1979). More recently, some cases of encephalopathy have been reported in patients who received valproic acid together with topiramate (Hamer et al., 2000; Solomon, 2000; Longin et al., 2002). One other postulated mechanism for valproic acid- induced encephalopathy is enhanced benzodiazepine receptor activity. In one case report, valproic acid-induced encephalopathy was reversible by using flumazenil and deteriorated with administration of midazolam (Steinhoff and Stodieck, 1993). Concomitant administration of valproic acid has been suggested to reduce the elimination of lorazepam and to induce coma (Lee et al., 2002). Reversible encephalopathy, slowing of electroencephalographic background, and myoclonic jerks also were observed when vigabatrin was added to carbamazepine (Salke-Kellermann et al., 1993). This effect may be the result of a pharmacodynamic interaction between the two medications.

"Unmasking of seizures"

Generalized tonic-clonic seizures may emerge in absence epilepsy after treatment with ethosuximide that does not protect against tonic-clonic seizures (Snead, 2005). However, it is difficult to differentiate an aggravating effect of ethosuximide and the natural course of absence epilepsy that often begins with absence seizures only to be followed by later tonic-clonic seizures.

Indirect effects of AEDs

Adverse effects may contribute to aggravation of seizures. Hyponatraemia induced by carbamazepine or oxcarbazepine may, in rare cases, cause seizures (Snead, 2005). Febrile seizures may be triggered by anhidrosis, an uncommon side effect of topiramate or zonisamide (Snead, 2005). Hyperammonaemia with valproate or sedation with phenobarbital are further examples of indirect seizure aggravation through adverse effects.

Spontaneous seizure fluctuation and AED withdrawal seizures

Seizure exacerbation due to drug withdrawal may be one further cause of seizure aggravation. Drug withdrawal seizures are difficult to distinguish from loss of protection or spontaneous fluctuation. However, even planned tapering and discontinuation of AEDs may lead to aggravation through loss of protection in as many as one in three previously seizure-free patients (Schmidt and Löscher, 2005).

Inappropriate Drug Choice

Inappropriate drug choice is a common clinical cause for seizure aggravation (*Table III*). Although carbamazepine and several other AEDs such as phenytoin, gabapentin, pregabalin, are effective for the control of partial seizures, they are inappropriate in specific types of generalized epilepsy, including patients with absence seizures, atypical absence seizures, myoclonic and astatic seizures. In addition, these AEDs have been implicated in aggravation when absence seizures, atypical absence seizures, myoclonic and astatic seizures emerge during the treatment of a patient thought to have partial epilepsy when treatment was started. Shields and Saslow (1983) reported five children with generalized tonic clonic and absence seizures, who developed myoclonic, atonic, and atypical absence seizures after carbamazepine treatment. This effect was reversible in four of five patients when carbamazepine was discontinued. Liporace et al. (1994) demonstrated new development or recrudescence of remote absence seizures in four adults with generalized epilepsy who were treated with carbamazepine. The effect was reversible after discontinuation of carbamazepine or addition of ethosuximide. In a case series of 59 children who were treated with carbamazepine, more abnormal electroencephalograms and mostly de novo spike and polyspike wave discharges developed in 44%, two thirds of whom experienced clinical seizure exacerbation (Talwar et al., 1994). Carbamazepine was shown by others to produce new seizure types such as myoclonic, atonic, partial, and atypical absence seizures (Shields and Saslow, 1983; Dhuna et al., 1991; Talwar et al., 1994; Parmeggiani et al., 1998; Prasad et al., 1998; Gansaeuer and Alsaadi, 2002; Kochen et al., 2002). This effect of carbamazepine may be related to toxic levels of its main metabolite (carbamazepine 10, 11-epoxide). Concomitant administration of carbamazepine with phenytoin or valproic acid causes accelerated carbamazepine epoxide formation and inhibition of carbamazepine epoxide degradation, respectively, which may result in toxic levels (So et al., 1994).

Other reports of aggravation through inappropriate use of AEDs include aggravation of juvenile myoclonic epilepsy with carbamazepine or phenytoin therapy. Among 150 consecutive patients with a diagnosis of juvenile myoclonic epilepsy discussed by Genton et al. (2000), 40 were treated with either carbamazepine or phenytoin. Of those, 68% in the carbamazepine group and 38% in the phenytoin group experienced seizure aggravation. A recent study from the same group demonstrated that oxcarbazepine can also exacerbate myoclonic and absence seizures in patients with idiopathic generalized epilepsy (Gelisse et al., 2004). They presented six patients with idiopathic generalized epilepsy, including juvenile myoclonic epilepsy and juvenile absence epilepsy, who were treated with oxcarbazepine (all monotherapy except for one case). Clear aggravation of myoclonic jerks, de novo myoclonic jerks, exacerbation of absence seizures, and absence status were reported in these patients. Discontinuation of oxcarbazepine resulted in immediate improvement in all cases.

Worsening or precipitation of absence and tonic-clonic seizures in patients treated with phenytoin is well known (Lerman, 1986; Patel and Crichton, 1968). Phenobarbital – which is effective against myoclonic seizures –, may trigger atypical absences in benign childhood epilepsy with centrotemporal spikes (Hamano et al., 2002). Lamotrigine induces worsening of convulsive and myoclonic seizures in

Table III. Inappropriate AED choice.

Carbamazepine for absence, juvenile myoclonic epilepsy, myoclonic seizures, Landau-Kleffner syndrome, atonic seizures
Oxcarbazepine for absence or juvenile myoclonic epilepsy
Phenytoin for absence and juvenile myoclonic epilepsy
Phenobarbital for absence or atypical absence
Tiagabine for absence or atypical absence
Vigabatrin for absence, atypical absence or juvenile myoclonic epilepsy
Lamotrigine for juvenile myoclonic epilepsy
Gabapentin for absence or juvenile myoclonic epilepsy

(Modified from Chaves and Sander, 2005; Sazger and Bourgeois, 2005; Snead 2005).

patients with severe myoclonic epilepsy. Guerrini et al. (1998) documented 21 patients with severe myoclonic epilepsy treated with lamotrigine, 80% of whom manifested worsening of myoclonic seizures or increase in convulsive seizures. Ninety-five percent exhibited improvement after discontinuation of lamotrigine. Negative myoclonus and paroxysmal electroencephalographic abnormalities were promptly reversible with discontinuation of lamotrigine in rolandic epilepsy (Cerminara et al., 2004).

In some other case series, tiagabine as add-on therapy was implicated in the development of nonconvulsive status (Ettinger et al., 1999), although this is controversial (Shinnar et al., 2001). There was no recurrence after discontinuation of tiagabine. Vigabatrin as add-on therapy may cause de novo appearance of myoclonic jerks in children or young adults with partial epilepsy, and has been reported to be associated with the onset of partial seizures in patients with symptomatic infantile spasms (Lortie et al., 1993). In adult patients with a history of absences and generalized tonic clonic seizures, seizures dramatically increased after the addition of vigabatrin (Panayiotopoulos et al., 1997; Cocito and Primavera, 1998). New onset of myoclonus has been shown in children with partial epilepsy treated with add-on gabapentin (Asconape et al., 1995, 2000; Scheyer et al., 1996; Vossler, 1996).

■ Potential mechanisms underlying aggravation of generalized epilepsies: experimental and clinical evidence

Seizure exacerbation seems to result from an adverse interaction between the mode of action of the drug and the pathogenic mechanisms underlying specific seizure types of, most commonly, idiopathic generalized epilepsies (Guerrini et al., 1998, Perucca et al., 1998). The pathogenesis of absence epilepsy of childhood has received the most attention (Snead, 1995; Mc Cormick and Contreras, 2001; Manning et al., 2003). Our understanding of the disease mechanism for other idiopathic generalized epilepsies including juvenile myoclonic epilepsies and epilepsies with generalized tonic-clonic seizures on awakening epilepsies is much more limited (Mc Cormick and Contreras, 2001), possibly because we have no adequate animal models (Löscher and Schmidt, 1988). Even for absence epilepsy of childhood, two different concepts exist. One is the classic view reviewed by Snead (1995) that the thalamus and a thalamo-cortical circuit, particularly the contribution of the ventrobasal thalamus and the reticular thalamic nucleus, the thalamocortical relay and the predominantly anterior and mesial frontal cerebral cortex are relevant for the generation and propagation of absence seizures *(Figure 1)*. However, a competing hypothesis by Bowery and coworkers (2003) suggested a specific site of seizure generation within the peri-oral region of the primary somato-sensory cortex (S1po). Drugs that exacerbate, or more rarely, produce *de novo* absence seizures in animal models or in the clinic can equally give insight into the underlying mechanisms of absence epilepsy.

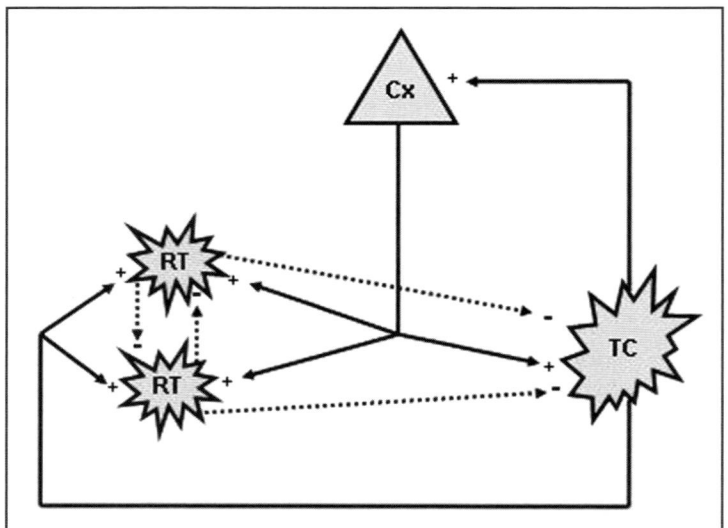

Figure 1. Aggravation of absence seizures by excess GABAergic activity.
Schematic representation of the cortico-thalamo-cortical circuit involved in generation of absence seizures with 3/sec. spike and wave discharges in the EEG. The interaction of the cerebral cortex and the thalamus, in conjunction with intrathalamic communication, can generate spike waves similar to those occurring during human absence seizure discharges (McCormick and Contreras, 2001). Activation of a low threshold Ca ++ current within TC neurons enables RT to produce a high frequency burst of action potentials. GABA is subsequently released onto TC neurons in the thalamic relay neurons, resulting in the production of a series of inhibitory polysynaptic potentials that increasingly remove the inactivation from the t-type Ca ++ channels. Excess GABA-mediated activity has been suggested to trigger absence seizures *via* an ability to elicit long-standing hyperpolarization, which is required to activate low threshold currents (Manning *et al.*, 2003). In addition, GABA-induced hyperpolarization of thalamic neurons enhances oscillatory thalamocortical activity, leading to more prominent and prolonged spike and-wave discharges (Vergnes *et al.*, 1984; Manning *et al.*, 2003).
Abbreviations: − = GABA inhibitory GABA synapses, + = excitatory glutamate synapse, Cx = cortical neuron, TC = thalamo-cortical neuron in the Ventrolateral Nucleus, RT = reticular thalamic neurons (after Steriade, 1999).

Experimental evidence

Aggravation and exacerbation of seizures by AEDs has been studied in animal models of epileptic seizures and of epilepsy (Coulter, 2005). Tiagabine, vigabatrin and barbiturate exacerbation of absence seizures has been replicated in models of absence epilepsy such as the GAERS or WAG/Rij rats (Löscher and Schmidt, 1998). In animal models of absence epilepsy, $GABA_B$ agonists produce an increase in seizure frequency by facilitating the de-inactivation of low threshold transient Ca^{++}- channels (T-channels), whereas GABA$_A$ agonists reduce absence seizure frequency (Hosford et al., 1992; Karlsson et al., 1992; Bittiger et al., 1993). The facilitation of thalamic oscillatory activity by GABAergic drugs appears to be mediated partly by GABA$_B$ receptors. GABA-induced hyperpolarization of thalamic neurons enhances oscillatory thalamocortical activity and promotion of the rebound oscillatory state, leading to more prominent and prolonged spike and-wave discharges (Vergnes et al., 1984; Mc Cormick and Contreras, 2001; Manning et al., 2003). Moreover, local microinjection of vigabatrin into the thalamic relay nuclei has been shown to increase the duration of spike wave discharges in GAERS (Liu et al., 1992). All these compounds are non-specific GABA agonists, and it has been suggested that the inhibitory postsynaptic potentials generated by the GABA agonists act as synchronizer of spike wave discharges, thus contributing to aggravation of absence seizures (see *Figure 1*). However, not all GABA agonists exacerbate spike wave discharges, for example benzodiazepines which are more specific GABA-agonists have not implicated to aggravate absence seizures. In fact, benzodiazepines are efficacious in the treatment of absence seizures and myoclonic seizures (Schmidt, 2006). Unfortunately, tolerance and sedation limit their clinical usefulness, except in treating status epilepticus (Schmidt, 2006). How can one explain why some GABA agonists exacerbate absence seizures while others (benzodiazepines) are efficacious? Spike waves discharges rely on GABAergic inhibition for synchronization. Agents that augment extracellular GABA levels such as vigabatrin or enhance GABAergic responses will exacerbate these seizures. However, agents that specifically increase GABAergic inhibition within nucleus reticularis thalami such as benzodiazepines will maintain AED efficacy (McCormick and Contreras, 2001). Phenobarbital facilitates the action of GABA *via* the modulation of GABA$_A$ Cl⁻ channel, appears to have a dual effect, suppressing absence seizures at lower doses but exacerbating them at high doses (Genton, 2000). With gabapentin, the situation is less clear, because this compound had no effect on newly diagnosed childhood absence epilepsy patients (Trudeau et al., 1996), although exacerbation of atypical absence seizures has been reported in a single case study (Vossler, 1996). There is equal uncertainty regarding an underlying mechanism of action for gabapentin. Designed as a structural analogue of GABA, it seems likely that its action is mediated by several means including modulation of certain types of Ca^{++} current, possibly through binding to the a2d extracelluar binding site, increased GABA synthesis in the brain, or decreasing glutamate mediated transmission *via* inhibition of branched chain amino acid aminotransferase (Taylor et al., 1998; Manning et al., 2003; Rogawski and Löscher, 2004). Pregabalin is another structural GABA analogue which has been suggested to share a similar mechanism of action as gabapentin (Rogawski and Löscher, 2004).

One further question is how voltage-gated sodium blocking AEDs may exacerbate absence seizures. The aggravating effects of phenytoin on absence seizures have been replicated in WAG/Rij rats where systemic administration of phenytoin doubled the spike wave discharges (van Luijtelaar et al., 2005). Emerging evidence suggests that carbamazepine may aggravate absences seizures in generalized absence epilepsy rats (GAERS) by acting on the ventrobasal thalamus *via* activation a GABA receptor mediated mechanism (O'Brien et al., 2005). In the report from Australia, seizure aggravation was noted in rats following microinjection of carbamazepine in the ventrobasal nucleus of the thalamus, while a control injection into the reticular nucleus did not result in aggravation. Furthermore they found that following administration of bicuculline, a GABA A antagonist, CBZ injection caused less aggravation. If these results which have been published only in abstract form are confirmed, CBZ-induced aggravation of absences seizures may be mediated by a GABAergic mechanism.

Clinical evidence

As shown in *Table I*, antiepileptic drugs that aggravate seizures are more likely to have primarily only one or two mechanisms of action, enhanced GABA-mediated transmission (vigabatrin, tiagabine) and, in the case of structural analogues of GABA (gabapentin, pregabalin) which have a less well defined mechanism, possibly involving increased synthesis of GABA (see above), or blockade of voltage-gated sodium channels (carbamazepine, oxcarbazepine, phenytoin, lamotrigine). As discussed above, carbamazepine may exert its proconvulsant activity by modifying $GABA_A$ receptor function (O'Brien et al., 2005). In contrast, AEDs with multiple mechanisms of actions (topiramate, valproic acid) are less likely to aggravate seizures (Hirsch and Genton, 2003; Sazgar and Bourgeois, 2005). In fact, Hirsch and Genton (2003) found no consistent evidence of pharmacodynamic seizure aggravation during treatment with valproate in the absence of clinical circumstances such as overdose, encephalopathy, hepatotoxicity or metabolic disorders. The authors concluded that valproate appears to have a very low potential for pharmacodynamic seizure aggravation. However, phenobarbital which also has a mixed mechanism of action involving blockade of high voltage activated calcium current, $GABA_A$ agonist action and blockade of AMPA current (Rogawski and Löscher, 2004), while it is effective for treatment of generalized myoclonic seizures, it seems to be ineffective or may even exacerbate absence seizures (Löscher and Schmidt, 1988). Although sedation may play a role in aggravation of absence seizures by phenobarbital, the exact mechanism of aggravation of absence seizures is still elusive. Finally, seizure exacerbation may also occur as a result of development of tolerance to the effect of antiepileptic drugs. A summary of the putative pharmacological mechanisms underlying seizure aggravation is given in *Table IV*.

Increased GABA-mediated transmission

Antiepileptic drugs that have been implicated to primarily enhance GABA-ergic neurotransmission, such as vigabatrin, tiagabine, and are at least structurally related to GABA such as gabapentin or pregabalin (S(+)-3-isobutyl GABA) do not appear to be effective in generalized epilepsies and may actually exacerbate generalized absence or myoclonic seizures. Treatment of patients with generalized epilepsy with GABA-ergic drugs is not recommended and may be considered an inappropriate use. The clinical observation that aggravation is seen more often in patients with overdosage or encephalopathy suggests that broadly speaking drugs at higher than well tolerated concentrations may perhaps shift to exert more GABAergic mechanisms. With inappropriate use of AEDs, patients with idiopathic generalized epilepsies are more vulnerable to GABAergic compounds because GABA may have bi-directional while in partial epilepsy, GABA-ergic mechanisms seem to exert a therapeutic role.

Table IV. Putative pharmacological mechanisms underlying seizure aggravation.

1. Increased GABA-mediated transmission (vigabatrin, tiagabine, and, possibly, at least in part, see text, gabapentin, pregabalin)
2. Blockade of voltage-gated sodium channels (carbamazepine, oxcarbazepine, lamotrigine, phenytoin)
3. Secondary effects of AEDs unrelated to their action at therapeutic concentration ranges
4. Homeostatic plasticity (relationship to AED mechanism of action uncertain)
5. Secondary loss of efficacy due to tolerance (GABA-mediated AEDs, blockers of voltage-gated sodium channels and AEDs with other mechanisms of action)

(modified from Sazger and Bourgeois, 2005).

Blockade of Voltage-Gated Sodium Channels
(Carbamazepine, Oxcarbazepine, Phenobarbital, Phenytoin, Lamotrigine)

Blockade of voltage-gated sodium channels by carbamazepine, oxcarbazepine, phenobarbital, phenytoin, and lamotrigine may be counterproductive in patients with absence or myoclonic seizures. The blockage of voltage-gated sodium channels may play a role in enhanced cortical inhibition underlying the slow wave component of the spike-wave complex and the appearance of negative myoclonus (Engel, 1995). Selective action of carbamazepine on brain structures responsible for generalized epileptiform discharges is suggested by findings in animal models of absence epilepsy and by electroencephalographic observations in patients. Exacerbation of seizures and epileptiform discharges by carbamazepine in epileptic patients is associated with slowing in the background activity (Rodin et al., 1976). As shown by Steriade and coworkers generalized slow waves on electroencephalogram may be generated by the same thalamocortical network responsible for spike-and-wave generation (Steriade et al., 1991; Curro Dossi et al., 1992). Therefore, an action of carbamazepine on the thalamocortical network may result in facilitation of generalized epileptogenesis (Sazger and Bourgeois, 2005).

Secondary effects of AEDs

Secondary effects of AEDs unrelated to their action at therapeutic concentration ranges may play a role in seizure exacerbation (Coulter, 2005). AEDs often have a wide range of clinically relevant concentration ranges. This may increase the probability that AEDs have secondary effects unrelated to their therapeutic actions. One example is ethosuximide with a primary action on T-type CA^{++} current block. However, a secondary action is a GABA antagonism (Coulter et al., 1990). Another example are benzodiazepines which in addition to their well-known GABAergic mechanism exhibit voltage – gated sodium blocking activity when used at higher doses for the treatment of status epilepticus (Schmidt, 2006). Unwanted secondary effects may exacerbate seizures, particularly when the drug is administered to patients where the primary action of the drug is unneeded. Thus, ethosuximide may exacerbate other generalized seizures because T-current effects are not relevant while secondary GABA antagonist effects are (Coulter, 2005).

Homeostatic plasticity

In addition, mechanism-independent effects which seem to be independent to their mechanism of action could be involved in seizure exacerbation. For example, the concept of homeostatic plasticity has been proposed to better understand seizure exacerbation (Coulter, 2005). According to the concept of homeostatic plasticity, neurons have an optimal activity range, and tonic enhancement or reduction in this optimal activity triggers multiple mechanism to reduce or enhance activity, respectively (Turrigiani and Nelson, 2004). According to these authors, homeostatic plasticity is a complex response which maintains synaptic weights. Plasticity involves the maintenance of relative efficacy of inhibitory and excitatory synapses by maintaining a balance between GABAergic and glutamatergic synaptic inputs (Turrigiani and Nelson, 2004). Such a system may not depend on which AED is given but rather how effective the AED is. Homeostatic plasticity could be a confounding factor to maintain efficacy and could theoretically lead to seizure exacerbation in various clinical situations and also when AEDs or other drugs are administered which enhance excitability.

Secondary loss of efficacy due to tolerance

Developing tolerance to antiepileptic drugs results in loss of their therapeutic effect and therefore aggravation of seizures. Tolerance after chronic exposure to certain medications is thought to be caused by up-regulation of receptor sensitivity or density. Alternately, the inhibitory action of a drug on a given system may trigger delayed reactive compensatory mechanisms, which may be the case in the generation of tolerance or withdrawal seizures. Development of tolerance, *i.e.*, the reduction in response to a drug after repeated administrations, is an adaptive response of the body to prolonged exposure to the drug, and tolerance to antiepileptic drugs (AEDs) is no exception (Löscher and Schmidt, 2006). Tolerance develops to some drug effects much more rapidly than to other effects. The extent of tolerance depends on the drug and individual (genetic?) factors. Tolerance may lead to attenuation of side effects but also to loss of efficacy of AEDs and is reversible after discontinuation of drug treatment. There are different experimental approaches to study tolerance in laboratory animals. Development of tolerance depends on the experimental model, drug, drug dosage, and duration of treatment, so that a battery of experimental protocols is needed to fully evaluate whether tolerance to effect occurs.

There are two major types of tolerance. Pharmacokinetic (metabolic) tolerance, which is due to induction of AED metabolising enzymes and has been shown for most first generation AEDs, but is easy to overcome by increasing dosage. Pharmacodynamic (functional) tolerance, which is due to "adaptation" of AED targets, *e.g.*, by loss of receptor sensitivity, and has been shown experimentally for all AEDs that lose activity during prolonged treatment. Functional tolerance may lead to complete loss of AED activity and cross-tolerance to other AEDs. There is convincing experimental evidence that almost all first, second and third generation AEDs lose their antiepileptic activity during prolonged treatment, although to a different extent (Löscher and Schmidt, 2006). Because of diverse confounding factors, detecting tolerance in patients with epilepsy is more difficult but can be done with careful assessment of decline at long-term individual patient response. After excluding confounding factors, tolerance to effect for most modern and old AEDs can be shown in small subgroups of responders by assessing individual or group response (Löscher and Schmidt, 2006). It should be noted that development of tolerance and also aggravation seems to occur more often during treatment with GABA-ergic drugs such as benzodiazepines or vigabatrin, tolerance does also develop with sodium blockers such as carbamazepine or phenytoin. Tolerance may also be disease-specific and may develop in certain severe epilepsy syndromes, such as in patients with Lennox-Gastaut syndrome (Genton and Dravet, 1998). Development of tolerance to the antiepileptic activity of an AED may be an important reason for seizure aggravation and failure of drug treatment in general (Löscher and Schmidt, 2006).

■ Discussion

AED-induced seizure aggravation can occur with virtually all antiepileptic medications. As the underlying mechanisms for anti-seizure effects of AEDs and the mechanisms of seizure generation for most generalized seizures – except perhaps for absence seizures – are not fully understood, the mechanisms involved in seizure aggravation cannot be explained with certainty. Nevertheless, it seems that AED-induced, non-specific overactivity of the GABAergic system may play an important role. Although there are several other causes of seizure exacerbation, AED-induced seizure exacerbation should be considered and the accuracy of diagnosis of the seizure type should be questioned whenever there is seizure worsening or the appearance of new seizure types after the introduction of any AED.

The following considerations will enable physicians to prevent or correct AED-induced seizure aggravation: (1) know the epileptic syndrome of your patient and the appropriate choice of medications to treat them; (2) avoid the use of GABA-ergic AEDs which are reported to consistently aggravate specific seizure types in generalized epilepsies; (3) prevent overtreatment. When the drug does not work or does more harm than good, discontinue it (Schmidt, 2002), (4) be aware of aggravation in patients at high risk for seizure-inducing effects of AEDs. These high-risk groups include infants, children and adolescents with specific epileptic syndromes, patients with cognitive deterioration, patients receiving polytherapy, those with high frequency of seizures or multiple seizure types before treatment, and patients with prominent or atypical epileptiform electroencephalographic activity (Sazger and Bourgeois, 2005). Antiepileptic drug-induced seizure exacerbation may be observed more frequently in certain epilepsy syndromes of infancy and childhood. These syndromes include Lennox-Gastaut, Landau-Kleffner, myoclonic-astatic epilepsy, severe myoclonic epilepsy of infancy, and electrical status epilepticus of sleep. When a definitive diagnosis is not reached, the use of antiepileptic medications with a broad spectrum of activity and with multiple mechanisms of action is less likely to cause seizure exacerbation. Nevertheless, seizure aggravation is not uncommon, and the possibility that it may be related to an AED always needs to be considered.

References

Asconape J, Diedrich A, DellaBadia J. Gabapentin-associated myoclonus. *Neurology* 1995; 45 (Suppl 4): A249-50.

Asconape J, Diedrich A, DellaBadia J. Myoclonus associated with the use of gabapentin. *Epilepsia* 2000; 41: 479-81.

Bauer J. Seizure-inducing effects of antiepileptic drugs: A review. *Acta Neurol Scand* 1996; 94: 367-77.

Biraben A, Allain H, Scarabin JM, Schuck S, Edan G. Exacerbation of juvenile myoclonic epilepsy with lamotrigine. *Neurology* 2000; 55: 1758.

Bittencourt PR, Richens A. Anticonvulsant-induced status epilepticus in Lennox-Gastaut syndrome. *Epilepsia* 1991; 22: 129-34.

Bittiger H, Froestl W, Mickel SJ, Olpe HR. $GABA_B$ receptor antagonists: From synthesis to therapeutic applications. *TIPS* 1993; 14: 391-4.

Bourgeois BF. Reducing overtreatment. *Epilepsy Res* 2002; 52: 53-60.

Carrazana EJ, Wheeler SD. Exacerbation of juvenile myoclonic epilepsy with lamotrigine. *Neurology* 2001; 56: 1424-5.

Cerminara C, Montanaro ML, Curatolo P, Seri S. Lamotrigine-induced seizure aggravation and negative myoclonus in idiopathic rolandic epilepsy. *Neurology* 2004; 63: 373-5.

Chaves J, Sander JW. Seizure aggravation in idiopathic generalized epilepsies. *Epilepsia* 2005; 46 (Suppl 9): 133-9.

Cocito L. Primavera A. Vigabatrin aggravates absences and absence status. *Neurology* 1998; 51: 1519-20.

Corda D, Gelisse P, Genton P, Dravet C, Baldy-Moulinier M. Incidence of drug-induced aggravation in benign epilepsy with centrotemporal spikes. *Epilepsia* 2001; 42: 754-9.

Coulter DA, Huguenard JR, Prince DA. Differential effects of petit mal anticonvulsants and convulsants on thalamic neurons: calcium current reduction. *British Journal of Pharmacology* 1990; 100 (4): 800-6.

Coulter DA. Experimental evidence and mechanisms of seizure aggravation: insight from animal models. In: Handout. Antiepileptic Therapy Symposium. Washington DC, 2005.

Cramer JO. Effect of antiepileptic drug compliance and withdrawal on seizures: unplanned and planned withdrawal. In: Handout. Antiepileptic Therapy Symposium. Washington DC, 2005.

Curro Dossi R, Nunez A. Steriade M. Electrophysiology of a low (0.5-4 HZ) intrinsic oscillation of cat thalamocortical neurons *in vivo*. *J Physiol* 1992; 447: 215-34.

Deckers CL, Genton P, Sills GJ, Schmidt D. Current limitations of antiepileptic drug therapy: a conference review. *Epilepsy Research* 2003; 53: 1-17.

Dhuna A, Pascual-Leone A, Talwar D. Exacerbation of partial seizures and onset of nonepileptic myoclonus with carbamazepine. *Epilepsia* 1991; 32: 275-8.

DiMario FJ Jr, Clancy RR. Paradoxical precipitation of tonic seizures by lorazepam in a child with atypical absence seizures. *Ped Neurol* 1988; 4: 249-51.

Elger CE, Bauer J, Schermann J, Widmer G. Aggravation of focal epileptic seizures by antiepileptic drugs. *Epilepsia* 1998; 39 (Suppl 3): S15-8.

Engel J Jr. Inhibitory mechanisms of epileptic seizure generation. *Adv Neurol* 1995; 67: 157-71.

Ettinger AB, Bernal OG, Andriola MR, *et al.* Two cases of nonconvulsive status epilepticus in association with tiagabine therapy. *Epilepsia* 1999; 40: 1159-62.

French JA, Kanner AM, Bautista J, American Academy of Neurology Therapeutics and Technology Assessment Subcommittee, American Academy of Neurology Quality Standards Subcommittee, American Epilepsy Society Quality Standards Subcommittee, American Epilepsy Society Therapeutics and

Technology Assessment Subcommittee. Efficacy and tolerability of the new antiepileptic drugs, I: Treatment of new-onset epilepsy: report of the TTA and QSS Subcommittees of the American Academy of Neurology and the American Epilepsy Society. *Neurology* 2004a; 62: 1252-60.

French JA, Kanner AM, Bautista J. American Academy of Neurology Therapeutics and Technology Assessment Subcommittee, American Academy of Neurology Quality Standards Subcommittee, American Epilepsy Society Therapeutics and Technology Assessment Subcommittee, American Epilepsy Society Quality Standards Subcommittee. Efficacy and tolerability of the new antiepileptic drugs, II: Treatment of refractory epilepsy: report of the TTA and QSS Subcommittees of the American Academy of Neurology and the American Epilepsy Society. *Neurology* 2004b; 62: 1261-73.

Gansaeuer M, Alsaadi TM. Carbamazepine-induced seizures: A case report and review of the literature. *Clin Electroencephalogr* 2002; 33: 174-7.

Gelisse P, Genton P, Kuate C, Pesenti A, Baldy-Moulinier M, Crespel A. Worsening of seizures by oxcarbazepine in juvenile idiopathic generalized epilepsies. *Epilepsia* 2004; 45: 282-6.

Genton P, Dravet C. Lennox Gastaut syndrome and other childhood epileptic encephalopathies. In: Engel J, Pedley TA, eds. *Epilepsy: A comprehensive textbook*. Vol. 3, 1998: 2355-66.

Genton P, Gelisse P, Thomas P, Dravet C. Do carbamazepine and phenytoin aggravate juvenile myoclonic epilepsy? *Neurology* 2000; 5: 1106-9.

Genton P, McMenamin J. Aggravation of seizures by antiepileptic drugs: What to do in clinical practice. *Epilepsia* 1998; 39 (Suppl 3): S26-9.

Genton P. When antiepileptic drugs aggravate epilepsy. *Brain Dev* 2000; 22: 75-80.

Guerrini R, Belmonte A, Genton P. Antiepileptic drug-induced worsening of seizures in children. *Epilepsia* 1998; 39 (Suppl 3): S2-10.

Guerrini R, Belmonte A, Parmeggiani L, Perucca E. Myoclonic status epilepticus following high-dosage lamotrigine therapy. *Brain Dev* 1999; 21: 420-41.

Guerrini R, Belmonte A, Strumia S, Hirsch E. Exacerbation of epileptic negative myoclonus by carbamazepine or phenobarbital in children with atypical benign rolandic epilepsy. *Epilepsia* 1995; 36 (Suppl 3): S65.

Guerrini R, Dravet C, Genton P, Belmonte A, Kaminska A, Dulac O. Lamotrigine and seizure aggravation in severe myoclonic epilepsy. *Epilepsia* 1998; 39: 508-12.

Hamano S. Mochizuki M. Morikawa T. Phenobarbital-induced atypical absence seizures in benign childhood epilepsy with centrotemporal spikes. *Seizure* 2002; 11: 201-4.

Hamer HM, Knake S, Schomburg U, Rosenow F. Valproate-induced hyperammonemic encephalopathy in the presence of topiramate. *Neurology* 2000; 54: 230-2.

Hirsch E. Genton P. Antiepileptic drug-induced pharmacodynamic aggravation of seizures: Does valproate have a lower potential? *CNS Drugs* 2003; 17: 633-40.

Horn CS, Ater SB, Hurst DL. Carbamazepine-exacerbated epilepsy in children and adolescents. *Pediatr Neurol* 1986; 2: 340-5.

Hosford DA, Clark S, Cao Z, *et al*. The role of $GABA_B$ receptor activation in absence seizures of lethargic (lh/lh) mice. *Science* 1992; 257: 398-401.

Janszky J, Rasonyi G, Halasz P, *et al*. Disabling erratic myoclonus during lamotrigine therapy with high serum level: Report of two cases. *Clin Neuropharmacol* 2000; 23: 86-9.

Karlsson G, Kolb C, Hausdorf A, Portet C, Schmutz M, Olpe HR. $GABA_B$ receptors in various *in vitro* and *in vivo* models of epilepsy: A study with the $GABA_B$ receptor blocker CGP-35348. *Neuroscience* 1992; 47: 63-8.

Kochen S, Giagante B, Oddo S. Spike-and-wave complexes and seizure exacerbation caused by carbamazepine. *Eur J Neurol* 2002; 9: 41-7.

Latour P, Biraben R, Polard E, *et al*. Drug induced encephalopathy in six epileptic patients: Topiramate, valproate, or both? *Hum Psychopharmacol Clin Exp* 2004; 19: 193-203.

Lee SA, Lee JK, Heo K. Coma probably induced by lorazepam-valproate interaction. *Seizure* 2002; 11: 124-5.

Lerman P. Seizures induced or aggravated by anticonvulsants. *Epilepsia* 1986; 27: 706-10.

Lerman-Sagie T, Watemberg N, Kramer U, Shahar E, Lerman P. Absence seizures aggravated by valproic acid. *Epilepsia* 2001; 42: 941-3.

Liu Z, Vergnes M, Depaulis A, Marescaux C, *et al*. Evidence for the critical role of GABAergic transmission within the thalamus in the genesis and control of absence seizures in the rat. *Brain Res* 1991; 545: 1-7.

Liporace JD, Sperling MR, Dichter MA. Absence seizures and carbamazepine in adults. *Epilepsia* 1994; 35: 1026-8.

Longin E, Teich M, Koelfen W, König S. Topiramate enhances the risk of valproate-associated side effects in three children. *Epilepsia* 2002; 43: 451-4.

Lortie A, Chiron C, Mumford J, Dulac O. The potential for increasing seizure frequency, relapse, and appearance of new seizure types with vigabatrin. *Neurology* 1993; 43 (11 Suppl 5): S24-7.

Löscher W, Schmidt D. Which animal models should be used in the search for new antiepileptic drugs? A proposal based on experimental and clinical considerations. *Epilepsy Res* 1988; 2: 145-81.

Löscher W, Schmidt D. Experimental and clinical evidence for loss of effect (tolerance) during prolonged treatment with antiepileptic drugs. *Epilepsia* 2006 (in press).

Manning JPA, Richards DA, Bowery NG. Pharmacology of absence epilepsy. *Trends in pharmacological science* 2003; 24: 542-9.

Marescaux C, Warter JM, Micheletti G, Rumbach L, Coquillat G, Kurtz D. Stuporous episodes during treatment with sodium valproate: Report of seven cases. *Epilepsia* 1982; 23: 297-305.

McCormick DA, Contreras D. On the cellular and network bases of epileptic seizures. *Annual Review of Physiology* 2001; 63: 815-46.

O'Brien TJ, Liu L, Wallengren C, Lohman R-J, Morris MJ. Carbamazepine aggravates absence seizures in GAERS rats by acting on the ventrobasal thalamus *via* a $GABA_A$ – mediated mechanism. *Epilepsia* 2005; 46 (Suppl 8): 296.

Osorio I, Burnstine R, Remler B, Manon-Espallat R, Reed RC. Phenytoin-induced seizures: A paradoxical effect at toxic concentrations in epileptic patients. *Epilepsia* 1989; 30: 230-40.

Panayiotopoulos CP, Agathonikou A, Sharoqi IA, Parker AP. Vigabatrin aggravates absences and absence status. *Neurology* 1997; 49: 1467.

Papini M, Pasquinelli A, Armellini M, Orlandi D. Alertness and incidence of seizures in patients with Lennox-Gastaut syndrome. *Epilepsia* 1984; 25: 161-7.

Parmeggiani A, Fraticelli E, Rossi PG. Exacerbation of epileptic seizures by carbamazepine: Report of 10 cases. *Seizure* 1998; 7: 479-83.

Patel H, Crichton JV. The neurologic hazards of diphenylhydantoin in childhood. *J Pediatr* 1968; 73: 676-84.

Perucca E, Gram L, Avanzini G, Dulac O. Antiepileptic drugs as a cause of worsening seizures. *Epilepsia* 1998; 39: 5-17.

Perucca E, Kwan P. Overtreatment in epilepsy: adverse consequences and mechanism. *Epilepsy Research* 2002; 52: 25-33.

Piccinelli P, Borgatti R, Perucca E, Tofani A, Donati G, Balottin U. Frontal nonconvulsive status epilepticus associated with high-dose tiagabine therapy in a child with familial bilateral perisylvian polymicrogyria. *Epilepsia* 2000; 41: 1485-8.

Prasad AN, Stefanelli M, Nagarajan L. Seizure exacerbation and developmental regression with carbamazepine. *Can J Neurol Sci* 1998; 25: 287-94.

Prior PF, Maclaine GN, Scott DF, Laurance BM. Tonic status epilepticus precipitated by intravenous diazepam in a child with petit mal status. *Epilepsia* 1971; 13: 467-72.

Rodin EA, Rim CS, Rennick PM. The effects of Tegretol on the EEG. *Electroencephalogr Clin Neurophysiol* 1976; 37: 329.

Rogawski MA, Löscher W. The neurobiology of antiepileptic drugs. *Nature Review Neuroscience* 2004; 5: 553-64.

Sackellares JC, Lee SI, Dreifuss FE. Stupor following administration of valproic acid to patients receiving other antiepileptic drugs. *Epilepsia* 1979; 20: 697-703.

Salke-Kellermann A, Baier H, Rambeck B, Boenigk HE, Wolf P. Acute encephalopathy with vigabatrin. *Lancet* 1993; 342: 185.

Sazgar M, Bourgeois BFD. Aggravation of epilepsy by antiepileptic drugs *Pediatr Neurol* 2005; 33: 227-34.

Scheyer RD, Assaf BA, Spencer SS, Mattson RH. Gabapentin related myoclonus. *Epilepsia* 1996; 37 (Suppl 5): 203.

Schmidt D, Löscher W. Drug resistance in epilepsy: putative neurobiologic and clinical mechanisms. *Epilepsia* 2005; 46: 858-77.

Schmidt D Wilensky A. Benzodiazepines. In: Engel J, Pedley T, eds. *Textbook of Epilepsy*. Philadelphia, USA: Lippincott Williams & Wilkins, Second edition (in press).

Schmidt D. Strategies to prevent overtreatment with antiepileptic drugs in patients with epilepsy. *Epilepsy Research* 2002; 52: 61-9.

Shields WD, Saslow E. Myoclonic, atonic, and absence seizures following institution of carbamazepine therapy in children. *Neurology* 1983; 33: 1487-9.

Shinnar S, Berg AT, Treiman DM, Hauser WA, Hesdorffer DC, Sackellares JC, Leppik I, Sillanpaa M, Sommerville KW. Status epilepticus and tiagabine therapy: review of safety data and epidemiologic comparisons. *Epilepsia* 2001; 42: 372-9.

Sillanpää M, Schmidt D. Natural history of treated childhood-onset epilepsy: prospective, long-term population-based study. *Brain* 2006; 129: 617-24.

Snead OC 3rd, Hosey LC. Exacerbation of seizures in children by carbamazepine. *N Engl J Med* 1985; 313: 916-21.

Snead OC. Basic mechanisms of generalized absence seizures. *Ann Neurol* 1995; 37: 146-57.

Snead OC. Seizure aggravation: clinical assessment and role of AEDs. In: Handout. *Antiepileptic Therapy Symposium*. Washington DC, 2005.

So EL, Ruggles KH, Cascino GD, Ahmann PA. Weatherford KW. Seizure exacerbation and status epilepticus related to carbamazepine-10,11-epoxide. *Ann Neurol* 1994; 35: 743-6.

Solomon GE. Valproate-induced hyperammonemic encephalopathy in the presence of topiramate. *Neurology* 2000; 55: 606.

Somerville ER. Aggravation of partial seizures by antiepileptic drugs: is there evidence from clinical trials? *Neurology* 2002; 59: 79-83.

Steinhoff BJ, Stodieck SR. Temporary abolition of seizure activity by flumazenil in a case of valproate-induced non-convulsive status epilepticus. *Seizure* 1993; 2: 261-5.

Steriade M, Oakson G, Diallo A. Cortically elicited spike-wave after discharges in thalamic neurons. *Electroencephal. Clin. Neurophysiol* 1976; 41: 641-4.

Talwar D, Arora MS, Sher PK. EEG changes and seizure exacerbation in young children treated with carbamazepine. *Epilepsia* 1994; 35: 1154-9.

Tassinari CA, Dravet C, Roger J, Cano JP, Gastaut H. Tonic status epilepticus precipitated by intravenous benzodiazepine in five patients with Lennox-Gastaut syndrome. *Epilepsia* 1972; 13: 421-35.

Tassinari CA, Gastaut H, Dravet C, Roger J. A paradoxal effect: Status epilepticus induced by benzodiazepines (Valium and Mogadon). *Electroencephalogr Clin Neurophysiol* 1971; 31: 182.

Taylor CP, Gee NS, Su TZ, Kocsis JD, Welty DF, Brown JP, Dooley DJ, Boden P, Singh L. Summary of mechanistic hypotheses of Gabapentin pharmacology. *Epilepsy Res* 1998; 29: 247-64.

Troupin AS, Ojemann LM. Paradoxical intoxication: A complication of anticonvulsant administration. *Epilepsia* 1975; 16: 753-8.

Trudeau V, Myers S, LaMoreaux L, Anhut H, Garofalo E, Ebersole J. Gabapentin in naive childhood absence epilepsy. Results from two double-blind, placebo-controlled, multicenter studies. *J Child Neurol* 1996; 11: 470-5.

Turrigiani GG, Nelson S. Homeostatic plasticity in the developing nervous system. *Nature Reviews Neuroscience* 2004; 5: 97-107.

Vallarta JM, Bell DB, Reichert A. Progressive encephalopathy due to chronic hydantoin intoxication. *Am J Dis Child* 1974; 128: 27-34.

Van Luijtelaar G, Azizova A, Onat F. The role of the cortex in absence epilepsy: focal and systemic effects of phenytoin. *Epilepsia* 2005; 46 (Suppl 8): 304.

Vergnes M, Marescaux C, Micheletti G, Depaulis A, Rumbach L, Warter JM. Enhancement of spike and wave discharges by GABAmimetic drugs in rats with spontaneous petit-mal-like epilepsy. *Neurosci Lett* 1984; 44: 911-4.

Völzke E, Doose H. Dipropylacetate (Depakine, Ergenyl) in the treatment of epilepsy. *Epilepsia* 1973; 14: 185-93.

Vossler DG. Exacerbation of seizures in Lennox-Gastaut syndrome by gabapentin. *Neurology* 1996; 46: 852-3.

Section VIII: Concluding remarks

Can we replace the terms "focal" and "generalized"?

Jerome Engel

Department of Neurology, David Geffen School of Medicine at UCLA, Los Angeles, USA

■ Historical background

Although Hippocrates (1967) and Galen (Temkin, 1945) recognized that epileptic seizures were due to disorders in the brain, their prophetic insights were followed by centuries of misconceptions about epilepsy due to prevalent beliefs in supernatural etiologies. The return to an understanding of natural causes of epilepsy began in eighteenth century France with the Traité de l'Épilepsie, published in 1770 by Simon André Tissot (1770). Tissot established the dichotomy between epilepsy due to a known brain injury, which he called "idiopathic", and that without a definite etiology, presumably due to an epileptic disposition, which he called "essential". We now use the terms "symptomatic" or "secondary" to describe Tissot's idiopathic epilepsies, and the terms "idiopathic" or "primary" to describe his essential epilepsies. The preservation of this dichotomy up to the current 1989 International Classification of the Epilepsies (Commission, 1989) is now as unsupportable as the dichotomy of "focal" *vs.* "generalized". Tissot was also responsible for distinguishing between generalized tonic-clonic seizures, which he called "grands acces", and minor, probably absence, seizures, which he called "petits acces". Another French physician, Esquirol (1938), introduced the terms "grand mal" and "petit mal" in 1865, which have been in common usage ever since.

Throughout the early part of the nineteenth century, epilepsy was considered to be a generalized disorder characterized by grand mal and petit mal seizures, commonly attributed to the medulla oblongata. L.F. Bravais (1827), in France, and Wilhelm Griesinger (1867), in Germany described focal seizures as epileptic phenomena, but it was John Hughlings Jackson (Taylor, 1958) and his colleagues David Ferrier (1873) and Victor Horsley (1886), at London's National Hospital for the Paralyzed and Epileptic at Queen Square, who deserve credit for developing the concept of focal epileptic seizures as manifestations of epilepsy. This team of a neurologist, a neurophysiologist, and a neurosurgeon argued that the mechanisms of epilepsy can be more easily identified by studying focal seizures than by studying generalized seizures. They localized the structural pathology responsible for specific forms of focal seizures, reproduced these focal ictal phenomena in monkeys by electrical stimulation of the cortex, and ultimately cured epilepsy by surgically removing localized epileptogenic brain tissue. From the late nineteenth century, many different types of epileptic seizures were recognized; the distinction between focal seizures and generalized seizures had particular clinical relevance, because the former could potentially be treated by surgical resection (Engel, 2005). At that time, differential diagnosis of focal seizures was accomplished almost entirely on the basis of ictal semiology and, indeed, Jackson helped to define early concepts of localization of function in the human brain by correlating the initial signs and symptoms of focal seizures with postmortem, or surgical, localization of structural cerebral pathology (Taylor, 1958). The introduction of cerebral angiography (Moniz, 1934) and pneumoencephalography (Dandy, 1919) made it possible to visualize, in vivo, structural etiologies of some focal seizures and furthered the importance of diagnosing focal epilepsies.

The advent of the EEG (Berger, 1929) contributed importantly to the development of the dichotomy between focal and generalized seizures. Gibbs, Gibbs, and Lennox (1938) identified characteristic generalized ictal EEG patterns that could differentiate between grand mal seizures, petit mal seizures, and psychomotor seizures; however, they utilized linked ears as a reference and were unable to detect localized epileptiform abnormalities. Jasper and Kershman (1941), however, used chain-linkage montages and pointed out that for some types of seizures, including psychomotor seizures, it was the location of the interictal and ictal discharges, and not their pattern, that was important for diagnosis. Subsequently, the EEG became the principal diagnostic approach, not only for distinguishing between generalized and focal epileptic disorders, but for localizing the epileptogenic abnormality in focal epilepsies when resective surgical treatment was considered (Engel, 2005). By this time, the old dichotomy of grand mal *vs.* petit mal seizures had been replaced by the dichotomy of focal *vs.* generalized seizures, which rapidly became solidly imbedded in the teachings of epileptology.

■ The ILAE classifications of seizures and epilepsies

Seizures

The 1970 International Classification of Epileptic Seizures (Gastaut, 1970) formalized the dichotomy between focal and generalized events that has continued into the current 1981 International Classification of Epileptic Seizures (Commission, 1981) (*Table I*). The term "partial", rather than "focal", was preferred in these classifications, however, in recognition of the fact that the epileptogenic abnormality can be quite distributed in some patients. The distinction between partial and generalized seizures was clearly defined; the former referred to ictal events for which behavioral or EEG evidence indicate that they begin in a part of the brain limited to one hemisphere, while the latter refered to ictal events which appear to begin on both sides of the brain simultaneously (Commission, 1981). Both classifications, however, recognized the occurrence of secondarily generalized seizures, a term which referred specifically to the evolution from a focal seizure to a generalized tonic-clonic seizure. There was

Table I. International Classification of Epileptic Seizures.

I. **Partial (focal, local) seizures**
   A. *Simple partial seizures*
      1. With motor signs
      2. With somatosensory or special sensory symptoms
      3. With autonomic symptoms or signs
      4. With psychic symptoms
   B. *Complex partial seizures*
      1. Simple partial onset followed by impairment of consciousness
      2. With impairment of consciousness at onset
   C. *Partial seizures evolving to secondarily generalized seizures*
      1. Simple partial seizures evolving to generalized seizures
      2. Complex partial seizures evolving to generalized seizures
      3. Simple partial seizures evolving to complex partial seizures evolving to generalized seizures
II. **Generalized seizures**
   A. *Absence seizures*
      1. Typical absences
      2. Atypical absences
   B. *Myoclonic seizures*
   C. *Clonic seizures*
   D. *Tonic seizures*
   E. *Tonic-clonic seizures*
   F. *Atonic seizures (astatic seizures)*
III. **Unclassified epileptic seizures**

From Commission on Classification and Terminology of the International League Against Epilepsy 1981. Used with permission.

no discussion of the inconsistency of the use of the term "generalized" to describe these focal onset tonic-clonic seizures when focal onset limbic seizures that evolved to involve both hemispheres equally were referred to as "complex partial". Furthermore, there was never any intention to imply that generalized seizures involved the entire brain, nor was there concern about the fact that some partial seizures could be bilateral.

Epilepsies

The 1970 International Classification of the Epilepsies (Merlis, 1970) fostered the belief that almost all epileptic disorders could be considered either partial, characterized by partial epileptic seizures with or without secondarily generalized seizures, or generalized, characterized by generalized seizures only. Partial epilepsies, therefore, were disorders where the epileptogenic abnormality was localized to part of one hemisphere, while generalized epilepsies were disorders where the abnormality was widespread and bilateral. This conceptual dichotomy was continued into the current 1989 International Classification of Epilepsies (Commission, 1989) *(Table II)*. A major difference between the 1970 and 1989 classifications is that the term "partial" was replaced with the term "localization-related", in order to avoid the misinterpretation of a partial epilepsy as part of an epilepsy syndrome. The terms "focal", "local", and "partial" epilepsy were considered, however, to be synonymous with localization-related epilepsy. Both the 1970 and 1989 classifications also contained the dichotomy of idiopathic (primary) and symptomatic (secondary) epilepsies, but whereas the 1970 classification only considered that generalized epilepsies could be idiopathic, the 1989 classification recognized the fact that some localization-related epilepsies are also

Table II. International Classification of Epilepsies, Epileptic Syndromes, and Related Seizure Disorders.

1. **Localization-related (focal, local, partial)**
   1.1 **Idiopathic (primary)**
      - Benign childhood epilepsy with centrotemporal spikes
      - Childhood epilepsy with occipital paroxysms
      - Primary reading epilepsy
   1.2 **Symptomatic (secondary)**
      - Temporal lobe epilepsies
      - Frontal lobe epilepsies
      - Parietal lobe epilepsies
      - Occipital lobe epilepsies
      - Chronic progressive epilepsia partialis continua of childhood
      - Syndromes characterized by seizures with specific modes of precipitation
   1.3 **Cryptogenic**, defined by:
      - Seizure type
      - Clinical features
      - Etiology
      - Anatomical localization
2. **Generalized**
   2.1 **Idiopathic (primary)**
      - Benign neonatal familial convulsions
      - Benign neonatal convulsions
      - Benign myoclonic epilepsy in infancy
      - Childhood absence epilepsy (pyknolepsy)
      - Juvenile absence epilepsy
      - Juvenile myoclonic epilepsy (impulsive petit mal)
      - Epilepsies with grand mal seizures (GTCS) on awakening
      - Other generalized idiopathic epilepsies
      - Epilepsies with seizures precipitated by specific modes of activation
   2.2 **Cryptogenic or symptomatic**
      - West syndrome (infantile spasms, Blitz-Nick-Salaam Krämpfe)
      - Lennox-Gastaut syndrome
      - Epilepsy with myoclonic-astatic seizures
      - Epilepsy with myoclonic absences
   2.3 **Symptomatic (secondary)**
      2.3.1 Nonspecific etiology
         - Early myoclonic encephalopathy
         - Early infantile epileptic encephalopathy with suppression bursts
         - Other symptomatic generalized epilepsies
      2.3.2 Specific syndromes
         - Epileptic seizures may complicate many disease states
3. **Undetermined epilepsies**
   3.1 **With both generalized and focal seizures**
      - Neonatal seizures
      - Severe myoclonic epilepsy in infancy
      - Epilepsy with continuous spike-waves during slow wave sleep
      - Acquired epileptic aphasia (Landau-Kleffner syndrome)
      - Other undetermined epilepsies
   3.2 **Without unequivocal generalized or focal features**
4. **Special syndromes**
   4.1 **Situation-related seizures** *(Gelegenheitsanfälle)*
      1. Febrile convulsions
      2. Isolated seizures or isolated status epilepticus
      3. Seizures occurring only when there is an acute or toxic event due to factors such as alcohol, drugs, eclampsia, nonketotic hyperglycemia

From Commission on Classification and Terminology of the International League Against Epilepsy 1989. Used with permission.

idiopathic, and referred to conditions that are probably symptomatic, without evidence, as "cryptogenic". The 1989 classification added a group of "Undetermined Epilepsies with both generalized and focal seizures, and without unequivocal generalized or focal features". This was, in fact, an admission that the focal/generalized dichotomy was by no means absolute.

Recent Recommendations

In a 2001 Report, the ILAE Task Force on Classification and Terminology (Engel, 2001), charged with the task of reevaluating the 1981 International Classification of Epileptic Seizures, and the 1989 International Classification of Epilepsies, noted that "the previous dichotomous classifications based on concepts of 'partial' or 'localization-related' vs. 'generalized' abnormalities created the false impression that epileptic seizures, or epilepsy syndromes, were due to either localized disturbances in one hemisphere, or disturbances involving the entire brain. A variety of conditions between focal and generalized epileptogenic dysfunctions include diffuse hemispheric abnormalities, multifocal abnormalities, and bilaterally symmetrical localized abnormalities. Although concepts of partial and generalized epileptogenicity have value, perhaps more with ictal events than to syndromes, it is neither appropriate nor useful to attempt to contain all seizures and syndromes within one or the other of these categorizations" (Engel, 2001). The Task Force Report proposed that the terms "partial" and "localization-related" be replaced with the older term "focal", because it remains in common use and is easier to apply, with the understanding that the term "focal" should not be construed to mean that the epileptogenic region is a small, well-delineated focus of neuronal pathology. This Report noted that "focal seizures, as well as focal syndromes, are almost always due to diffuse, and at times widespread, areas of cerebral dysfunction" (Engel, 2001). For this reason, it was concluded that a new, more rational classification would probably not include the focal/generalized dichotomy.

Rather than propose a new classification, the 2001 ILAE Classification Report (Engel, 2001) proposed a diagnostic scheme for use in describing individual patients. The scheme consisted of five axes, the first of which was a description of ictal semiology; the second was seizure type as a diagnostic entity; the third was syndrome diagnosis; the fourth was etiology; and the fifth was impairment. The concept of a seizure as a diagnostic entity differed from previous classifications where epileptic seizures were defined on the basis of ictal phenomenology and EEG features alone. The new concept of epileptic seizure types as diagnostic entities is based on pathophysiological mechanisms and anatomical substrates (which are better understood now than they were in 1981), and is meant to have etiologic, therapeutic, and prognostic implications that could be used for planning diagnostic evaluations and therapeutic approaches when an epilepsy syndrome can not be diagnosed.

In a more recent Report (Engel, 2006), a Core Group of the ILAE Classification Task Force set forth a proposal for identifying specific epileptic seizure types and epilepsy syndromes as discrete diagnostic entities, patterned after biological classifications based on natural classes (Ax, 1996). This report lists recognized seizure types and syndromes and noted "although the dichotomy of focal (partial) vs. generalized has been criticized, and we have recommended in an earlier report that these terms should eventually be discarded because no seizures or syndromes are truly generalized, nor is it likely that many, if any, seizures or syndromes are due to a discretely focal epileptogenic process, the Core Group has recognized the value of distinguishing epileptic seizures that begin in a part of one hemisphere, from those that appear to begin in both hemispheres at the same time. The Core Group, however, has been unable to come up with simple terms to describe these two situations. Given the prevalent usage, and the therapeutic implications, of the terms 'focal and generalized', we have decided to retain them, with the understanding that the former does not necessarily imply that the epileptogenic region is limited to a small circumscribed area, nor does the latter imply that the entire brain is involved in initiation of the epileptogenic process" (Engel, 2006). With respect to the list of epilepsy syndromes, the Report noted that "not all syndromes can be easily classified as either focal or generalized or as either symptomatic or idiopathic, and there is no need to do so. These terms are used here with respect to specific syndromes only when they have historical or clinical value" (Engel, 2006).

■ Arguments against the use of a focal/generalized dichotomy

Seizures

The 1981 (current) International Classification of Epileptic Seizures was purportedly based entirely on ictal semiology and EEG, because information at the time was inadequate to base it on pathophysiological and anatomical considerations (Commission, 1981). Seizures categorized as partial can begin with clearly focal signs, such as clonic motor movements of the hand and face, but the bilateral motor movements of classic supplementary motor seizures certainly cannot be considered focal (Ajmone-Marsan and Ralston, 1957). Complicated multimodal sensory auras, often associated with emotional experiences such as fear, also appear to require relatively large areas of the brain for their manifestation (Halgren et al., 1978). Although it is assumed that complex partial seizures (that is, focal seizures with impaired consciousness) begin unilaterally, their typical signs and symptoms require bilateral brain involvement (Williamson and Engel, 1997); consequently, from the perspective of ictal semiology, there is nothing focal about the onset of complex partial seizures that are not preceded by auras. Similarly, there is nothing focal about the ictal semiology of secondarily generalized seizures that originate in so-called silent areas of the brain. If an ictal event is deemed generalized from the perspective of ictal semiology merely because there are no focal features, then there are no grounds for distinction between partial and generalized ictal events based on ictal semiology alone. On the other hand, generalized spasms can result from focal lesions, and generalized seizures can have focal features, even in the idiopathic epilepsies (Ferrie, 2005).

The diagnosis of partial seizures also requires consideration of interictal and ictal EEG features. Here again, however, there is no clear focal/generalized dichotomy, but, rather, a wide diversity of patterns. Interictally, patients can display truly focal interictal spikes on EEG or, as is often the case with mesial temporal lobe epilepsy, interictal spikes can be bilaterally independent (Williamson and Engel, 1997). Focal epileptogenic abnormalities can give rise to secondary bilateral synchrony, which in some cases is the only manifestation of a so-called localization-related epilepsy disorder (Blume and Pillay, 1985). Multifocal interictal spike discharges are characteristic of patients with diffuse brain damage and are typically associated with generalized seizures (Noriega-Sanchez and Markand, 1976). It is well known that patients with idiopathic absence epilepsies can have focal interictal EEG spikes (Ferrie, 2005).

Ictal EEG patterns display a similar diversity. Some seizures can clearly begin with a focal ictal EEG onset; however, even when a discrete structural abnormality is present, as in the case of mesial temporal lobe epilepsy with hippocampal sclerosis, there is increasing evidence that wide areas of brain abnormality are necessary for ictal events to manifest (Wieser et al., 2004). Perhaps the semiological epitome of a focal seizure is epilepsia partialis continua. Whereas some of these events can be truly focal, due to discrete structural lesions, they more commonly occur in association with Rasmussen's encephalitis, where the ictal EEG is characterized by diffuse hemispheric disturbances on EEG, typically bilateral theta and delta activity with no focal features at all (Engel et al., 1983). Again this supports the notion that large areas of brain dysfunction are necessary for at least some types of focal seizures to manifest. Complex partial status epilepticus, particularly arising from frontal lobe, is characterized by bilaterally synchronous spike-and-wave discharges which often cannot be distinguished electrographically from atypical absences (Williamson et al., 1985). There may, in fact, be a relationship between some types of frontal lobe seizures and absences in patients with symptomatic generalized epilepsies. As with seizure semiology, therefore, there is no basis for designating ictal events as generalized based on the absence of focal or lateralizing features. Conversely, whereas seizures classified as generalized are characterized by ictal discharges that are bilaterally synchronous, in most cases they do not involve all parts of the brain equally. Many so-called generalized seizures show frontal predominance on the ictal EEG. Furthermore, seizures that appear to be electroclinically generalized in infants and young children, such as spasms, can be due to focal lesions (Shields et al.). There would, therefore, appear to be little basis to argue from ictal electrographic data that these events are generalized and that certain frontal lobe seizures, complex partial seizures, and epilepsia partialis continua are not. Obviously the differential diagnosis involves more than just seizure semiology and EEG.

The recent ILAE Report on classification (Engel, 2006) proposed a number of criteria for recognizing epileptic seizure types as discrete diagnostic entities that, like syndromes, would have etiologic, therapeutic, and prognostic implications. These criteria are pathophysiologic mechanisms, neuronal substrates, responses to AEDs, ictal EEG patterns, propagation patterns and postictal features, and the epilepsy syndromes with which they are associated. The Report lists recognized seizure types based on these criteria *(Table III)* and divides them into those with generalized onset and those with focal onset. This represents a subtle difference from the focal/generalized dichotomy of prior classifications where seizures were merely called "partial" or "generalized", even though the definition of these terms always referred only to onset. Focal onset seizures are further divided into local seizure types, which remain in the area of

Table III. Seizure types.

Self-limited epileptic seizures
I. Generalized onset
    A. Seizures with tonic and/or clonic manifestations
        1. Tonic-clonic seizures
        2. Clonic seizures
        3. Tonic seizures
    B. Absences
        1. Typical absences
        2. Atypical absences
        3. Myoclonic absences
    C. Myoclonic seizure types
        1. Myoclonic seizures
        2. Myoclonic astatic seizures
        3. Eyelid myoclonia
    D. Epileptic spasms
    E. Atonic seizures
II. Focal onset (partial)
    A. Local
        1. Neocortical
            a. Without local spread
                1) Focal clonic seizures
                2) Focal myoclonic seizures
                3) Inhibitory motor seizures
                4) Focal sensory seizures with elementary symptoms
                5) Aphasic seizures
            b. With local spread
                1) Jacksonian march seizures
                2) Focal (asymmetrical) tonic seizures
                3) Focal sensory seizures with experiential symptoms
        2. Hippocampal and parahippocampal
    B. With ipsilateral propagation to:
        1. Neocortical areas (includes hemiclonic seizures)
        2. Limbic areas (includes gelastic seizures)
    C. With contralateral spread to:
        1. Neocortical areas (hyperkinetic seizures)
        2. Limbic areas (dyscognitive seizures with or without automatisms [psychomotor])
    D. Secondarily generalized
        1. Tonic-clonic seizures
        2. Absence seizures
        3. Epileptic spasms (unverified)
III. Neonatal seizures

Status epilepticus
I. Epilepsia partialis continua (EPC)
    A. As occurs with Rasmussen syndrome
    B. As occurs with focal lesions
    C. As a component of inborn errors of metabolism
II. Supplementary motor area (SMA) status epilepticus
III. Aura continua
IV. Dyscognitive focal (psychomotor, complex partial) status epilepticus
    A. Mesial temporal
    B. Neocortical
V. Tonic-clonic status epilepticus
VI. Absence status epilepticus
    A. Typical and atypical absence status epilepticus
    B. Myoclonic absence status epilepticus
VII. Myoclonic status epilepticus
VIII. Tonic status epilepticus
IX. Subtle status epilepticus

From Engel 2006. Used with permission.

generation, or demonstrate local spread, such as Jacksonian march seizures; those with long-tract ipsilateral propagation; those with contralateral propagation; and secondarily generalized seizures. Secondarily generalized seizures include absences as well as tonic-clonic seizures, and perhaps also spasms. These events all clearly involve subcortical as well as cortical mechanisms (Fromm et al., 1987; Holmes and Vigevano, 1997; McCormick and Contreras, 2001), whereas subcortical contributions to other bilateral ictal events such as atypical absences, hyperkinetic seizures, and limbic seizures with impaired consciousness are less well defined. The term "generalized" here, and in the classification of generalized onset seizures, is not meant to imply that these ictal events involve the entire brain, either at onset or subsequently. The Core Group of the Task Force, however, was unable to find a better word to describe the diffuse phenomena that characterize these seizure types and maintained the term "generalized" because of its common usage and therapeutic utility (Engel, 2006).

Syndromes

The 1989 International Classification of a Epilepsies defines a syndrome as "an epileptic disorder characterized by a cluster of signs and symptoms customarily occurring together; these include such items as type of seizure, etiology, anatomy, precipitating factors, age of onset, severity, chronicity, diurnal and circadian cycling, and sometimes prognosis. However, in contradistinction to a disease, a syndrome does not necessarily have a common etiology and prognosis (Commission, 1989). The rationale for listing syndromes as localization-related was based on "seizure semiology or findings at an investigation (which) disclose a localized origin of the seizures". It was further noted that "this includes not only patients with small circumscribed constant epileptogenic lesions..., but also patients with less well-defined lesions, whose seizures may originate from variable loci. In most symptomatic localization-related epilepsies, the epileptogenic lesions can be traced to one part of one cerebral hemisphere, but in idiopathic age-related epilepsies with focal seizures, corresponding regions of both hemispheres may be functionally involved" (Commission, 1989). This is contrasted with syndromes listed as generalized epilepsies which are defined as "epileptic disorders with generalized seizures, i.e., 'seizures in which the first clinical changes indicate initial involvement of both hemispheres'... the ictal encephalographic patterns initially are bilateral" (Commission, 1989). Because these definitions were anchored in the seizure types characterizing the syndromes, it would seem that the same arguments against a clear dichotomy between partial and generalized seizures in the 1981 International Classification of Epileptic Seizures (Commission, 1981) would apply to an argument against a clear dichotomy between localization-related and generalized epilepsies with respect to syndromes listed in the 1989 International Classification of Epilepsies (Commission, 1989).

The 2001 ILAE classification report (Engel, 2001) defined an epilepsy syndrome as "a complex of signs and symptoms that define a unique epilepsy condition. This must involve more than just seizure type; thus frontal lobe seizures per se, for instance, do not constitute a syndrome". An epilepsy syndrome was distinguished from an epilepsy disease, defined as "a pathologic condition with a single specific well-defined etiology. Thus, Progressive myoclonus epilepsy is a syndrome, but Unverricht-Lundborg is a disease" (Engel, 2001). The recent ILAE Report (Engel, 2006) further develops the concept of syndromes as discrete diagnostic entities by establishing criteria for recognizing conditions as unique natural classes. The criteria are not only the epileptic seizure types associated with the condition, but age of onset, progressive nature, interictal EEG, associated interictal signs and symptoms, pathophysiologic mechanisms, anatomical substrates and etiological categories, and genetic bases. A list of recognized syndromes was included (*Table IV*), organized by age rather than according to the localization-related/generalized and idiopathic/symptomatic dichotomies of the 1989 classification (Commission, 1989). This Report (Engel, 2006), however, acknowledged that there *was* value in recognizing some syndromes as focal or generalized, and some syndromes as idiopathic or symptomatic, but that there is no need to use these concepts to force syndromes into one category or another. The terms "focal", "generalized", and "symptomatic" rarely appear in the names of syndromes listed in *table IV*, and the term "idiopathic" does not occur at all, although the concept of Idiopathic generalized epilepsies is preserved. The list of syndromes in *table IV*, however, is still not a classification, and no ILAE recommendations have been made concerning a more useful approach to *organizing* identified epilepsy syndromes that would improve upon the 1989 focal/generalized and symptomatic/idiopathic dichotomies. In fact, the Classification Core Group (Engel, 2006) made the following statement regarding the 1981 Classification of Epileptic Seizures (Commission, 1981) and the 1989 Classification of Epilepsies (Commission, 1989): "It was a unanimous early agreement of the group that these two current classifications are generally accepted and workable, and that they should not be discarded unless, and until, a clearly better classification has been devised, although some modifications to the current classifications are anticipated" (Engel, 2006).

■ Can the terms focal and generalized be replaced?

Clearly, the difficulties that the ILAE has had in replacing the largely inaccurate concepts of focal and generalized seizures and focal and generalized epilepsies relates to the unquestionable clinical value of these terms. At least since the 1970 classifications of seizures and of epilepsies, the diagnosis of a partial seizure and a partial syndrome immediately raises the issue of localized pathology that needed to be identified using detailed diagnostic approaches, because specific treatment might be needed for focal brain lesions such as neoplasms and infections, or patients could be candidates for surgical therapy. Generalized seizures and epilepsies, on the other hand, implied benign idiopathic conditions that responded to certain medications but not others, with the exception of easily diagnosed symptomatic generalized epilepsies such as Early myoclonic encephalopathy and Ohtahara syndrome, West syndrome, and Lennox-Gastaut syndrome. This concept became blurred with the later recognition that partial epilepsies could be idiopathic and, more recently, the recognition that idiopathic epilepsies such as Severe myoclonic epilepsy in infancy (Dravet syndrome), and Landau-Kleffner syndrome, can be very malignant. Nevertheless, both the focal/generalized dichotomy and the idiopathic/symptomatic dichotomy have provided a useful framework for non-epileptologists to understand the etiologic, therapeutic, and

Table IV. Epilepsy syndromes by age of onset and related conditions.

Neonatal period
    Benign familial neonatal seizures (BFNS)
    Early myoclonic encephalopathy (EME)
    Ohtahara syndrome
Infancy
    Migrating partial seizures of infancy
    West syndrome
    Myoclonic epilepsy in infancy (MEI)
    Benign infantile seizures
    Dravet syndrome
    Myoclonic encephalopathy in nonprogressive disorders
Childhood
    Early onset benign childhood occipital epilepsy (Panayiotopoulos type)
    Epilepsy with myoclonic astatic seizures
    Benign childhood epilepsy with centrotemporal spikes (BCECTS)
    Late onset childhood occipital epilepsy (Gastaut type)
    Epilepsy with myoclonic absences
    Lennox-Gastaut syndrome
    Epileptic encephalopathy with continuous spike-and-wave during sleep (CSWS) including
        Landau-Kleffner syndrome (LKS)
    Childhood absence epilepsy (CAE)
Adolescence
    Juvenile absence epilepsy (JAE)
    Juvenile myoclonic epilepsy (JME)
    Epilepsy with generalized tonic-clonic seizures only
    Progressive myoclonus epilepsies (PME)
Less Specific Age Relationships
    Autosomal-dominant nocturnal frontal lobe epilepsy (ADNFLE)
    Familial temporal lobe epilepsies
    Mesial temporal lobe epilepsy with hippocampal sclerosis (MTLE with HS)
    Rasmussen syndrome
    Gelastic seizures with hypothalamic hamartoma
Special Epilepsy Conditions
    Symptomatic focal epilepsies not otherwise specified
    Reflex epilepsies
    Febrile seizures plus (FS+)
    Familial focal epilepsy with variable foci
Conditions with epileptic seizures that do not require a diagnosis of epilepsy
    Benign (non-familial) neonatal seizures (BNS)
    Febrile seizures (FS)

From Engel 2006. Used with permission.

prognostic issues associated with a growing number of diverse epilepsy conditions. As inaccurate as these terms may be, no one as yet has been able to suggest alternative terminology that provides the same practical diagnostic utility.

Given the foregoing discussion, it is clear that there is no pathophysiologic or anatomic evidence for the existence of either focal or generalized epileptic seizures or epilepsy syndromes, and that a strict dichotomous categorization is unsupportable. What are the alternatives? The chapters in this book provide important clinical and basic observations that should help us devise much more intellectually satisfying approaches to conceptualizing ictal phenomena and the epilepsy syndromes with which they are associated. One view occasionally expressed is that ictal electroclinical phenomena should be viewed along a continuum, rather than as absolutely focal, or absolutely generalized. Although this perspective reinforces the obvious conclusion that many seizures and syndromes have both focal and generalized features, attempting to force every seizure and syndrome into a continuum is as unacceptable as attempting to force them all into a dichotomy. There are many types of seizures and syndromes that need to be identified and defined individually, and then related to some, but not necessarily all, other seizures and syndromes. For instance, one could devise a number of ways to describe a bowl of fruit along a continuum, by color perhaps, or sour *vs.* sweet, but whereas the tangerines in the bowl might be closely related to the oranges, they have nothing to do with the apples, bananas, or kiwis, other than the fact that they are all fruit, nor is there much else to relate these three other fruits with each other. A more useful construct that has arisen from the Rome meeting, and is discussed in the preceding chapters, is the fact that all epileptic seizures can be viewed as network phenomena, *i.e.*, ictal manifestations reflect aberrant activity within neuronal networks that can be restricted, or distributed. Syndromes represent specific pathological disturbances either within these networks, or in systems that access these networks.

Seizures

Chapters in this book discuss cortico-thalamic and other networks that are important for the generation of typical absence seizures, and brain stem networks that are responsible for the manifestation of what we now refer to as generalized tonic-clonic seizures. Among the focal ictal events that are not specifically discussed in these chapters are limbic seizures, which involve networks that have, to a large extent, been identified, and neocortical seizures that involve a variety of more restricted, or sometimes distributed, networks. Secondarily generalized focal seizures, on the other hand, are discussed in this volume, and it is clear that their neuronal networks cannot be identical to those responsible for primarily generalized seizures, because observations of patients, as well as kindled rats, reveal that the seizures are asymmetrical and, under certain experimental conditions, can even be unilateral. Thus, the neuronal networks responsible for Stage 4 and 5 kindled seizures, as well as for secondarily generalized seizures commonly observed in patients on telemetry units, still need to be identified and defined. Similarly, the electroclinically bilateral spike-and-wave stupor that arises from frontal lobe lesions, the infantile spasms seen in infants and young children with localized structural abnormalities that resolve with resection, and other so-called secondarily generalized epileptic phenomena seen in children with catastrophic epilepsies, must reflect characteristic neuronal networks distinct from those responsible for primarily generalized tonic-clonic seizures and typical absences.

Other ictal events currently referred to as generalized that are discussed in the preceding chapters remain poorly understood. The distinction between myoclonic and clonic seizures, for instance, is not well-defined, and the relationships between generalized, multifocal, and focal myoclonic phenomena remain obscure. There are no good animal models for generalized myoclonic or atonic seizures, and these would seem to be important if the neuronal networks responsible for these diverse and often disabling ictal events are to be elucidated, given that patients with these seizure types rarely undergo invasive presurgical investigations. It is possible that myoclonic and atonic seizures, as well as the tonic-clonic seizures and atypical absences, that occur with symptomatic generalized epilepsies such as the Lennox-Gastaut syndrome, involve networks more related to those that give rise to secondarily generalized seizures than to primarily generalized seizures.

Functional imaging will play an increasingly important role in the anatomical delineation of ictal neuronal networks, although interpretation of the functional magnetic resonance imaging (fMRI), single photon emission computed tomography (SPECT), and positron emission tomography (PET) data discussed in the preceding chapters requires caution. Most of these studies detect changes in cerebral metabolism or perfusion that are altered in relationship to neuronal activity, predominantly postsynaptic potentials, without regard for whether these events are excitatory or inhibitory. Furthermore, hypersynchrony, which is the hallmark of many ictal phenomena, reflects changes in the pattern, rather than the amount, of synaptic input, so that metabolism and perfusion can be unchanged, or even reduced, in areas where this activity predominates.

Among the subcortical structures that have been identified in functional imaging of clinical and experimental epilepsy, but are not clearly part of any defined epileptogenic networks, is the cerebellum. Several chapters in this book mention the cerebellum in this regard, and it would seem an important priority to better define whether, and if so how, cerebellar influences generate or modulate epileptic phenomena, particularly given the fact that the therapeutic value of cerebellar stimulation has never been definitively disproved (Cooper et al., 1973).

An important question that appears unresolved from the chapters in this book is whether epileptic seizures necessarily involve cerebral cortex. There is no longer any doubt that subcortical structures are required for the manifestation of many, if not perhaps all, ictal events (which goes without saying, given that peripheral nerve and muscle are necessary for motor manifestations), and there also is no doubt that some seizures can be elicited experimentally by directly affecting subcortical structures, including spinal cord. This does not, however, mean that cortical disturbances are not always necessary for accessing these subcortical networks in human epilepsies. Consequently, some degree of cortical pathology could still be an essential component of all the conditions we currently consider to be epilepsy.

Another aspect of the network concept of seizures is the recognition that multiple networks can be involved in sequence in order to give rise to the evolutionary features of certain types of ictal events. This can be easily studied in animal models, such as kindling, where Stage 1-3 ictal events are not necessarily followed by Stage 4 and 5 seizures (Racine, 1972). Interactions between seizure types could also provide clues concerning overlapping networks that may have agonistic or antagonistic effects. For instance, the observation that amygdala kindling is retarded in rats with genetic absence epilepsy, and that it is the secondarily generalized and not the limbic manifestations that are delayed, suggests negative interactions at the subcortical level (Aker et al., 2006). On the other hand, Papio papio baboons with photosensitive epilepsy undergo amygdala kindling much more rapidly than non-photosensitive rhesus monkeys, suggesting a positive interaction (Wada and Osawa, 1976). This latter phenomenon could explain the observation that patients with temporal lobe epilepsy who have a family history of idiopathic epilepsy do better surgically (Andermann, 1980); due to their lower epileptogenic threshold, the establishment of refractory focal epilepsy would require relatively small lesions that can be easily resected.

Syndromes

The ILAE considers epilepsy syndromes to be "a complex of signs and symptoms that define a unique epilepsy condition" (Engel, 2001). Paramount among the criteria that are now being used to define epilepsy syndromes is the seizure type(s) with which each is associated (Engel, 2006). Whereas a description of the neuronal networks responsible for the electroclinical manifestations of ictal events is crucial for defining specific epileptic seizure types, syndromes require reference to the location of an enduring pathological disturbance. This can be within an abnormal ictal neuronal network or in an area of brain that elicits no clinical manifestations until it accesses a distant neuronal network that is an integral part of the normal nervous system. Consequently, different epilepsy syndromes or epilepsy diseases could give rise to identical seizure types, as a result of inherent pathophysiologic disturbances that involve uniquely different parts of the same ictal neuronal network, or its afferent structures. These enduring syndromic disturbances must be defined as distinct and separate from the transient pathophysiologic events that give rise to the ictal manifestations.

■ Conclusions

Given this discussion, the question at the present time is not whether the terms "focal" and "generalized" are correct (they aren't), but whether their clinical utility justifies their continued use despite the fact that they are descriptively inaccurate. This seems to be the case, at least until a better approach can be devised. Broad principles apply as a useful construct, as long as the exceptions to the rules are understood. The most important near-term objective, therefore, may not be to find better terms to replace the concepts of focal and generalized seizures and epilepsies, but to make sure that physicians understand all the subtleties of individual conditions, irrespective of how they might be classified.

Acknowledgments

Original research reported by the author was supported in part by Grants NS-02808, NS-15654, NS-33310, and GM-24839, from the National Institutes of Health, and Contract DE-AC03-76-SF00012 from the Department of Energy.

References

Ajmone-Marsan C, Ralston BL. *The Epileptic Seizure, Its Functional Morphology and Diagnostic Significance; A Clinical-Electrographic Analysis of Metrazol-Induced Attacks*. Charles C. Thomas: Springfield, IL: 1957.

Aker RG, Yananli HR, Gurbanova AA, Ozkaynakci AE, Ates N, Luijtelaar G, Onat FY. Amygdala kindling in the WAG/Rij rat model of absence epilepsy. *Epilepsia* 2006; 47: 33-40.

Andermann E. Multifactorial inheritance in the epilepsies. In: Canger R, Angeleri F, Penry JK, eds. *Advances in Epileptology, XIth Epilepsy International Symposium.* New York: Raven Press, 1980: 297-309.

Ax P. *Multicellular Animals: A New Approach to the Phylogenetic Order of Nature.* Berlin: Springer-Verlag, 1996: 9-21.

Berger H. Uber das Flektrenkephalogram des Menschen. *Arch Psychiatr Nervenkr* 1929; 87: 527-70.

Blume WT, Pillay N. Electrographic and clinical correlates of secondary, bilateral synchrony. *Epilepsia* 1985; 26: 636-41.

Bravais LF. Recherches sur les symptômes et le traitement de l'épilepsie hémiplégique. Paris (Thése de Paris No 118), 1827.

Commission on Classification and Terminology of the International League Against Epilepsy. Proposal for revised clinical and electroencephalographic classification of epileptic seizures. *Epilepsia* 1981; 22: 489-501.

Commission on Classification and Terminology of the International League Against Epilepsy. Proposal for revised classification of epilepsies and epileptic syndromes. *Epilepsia* 1989; 30: 389-99.

Cooper IS, Crighel E, Amin I. Clinical and physiological effects of stimulation of the paleocerebellum in humans. *J Am Geriatr Soc* 1973; 21: 40-3.

Dandy WE. Roentgenography of the brain after injection of air into the spinal canal. *Ann Surg* 1919; 70: 397-403.

Engel J Jr. A proposed diagnostic scheme for people with epileptic seizures and with epilepsy: Report of the ILAE Task Force on Classification and Terminology. *Epilepsia* 2001; 42: 796-803.

Engel J Jr. The emergence of neurosurgical approaches to the treatment of epilepsy. In: Waxman S, ed. *From Neuroscience to Neurology: Neuroscience, Molecular Medicine, and the Therapeutic Transformation of Neurology.* Amsterdam: Elsevier, 2005: 81-105.

Engel J Jr. Report of the ILAE Classification Core Group. *Epilepsia* 2006; 47 (in press).

Engel J Jr, Kuhl DE, Phelps ME, Rausch R, Nuwer M. Local cerebral metabolism during partial seizures. *Neurology* 1983; 33: 400-13.

Esquirol E. *Des maladies mentales*, 2 vols. Paris: 1838.

Ferrie CD. Idiopathic generalized epilepsies imitating focal epilepsies. *Epilepsia* 2005; 46: 91-5.

Ferrier D. Experimental researches in cerebral physiology and pathology. *The West Riding Lunatic Asylum Medical Reports* 1873; 3: 30-96.

Fromm GH, Faingold CL, Browning RL, Burnham WM. *Epilepsy and the Reticular Formation: The Role of the Reticular Core in Convulsive Seizures.* New York: Alan R. Liss, 1987.

Gastaut H. Clinical and electroencephalographical classification of epileptic seizures. *Epilepsia* 1970: 11: 102-13.

Gibbs FA, Gibbs EL, Lennox WG. Cerebral dysrhythmias of epilepsy. *Arch Neurol Psychiatr* 1938; 39: 298-314.

Griesinger W. *Mental Pathology and Therapeutics.* Robertson CL, Rutherford J, translators. London: New Sydenham Society, 1867.

Halgren E, Walter RD, Cherlow DG, Crandall PH. Mental phenomena evoked by electrical stimulation of the human hippocampal formation and amygdala. *Brain* 1978; 101: 83-117.

Hippocrates. The sacred disease. In: Page TE, Capps E, Rouse WHD, Post LA, Warmington EH (WHS Jones transl), eds. *Hippocrates*, vol. II. Cambridge, MA: Harvard University Press, 1967: 127-84.

Holmes GL, Vigevano F. Infantile spasms. In: Engel J Jr, Pedley TA, eds. *Epilepsy: A Comprehensive Textbook.* Philadelphia: Lippincott-Raven, 1997: 627-42.

Horsley V. Brain surgery. *Br Med J* 1886; 2: 670-5.

Jasper H, Kershman J. Electroencephalographic classification of the epilepsies. *Arch Neurol Psychiatr* 1941; 45: 903-43.

McCormick DA, Contreras D. On the cellular and network bases of epileptic seizures. *Ann Rev Physiol* 2001; 63: 815-46.

Merlis JK. Proposal for an international classification of the epilepsies. *Epilepsia* 1970; 11: 114-9.

Moniz E. *L'angiographie cérébrale*. Paris: Masson et Cie, 1934.

Noriega-Sanchez A, Markand ON. Clinical and electroencephalographic correlation of independent multifocal spike discharges. *Neurology* 1976; 26: 667-72.

Racine RJ. Modification of seizure activity by electrical stimulation. II. Motor seizure. *Electroencephalogr Clin Neurophysiol* 1972; 32: 281-94.

Taylor J. *Selected Writings of John Hughlings Jackson*, vol. 1. New York: Basic Books Inc, 1958.

Temkin O. *The Falling Sickness*. Baltimore: Johns Hopkins Press, 1945.

Tissot SA. Traité de l'épilepsie, faisant le tome troisième du traité des nerfs et de leurs maladies. Paris: 1770.

Wada JA, Osawa T. Spontaneous recurrent seizure state induced by daily electrical amygdaloid stimulation in Senegalese baboons, *Papio papio*. *Neurology* 1976; 26: 273-86.

Wieser HG, Özkara Ç, Engel J Jr, Hauser AW, Moshé SL, Avanzini G, Helmstaedter C, Henry TR, Sperling MR. Mesial temporal lobe epilepsy with hippocampal sclerosis: Report of the ILAE Commission on Neurosurgery of Epilepsy. *Epilepsia* 2004; 45: 695-714.

Williamson PD, Engel J Jr. Complex partial seizures. In: Engel J Jr, Pedley TA. *Epilepsy: A Comprehensive Textbook*. Philadelphia: Lippincott-Raven, 1997: 557-66.

Williamson PD, Spencer DD, Spencer SS, Novelly RA, Mattson RH. Complex partial status epilepticus: A depth electrode study. *Ann Neurol* 1985; 28: 647-54.

Achevé d'imprimer par Corlet, Imprimeur, S.A.
14110 Condé-sur-Noireau
N° d'Imprimeur : 92461 - Dépôt légal : juillet 2006

Imprimé en France